P9-CMZ-358

Childhood Diseases and Disorders SOURCEBOOK

Fourth Edition

Health Reference Series

Fourth Edition

Childhood Diseases and Disorders SOURCEBOOK

Basic Consumer Health Information about the Physical, Mental, and Developmental Health of Pre-Adolescent Children, Including Facts about Infectious Diseases, Asthma and Allergies, Cancer, Diabetes, Growth Disorders, and Conditions Affecting the Blood, Heart, Ear, Nose, Throat, Gastrointestinal Tract, Kidney, Liver, Bones, Muscles, Brain, Lungs, Skin, and Eyes

Along with Information about Vaccines, Medications, Wellness Promotion, a Glossary of Related Terms, and a List of Resources for Parents and Caregivers

OMNIGRAPHICS

615 Griswold, Ste. 901, Detroit, MI 48226

* * *

Health Reference Series
Keith Jones, *Managing Editor*

***

OMNIGRAPHICS
A PART OF RELEVANT INFORMATION

***

ISBN 978-0-7808-1538-4
E-ISBN 978-0-7808-1539-1

Library of Congress Cataloging-in-Publication Data

Names: Omnigraphics, Inc., issuing body.

Title: Childhood diseases and disorders sourcebook: basic consumer health information about the physical, mental, and developmental health of pre-adolescent children, including facts about infectious diseases, asthma and allergies, cancer, diabetes, growth disorders, and conditions affecting the blood, heart, ear, nose, throat, gastrointestinal tract, kidney, liver, bones, muscles, brain, lungs, skin, and eyes; along with information about vaccines, medications, wellness promotion, a glossary of related terms, and a list of resources for parents and caregivers.

Description: Fourth edition. | Detroit, MI: Omnigraphics, [2017] | Series: Health reference series | Includes bibliographical references and index.

Identifiers: LCCN 2016042334 (print) | LCCN 2016042944 (ebook) | ISBN 9780780815384 (hardcover: alk. paper) | ISBN 9780780815391 (ebook) |ISBN 9780780815391 (eBook)

Subjects: LCSH: Pediatrics. | Children--Health and hygiene. |Children--Diseases.

Classification: LCC RJ61.C5427 2017 (print) | LCC RJ61 (ebook) | DDC 618.92--dc23

LC record available at https://lccn.loc.gov/2016042334

This book is printed on acid-free paper meeting the ANSI Z39.48 Standard. The infinity symbol that appears above indicates that the paper in this book meets that standard.

Printed in the United States

Table of Contents

Part II: Childhood Infections and Related Concerns

Part III: Medical Conditions Appearing in Childhood

Part IV: Developmental and Pediatric Mental Health Concerns

Part V: Additional Help and Information

Preface

About This Book

According to the Centers for Disease Control and Prevention (CDC), 83.8% of school-age children were reported in good or very good health. However, even healthy children often face illnesses and injuries. Other children sometimes suffer from chronic diseases that limit their daily activities or threaten future health. In addition, 17.4% of school-age children are considered obese. These matters, along with environmental hazards, lack of physical activity, poor diet, and other dangers, create concern for the well-being of our nation's children.

Childhood Diseases and Disorders Sourcebook, Fourth Edition, provides up-to-date information about common disorders that affect the physical, mental, and developmental health of school-age children. It discusses infectious diseases, asthma and allergies, cancer, diabetes, growth and developmental disorders, mental health and conduct disorders, and conditions affecting the blood, brain, muscles and bones, skin, and internal organs. Included are guidelines for promoting wellness and preventing injuries, along with a glossary of related terms and a list of organizations providing further information.

How to Use This Book

This book is divided into parts and chapters. Parts focus on broad areas of interest. Chapters are devoted to single topics within a part.

Part I: Introduction to Children's Health and Safety provides basic information on routine and emergency medical care for children, as well as guidelines for childhood vaccination and medication. It also discusses childhood obesity, secondhand smoking, and other health problems.

Part II: Childhood Infections and Related Concerns focuses on foodborne, bacterial, viral, and parasitic and fungal infections that can occur in childhood as well as other diseases associated with infections.

Part III: Medical Conditions Appearing in Childhood describes conditions and disorders that are generally diagnosed during childhood. This part provides facts about allergies, cancer, diabetes, growth disorders, and disorders affecting the blood and heart, ear, nose, and throat, gastrointestinal tract, endocrine system, kidneys, liver, muscles and bones, brain, lungs, skin, and eyes.

Part IV: Developmental and Pediatric Mental Health Concerns details mental health disorders than can affect children, as well as common developmental and learning disabilities.

Part V: Additional Help and Information provides a glossary of terms related to childhood diseases and disorders and concludes with a list of resources for parents and caregivers.

Bibliographic Note

This volume contains documents and excerpts from publications issued by the following U.S. government agencies:

Agency for Healthcare Research and Quality (AHRQ); Center for Parent Information and Resources (CPIR); Centers for Disease Control and Prevention (CDC); Education Resources Information Center (ERIC); *Eunice Kennedy Shriver* National Institute of Child Health and Human Development (NICHD); Federal Emergency Management Agency (FEMA); Federal Trade Commission (FTC); Genetic and Rare Diseases (GARD) Information Center; Genetics Home Reference (GHR); Maternal and Child Health Bureau (MCHB); National Cancer Institute (NCI); National Center for Complementary and Integrative Health (NCCIH); National Eye Institute (NEI); National Heart, Lung, and Blood Institute (NHLBI); National Human Genome Research Institute (NHGRI); National Institute of Allergy and Infectious Diseases (NIAID); National Institute of Arthritis and Musculoskeletal and Skin Diseases (NIAMS); National Institute of Diabetes and Digestive and Kidney Diseases (NIDDK); National Institute of Mental

Health (NIMH); National Institute of Neurological Disorders and Stroke (NINDS); National Institute on Aging (NIA); National Institute on Deafness and Other Communication Disorders (NIDCD); National Institutes of Health (NIH); Office of Dietary Supplements (ODS); Office of Disease Prevention and Health Promotion (ODPHP); Office on Women's Health (OWH); U.S. Department of Agriculture (USDA); U.S. Department of Education (ED); U.S. Department of Health and Human Services (HHS); U.S. Department of Veterans Affairs (VA); U.S. Food and Drug Administration (FDA); and WhiteHouse.gov.

In addition, this volume contains copyrighted documents from the following organization: The Nemours Foundation

It may also contain original material produced by Omnigraphics and reviewed by medical consultants.

About the Health Reference Series

The *Health Reference Series* is designed to provide basic medical information for patients, families, caregivers, and the general public. Each volume takes a particular topic and provides comprehensive coverage. This is especially important for people who may be dealing with a newly diagnosed disease or a chronic disorder in themselves or in a family member. People looking for preventive guidance, information about disease warning signs, medical statistics, and risk factors for health problems will also find answers to their questions in the *Health Reference Series*. The *Series*, however, is not intended to serve as a tool for diagnosing illness, in prescribing treatments, or as a substitute for the physician/patient relationship. All people concerned about medical symptoms or the possibility of disease are encouraged to seek professional care from an appropriate healthcare provider.

A Note about Spelling and Style

Health Reference Series editors use *Stedman's Medical Dictionary* as an authority for questions related to the spelling of medical terms and the *Chicago Manual of Style* for questions related to grammatical structures, punctuation, and other editorial concerns. Consistent adherence is not always possible, however, because the individual volumes within the *Series* include many documents from a wide variety of different producers, and the editor's primary goal is to present material from each source as accurately as is possible. This sometimes means that information in different chapters or sections may follow other guidelines and alternate spelling authorities.

Medical Review

Omnigraphics contracts with a team of qualified, senior medical professionals who serve as medical consultants for the *Health Reference Series*. As necessary, medical consultants review reprinted and originally written material for currency and accuracy. Citations including the phrase, "Reviewed (month, year)" indicate material reviewed by this team. Medical consultation services are provided to the *Health Reference Series* editors by:

Dr. Senthil Selvan, MBBS, DCH, MD
Dr. K. Sivanandham, MBBS, DCH, MS (Research), PhD

Our Advisory Board

We would like to thank the following board members for providing initial guidance on the development of this series:

- Dr. Lynda Baker, Associate Professor of Library and Information Science, Wayne State University, Detroit, MI
- Nancy Bulgarelli, William Beaumont Hospital Library, Royal Oak, MI
- Karen Imarisio, Bloomfield Township Public Library, Bloomfield Township, MI
- Karen Morgan, Mardigian Library, University of Michigan-Dearborn, Dearborn, MI
- Rosemary Orlando, St. Clair Shores Public Library, St. Clair Shores, MI

Health Reference Series *Update Policy*

The inaugural book in the *Health Reference Series* was the first edition of *Cancer Sourcebook* published in 1989. Since then, the *Series* has been enthusiastically received by librarians and in the medical community. In order to maintain the standard of providing high-quality health information for the layperson the editorial staff at Omnigraphics felt it was necessary to implement a policy of updating volumes when warranted.

Medical researchers have been making tremendous strides, and it is the purpose of the *Health Reference Series* to stay current with the most recent advances. Each decision to update a volume is made on an individual basis. Some of the considerations include how much new information is available and the feedback we receive from people who use the books. If there is a topic you would like to see added to the update list, or an area of medical concern you feel has not been adequately addressed, please write to:

Managing Editor
Health Reference Series
Omnigraphics
615 Griswold, Ste. 901
Detroit, MI 48226

Part One

Introduction to Children's Health and Safety

Chapter 1

Child Health Statistics

Survey on Health and Well-Being of Children

Since 2003, the National Survey of Children' Health (NSCH) has presented in-depth National and State-level data on the health and well-being of children in their families and communities. The survey, conducted in 2011–2012, provides a snapshot of children's physical, mental, and developmental health status; access to healthcare; activities at school, outside of school, and at home; and their safety and security in their neighborhoods and at school.

Findings from the Survey

The survey found that, in general, children are healthy and receive regular healthcare. Overall, 84.2 percent of children are reported to be in excellent or very good health, 94.5 percent had health insurance at the time of the survey, and 84.4 percent receive an annual preventive healthcare checkup. Most young children (79.2 percent of children aged 0–5 years) were reported to have ever been breastfed, and 81.6

This chapter contains text excerpted from the following sources: Text beginning with the heading "Survey on Health and Well-Being of Children" is excerpted from "The Health and Well-Being of Children: A Portrait of States and the Nation 2011–2012," Maternal and Child Health Bureau (MCHB), U.S. Department of Health and Human Services (HHS), June 2014; text beginning with the heading "Child Health Status" is excerpted from "The Health and Well-Being of Children: A Portrait of States and the Nation 2011–2012," Maternal and Child Health Bureau (MCHB), U.S. Department of Health and Human Services (HHS), June 2014.

percent of school age children miss a week of school or less each year due to illness.

Many aspects of children's home and family environment support their health and development. Eighty-four percent of school-aged children read for pleasure on a typical day, a habit that can improve their school performance and support their intellectual development, and more than three quarters (78.4 percent) share meals with their families most days of the week. A new indicator in this round of the survey measures whether children are flourishing, based on their ability to interact positively with their families and communities. Overall, 73.2 percent of young children (aged 6 months–5 years) met all of the survey's criteria for flourishing, as did 47.7 percent of older children (aged 6–17 years).

Most parents express confidence in their communities as well: 82.1 percent of children live in neighborhoods that their parents find to be supportive of them, the parents of 86.6 percent report that their children are safe in their neighborhood, and 92.6 percent were reported to be safe at school. These statistics represent good news about children's prospects for healthy development.

Just as a child's family environments influence their health, so too can a child's health affect the wellbeing of the family. The needs of children who have asthma or other special healthcare needs, including emotional and behavioral problems, can place demands on their families due to the time and expense required for their care. Nearly one-quarter of children (23.6 percent) are reported to have at least one of a list of 18 chronic conditions, and of these children, 49.8 percent have a condition that is moderate or severe in its impact, in the view of their parents.

The survey also shows areas of children's health and healthcare services where room remains for improvement. While a large majority of children receive annual preventive healthcare visits, fewer receive annual preventive dental care; only 77.2 percent of children received a preventive dental visit in the previous year. In addition, many children with developmental, behavioral or emotional conditions need mental health services, but only 61 percent of these children receive any such services, according to their parents.

Another measure of children's access to appropriate healthcare is whether or not they have a "medical home," a regular source of medical care that meets the standards of accessibility, continuousness, comprehensiveness, coordination, compassion, and cultural sensitivity. The parents of just over half of children (54.4 percent) report that their children's care meets this standard. Among children with special healthcare needs, defined as those who have a chronic physical, developmental, behavioral or emotional condition and who also require health and related services of a type or amount beyond that required by children generally, fewer than half (46.8 percent) received care from a medical home.

While children's family environments appear to support their development, some parents may not be able to provide a healthy, stimulating environment for young children. For example, nearly one quarter (24.1 percent) of children live in a household with a smoker. Added to this round of the survey is a series of questions about adverse experiences that a child may have faced, such as experiencing poverty or divorce, witnessing domestic violence, or living with someone with a mental illness or problems with alcohol or drugs. Overall, 47.9 percent of children have had at least one of these adverse experiences in their lifetimes.

Some groups of children are at higher risk of health problems and barriers to healthcare as well. Children in low-income households are less likely to be in excellent or very good health, miss more days of school due to illness, and are more likely to be overweight or obese than children in higher-income households. Low-income children are less likely to be read to daily, more likely to live in households where someone smokes, more likely to repeat a grade in school, and more likely to live in neighborhoods that do not feel safe or supportive, and their parents are more likely to report parenting stress. These circumstances may combine to put children in low-income households at a health, developmental, and educational disadvantage.

Children from low-income households are less likely than children from higher-income households to do volunteer work or community service, to work for pay, to read for pleasure on a typical weekday, or to participate in activities outside of school like sports teams, Scouts, and religious groups.

These activities, among others, can enrich the lives of children, their families, and communities. Having adequate and continuous health insurance can help to assure access to needed healthcare. Children without health insurance are less likely to receive preventive medical and dental care, receive all of the mental health services they need, and to have a medical home. Another population of children who may be especially vulnerable is children with special healthcare needs; compared to other children, children with special healthcare needs are more likely to have conditions that have a moderate or severe impact on their families, and more likely to have injuries that require medical care, and miss more days of school each year. However, these children are also more likely to have health insurance and less likely to have a gap in coverage over the course of a year than are children without special healthcare needs.

Child Health Status

The National Survey of Children's Health (NSCH) measures children's health status, their healthcare, and their activities in and outside of school. Taken together, these measures provide a snapshot of children's health and well-being that represents a range of aspects of their lives. Children's health status was measured through parents' or caregivers' reports of their children's overall health, as well as whether they currently have specific conditions, such as asthma, autism spectrum disorders, learning disabilities, and attention deficit/hyperactivity disorder.

In addition, parents were asked about their concerns regarding their children's development and behavior, whether their child was screened for problems in these areas, and whether those who needed mental health services received them. Children's access to healthcare and parents' satisfaction with the healthcare that their children receive were measured through questions about children's health insurance coverage, their use of preventive medical and dental services, and their access to needed mental health services.

Several survey questions were combined to assess whether children had a "medical home," a source of primary care that is accessible, family-centered, continuous, comprehensive, coordinated, compassionate, and culturally effective. Children's participation in activities in school and in the community represents another important aspect of their well-being. The survey addressed whether young children often played with children their own age, and whether school-aged children were engaged in school and had ever repeated a grade. In addition, parents were asked about their children's participation in activities such as reading for pleasure, volunteering and working for pay, as well as other activities outside of school.

The general state of a child's health, as perceived by his or her parents, is a useful measure of the child's overall health and ability to function. This is, however, only a general measure of a child's health, as parents may have a positive view of their child's health even in the presence of significant health issues. Parents were asked to rate their child's health status as excellent, very good, good, fair, or poor. Overall, the parents of 84.2 percent of children reported that their child's health was excellent or very good. This proportion did not vary by the sex of the child. Younger children are slightly more likely to be reported to be in excellent or very good health than are school-aged children or adolescents.

Of children aged 5 years and under, 85.9 percent were reported to be in excellent or very good health, compared to 83.3 percent of older children. Children in low-income households are much more likely to have poorer reported health status than children with higher household incomes. Only 69.5 percent of children with household incomes below the Federal poverty level (FPL; $22,350 for a family of 4 in 2011) were reported to be in excellent or very good health, compared to 81.0 percent of children with household incomes between 100 and 199 percent of the FPL. Among children with household incomes between 200 and 399 percent of the FPL, 89.4 percent were in excellent or very good health, as were 93.1 percent of children with household incomes of 400 percent of the FPL or more. A child whose mother is herself in excellent or very good health appears to be more likely to be reported to be in excellent or very good health. Of children whose mothers were reported to be in excellent mental, emotional, and physical health, 93.6 percent were themselves reported to be in excellent or very good health; of children whose mothers' health was poor, only 59.7 percent were in excellent or very good health.

Chapter 2

Preparing Your Child for Visits to the Doctor

When they know they're "going to the doctor," many kids worry a bit about the visit. Whether they're going to see their primary care doctor or a specialist for a routine exam, illness, or special problem, kids are likely to have fears, and some may even feel guilty. Some fears and guilty feelings surface easily, so that kids can talk about them. Others are kept secret and remain unspoken. Here's how to help your child express these fears and overcome them.

Common Fears and Concerns about Medical Exams

Things that often top kids' lists of concerns about going to the doctor include:

- **Separation.** Kids often fear that their parents may leave them in the exam room and wait in another room. The fear of separation from the parent during mysterious examinations is most common in kids under 7 years old, but can be frightening to older kids through ages 12 or 13.
- **Pain.** Kids may worry that a part of the exam or a medical procedure will hurt. They especially fear they may need an injection, particularly kids ages 6 through 12.

Text in this chapter is excerpted from "Preparing Your Child for Visits to the Doctor," © 1995–2016. The Nemours Foundation/KidsHealth®. Reprinted with permission.

- **The doctor.** Some kids' concerns may be about the doctor's manner. A kid may misinterpret qualities such as speed, efficiency, or a detached attitude and view them as sternness, dislike, or rejection.
- **The unknown.** Kids sometimes worry that a medical problem is much worse than their parents are telling them. Some who have simple problems suspect they may need surgery or hospitalization; some who are ill worry that they may die.

Also, kids often have feelings of guilt: They may believe that their illness or condition is punishment for something they've done or neglected to do. Kids who feel guilty also might believe that examinations and medical procedures are part of their punishment.

How to Help

Encourage your kids to express their fears, and then address them in words that they understand and aren't likely to misinterpret. Here are some practical ways to do this:

Explain the Purpose of the Visit

If the upcoming appointment is for a regular health checkup, explain that it's "a well-child visit. The doctor will check on how you're growing and developing, and also ask questions and examine you to make sure that your body is healthy. And you'll get a chance to ask any questions you want to about your body and your health." Also, stress that all healthy kids go to the doctor for such visits.

If the visit is to diagnose and treat an illness or other condition, explain—in very non-scary language—that the doctor "needs to examine you to find out how to fix this and help you get better."

It's wise to prepare kids by giving them advance notice of a visit so it's not a surprise. When explaining the purpose of the visit, talk about the doctor in a positive way to help promote the relationship between your child and the doctor.

Address Any Guilty Feelings

A child who is going to the doctor because of an illness or other condition might have unspoken feelings of guilt about it. Discuss the illness or condition in neutral language and reassure your child: "This isn't caused by anything you did or forgot to do. Illnesses like this happen to many kids. Aren't we lucky to have doctors who can find the causes and who know how to help us get well?"

If you, your spouse, other relatives, or friends had (or have) the same condition, share this information. Knowing that others have been through the same thing can help ease a child's guilt and fear.

If your child needs a doctor's attention because of a condition that resulted in ridicule or rejection by other kids (or even by adults), you'll need to double your efforts to relieve shame and blame. Head lice, embarrassing scratching caused by pinworm, and involuntary daytime wetting or bedwetting are examples of conditions that are often misunderstood by others.

Even if you've been very supportive, reassure your child again, before the visit to the doctor, that the condition is not his or her fault and that many kids have had it.

Of course, if your child has suffered an injury after disregarding safety rules, it's wise to point out (as matter-of-factly as possible) the cause-and-effect relationship between the action and the injury. However, you should still try to relieve guilt. You could say, "You probably didn't understand the danger involved in doing that, but I'm sure you understand now, and I know you won't do it that way again." If your child repeatedly disobeys rules and becomes injured, speak to your doctor. This sort of worrisome behavior pattern needs a closer look.

In any of these cases, though, be sure to explain, especially to young kids, that going to the doctor for an examination is not a punishment. Help your kids understand that adults go to doctors just like kids do and that the doctor's job is to help people stay healthy and fix any problems.

Tell Kids What to Expect during a Routine Exam

Children learn best during play, and this may be a time when they feel most comfortable asking any questions regarding fears they may have. You can use a doll or teddy bear to show a young child how the nurse will measure height and weight or demonstrate parts of the routine exam. Many children's books are available to help illustrate the doctor visit. It also helps to use role-playing to show how the doctor might:

- use a blood pressure cuff to "hug the arm"
- look in the mouth (and will need to hold the tongue down with a special stick for just a few seconds to see the throat)
- look at the eyes and into the ears

- listen to the chest and back with a stethoscope
- tap or press on the tummy to listen to or feel what's inside
- look quickly to see that the "private areas" are healthy
- tap on the knees
- look at the feet

It's important for parents to let their kids know that what they've taught them about the privacy of their bodies is still true, but that doctors, nurses, and parents must sometimes examine all parts of the body. Emphasize, though, that these people are the only exceptions. And reassure your child that you will be in the exam room with him or her.

Tell Kids What to Expect during Other Exams

If your child is going to the doctor because of an illness or medical condition or is going to visit a specialist, you might not even know what to expect during the exam.

When you're calling to make the appointment, you can ask to speak to the doctor or a nurse to find out, in a general way, what will take place during the office visit and exam. Then you can explain some of the procedures and their purpose in gentle language, appropriate to your child's age level. Your child will feel more secure understanding what's going to take place and why it's necessary.

Be honest, but not brutally honest. Let your child know if a procedure is going to be somewhat embarrassing, uncomfortable, or even painful, but don't go into alarming detail.

Reassure your child that you'll be there and that the procedure is truly necessary to fix—or find out how to fix—the problem. (Adolescents may prefer to be examined without a parent or with only a same-sex parent or same-sex chaperone present. That preference should be honored.)

Kids can cope with discomfort or pain more easily if they're forewarned, and they'll learn to trust you if you're honest with them. If you don't know much about the illness or condition, admit that but reassure your child that you'll both be able to ask the doctor questions about it. Write down your child's questions.

If a blood sample will be taken during or after the examination, be careful how you explain this. Some young kids worry that "taking blood" means that all their blood will be taken. Let your child know that the body contains a great deal of blood and that only a very little bit of it (usually no more than 1 or 2 teaspoons [about 10 milliliters]) will be taken for testing.

Again, make certain that your child understands that the visit, with its embarrassing or uncomfortable procedures, is not a punishment for any misbehavior or disobedience.

Involve Your Child in the Process

- **Gathering information for the doctor.** If the situation isn't an emergency, let your child contribute to a list of symptoms that you create for the doctor. Include all symptoms you've observed, no matter how unrelated they may seem to the problem at hand. Also, before the visit, prepare a list of your child's previous illnesses and medical conditions and a history of illnesses and medical conditions among close members of the family (parents, siblings, grandparents, aunts, and uncles).
- **Writing down questions.** Ask your child to think of questions to ask the doctor. Write them down and give them to the doctor. Or, if kids are old enough, they can write down and ask the questions themselves. If the problem has happened before, list the things that have worked and the things that haven't worked in previous treatment. Kids will be reassured by your active role in their medical care and will learn from your example. And you'll be prepared to give the doctor information vital to making an informed diagnosis.

Choose a Doctor Who Relates Well to Kids

Because your doctor is your best ally in helping your kids cope with health examinations, it's important to carefully select a doctor. Of course, you want one who's knowledgeable and competent. However, you also want a doctor who understands kids' needs and fears and who communicates easily with them in a friendly manner, without talking down to them.

In the course of a physical exam, the doctor inspects, taps, and probes various parts of the body—procedures that may be embarrassing (or even physically uncomfortable) for kids. A good relationship between doctor and patient can minimize these feelings.

If your child's doctor seems critical, uncommunicative, disinterested, or unsympathetic, do not be afraid to change doctors. Ask for recommendations from other parents in your area or from other doctors whose opinions you trust.

If your child's illness or condition requires a specialist, ask your doctor to recommend someone who's knowledgeable, experienced, and friendly. After all, adults want these characteristics in their own doctors, so as a parent you should be your child's advocate in seeking medical care.

Chapter 3

How to Give Medicine to Children

Common Questions on Giving Medications to Children

Should OTC Medications Be Given to a Child?

Parents need to weigh the benefit of treating the child's symptoms against the risk of any adverse affects of the drugs. For the common cold, for example, the symptoms will run their course. Remember, over-the-counter (OTC) cough and cold products do not treat the underlying cause of the problem. They treat the symptoms. Read the labels to make sure the product is appropriate for your child's age. Just because a product's box says that it is intended for children does not mean it is intended for children of all ages. Also, be sure that you understand the possible side effects so you can be aware that it may not be the disease that is causing a symptom.

This chapter contains text excerpted from the following sources: Text beginning with the heading "Common Questions on Giving Medications to Children" is excerpted from "Giving Medication to Children," U.S. Food and Drug Administration (FDA), June 9, 2009. Reviewed October 2016; Text under the heading "Kids Aren't Just Small Adults: Medicines, Children, and the Care Every Child Deserves" is excerpted from "Kids Aren't Just Small Adults—Medicines, Children, and the Care Every Child Deserves," U.S. Food and Drug Administration (FDA), August 28, 2013.

Kids Aren't Just Small Adults: Medicines, Children, and the Care Every Child Deserves

Use care when giving any medicine to an infant or a child. Even OTC medicines that you buy are serious medicines. The following is advice for giving OTC medicine to your child, from the FDA and the makers of OTC medicines:

1. **Always read and follow the Drug Facts label on your OTC medicine.** This is important for choosing and safely using all OTC medicines. Read the label every time, before you give the medicine. Be sure you clearly understand how much medicine to give and when the medicine can be taken again.
2. **Know the "active ingredient" in your child's medicine.** This is what makes the medicine work and is always listed at the top of the Drug Facts label. Sometimes an active ingredient can treat more than one medical condition. For that reason, the same active ingredient can be found in many different medicines that are used to treat different symptoms. For example, a medicine for a cold and a medicine for a headache could each contain the same active ingredient. So, if you're treating a cold and a headache with two medicines and both have the same active ingredient, you could be giving two times the normal dose. If you're confused about your child's medicines, check with a doctor, nurse, or pharmacist.
3. **Give the right medicine, in the right amount, to your child.** Not all medicines are right for an infant or a child. Medicines with the same brand name can be sold in many different strengths, such as infant, children, and adult formulas. The amount and directions are also different for children of different ages or weights. Always use the right medicine and follow the directions exactly. Never use more medicine than directed, even if your child seems sicker than the last time.
4. **Talk to your doctor, pharmacist, or nurse to find out what mixes well and what doesn't.** Medicines, vitamins, supplements, foods, and beverages don't always mix well with each other. Your healthcare professional can help.
5. **Use the dosing tool that comes with the medicine, such as a dropper or a dosing cup.** A different dosing tool, or a kitchen spoon, could hold the wrong amount of medicine.

6. **Know the difference between a tablespoon (tbsp.) and a teaspoon (tsp.)** Do not confuse them! A tablespoon holds three times as much medicine as a teaspoon. On measuring tools, a teaspoon (tsp.) is equal to "5 cc" or "5 mL."

7. **Know your child's weight.** Directions on some OTC medicines are based on weight. Never guess the amount of medicine to give to your child or try to figure it out from the adult dose instructions. If a dose is not listed for your child's age or weight, call your doctor or other members of your healthcare team.

8. **Prevent a poison emergency by always using a child-resistant cap.** Re-lock the cap after each use. Be especially careful with any products that contain iron; they are the leading cause of poisoning deaths in young children.

9. **Store all medicines in a safe place.** Today's medicines are tasty, colorful, and many can be chewed. Kids may think that these products are candy. To prevent an overdose or poisoning emergency, store all medicines and vitamins in a safe place out of your child's (and even your pet's) sight and reach. If your child takes too much, call the Poison Center Hotline at 1-800-222-1222 (open 24 hours every day, 7 days a week) or call 9-1-1.

10. **Check the medicine three times.** First, check the outside packaging for such things as cuts, slices, or tears. Second, once you are at home, check the label on the inside package to be sure you have the right medicine. Make sure the lid and seal are not broken. Third, check the color, shape, size, and smell of the medicine. If you notice anything different or unusual, talk to a pharmacist or another healthcare professional.

Chapter 4

Recommended Childhood Vaccinations

Vaccines for Children

Vaccines have contributed to a significant reduction in many childhood infectious diseases, such as diphtheria, measles, and *Haemophilus influenzae* type b (Hib). Some infectious diseases, such as polio and smallpox, have been eliminated in the United States due to effective vaccines. It is now rare for children in the United States to experience the devastating and often deadly effects of these diseases that were once common in the United States and other countries with high vaccination coverage.

Types of Routinely Administered Vaccines for Children

Vaccines work by preparing the body's immune system for future attacks by a certain disease, caused by either viruses or bacteria. Vaccines contain weakened bacteria or viruses, or parts of bacteria or viruses, and mimic these disease-causing agents (which are called antigens). As a result of vaccination, the body's immune system thinks the antigens from the vaccine are foreign and shouldn't be in the body, but

---

This chapter includes text excerpted from "Vaccines for Children—a Guide for Parents and Caregivers," U.S. Food and Drug Administration (FDA), September 2016.

the antigens don't cause disease in the person receiving the vaccine. After receiving the vaccine, if the virus or bacteria that cause the real disease then enters the body in the future, the immune system is prepared and responds quickly and forcefully to attack the disease-causing agent to prevent the person from getting sick. Vaccines are frequently given by injection (a shot), but some are given by mouth and one is sprayed into the nose.

There are various types of vaccines that are routinely given to children:

- **Attenuated (weakened) live viruses:** These vaccines contain a live virus that has been weakened during the manufacturing process so that they do not cause the actual disease in the person being vaccinated. However, because they contain a small amount of the weakened live virus, people with weakened immune systems should talk to their healthcare provider before receiving them. Examples include vaccines that prevent chickenpox and rotavirus and measles, mumps and rubella.
- **Inactivated (killed) viruses:** These vaccines contain a virus that has been killed so as not to cause disease, but the body still recognizes it and stimulates production of antibodies against the disease. They can be given to individuals with weakened immune systems. Examples include vaccines to prevent polio and hepatitis A.
- **Subunits:** In some cases, the entire virus or bacteria is not required for an immune response to prevent disease; just the important parts, a portion or a "subunit" of the disease-causing bacteria or virus is needed to provide protection. The vaccine to prevent influenza (the flu) that is given as a shot is an example of a subunit vaccine, because it is made with parts of the influenza virus.
- **Toxoids:** Some bacteria cause illness in people by secreting a poison (a toxin). Scientists discovered that weakening the toxins, so that they are "detoxified" does not cause illness. Examples of vaccines that contain toxoids include those to prevent tetanus and diphtheria disease.
- **Recombinant:** These vaccines are made by genetic engineering, the process and method of manipulating the genetic material of an organism. An example of this type of vaccine is those that prevent certain diseases caused by the human papillomavirus

(HPV), such as cervical cancer. In this case, the genes that code for a specific protein from each of the virus types of HPV included in the vaccine are expressed in yeast to create large quantities of the protein. The protein that is produced is purified and then used to make the vaccine. Because the vaccine only contains a protein, and not the entire virus, the vaccine cannot cause the HPV infection. It is the body's immune response to the recombinant protein(s) that then protects against infection by the naturally occurring virus.

- **Polysaccharides:** To protect against certain disease-causing bacteria, the main antigens in vaccine are sugar-like substances called polysaccharides; these are purified from the bacteria to make polysaccharide vaccines. However, vaccines composed solely of purified polysaccharides are only effective in older children and adults. Pneumovax 23, a vaccine for the prevention of pneumococcal disease caused by 23 different strains, is an example of a polysaccharide vaccine.
- **Conjugates:** Vaccines made only with polysaccharides do not work very well in young children because their immune system has not fully developed. To make vaccines that protect young children against diseases caused by certain bacteria, the polysaccharides are connected to a protein so that the immune system can recognize and respond to the polysaccharide. The protein acts as a "carrier" for the part of the vaccine that will make protective antibodies in the body. Examples of conjugate vaccines include those to prevent invasive disease caused by *Haemophilus influenzae type b (Hib).*

Steps to Take When Your Child is Vaccinated

- **Review the vaccine information sheets**

  These sheets explain both the benefits and risks of a vaccine. Healthcare providers are required by law to provide them.

- **Talk to your healthcare provider about the benefits and risks of vaccines**

  Learn the facts about the benefits and risks of vaccines, along with the potential consequences of not vaccinating against diseases. Some parents and caregivers are surprised to learn that children can be harmed or die of measles, diphtheria, pertussis, and other vaccine-preventable diseases.

- **Conditions to make your healthcare provider aware of before vaccination**

  This might include being sick or having a history of certain allergic or other adverse reactions to previous vaccinations or their components. For example, eggs are used to grow many influenza (flu) vaccines; therefore, it is important to inform the healthcare provider if a child is severely allergic to eggs.

  The packaging of some vaccines that are supplied in vials or prefilled syringes may contain natural rubber latex, which may cause allergic reactions in latex-sensitive individuals; therefore, an allergy to latex is helpful to inform healthcare providers of beforehand.

  It is also particularly important to discuss with your healthcare provider which vaccines should or should not be given to children who have weakened immune systems.

- **Report adverse reactions**

  Adverse reactions and other problems related to vaccines should be reported to the Vaccine Adverse Event Reporting System, which is maintained by FDA and the Centers for Disease Control and Prevention (CDC). For a copy of the vaccine reporting form, call 1-800-822-7967, or report online to www.vaers.hhs.gov

Routinely Administered Vaccines for Children

Some of the most commonly administered vaccines are briefly discussed below.

Diphtheria and Tetanus Toxoids and Acellular Pertussis Adsorbed (DTaP)

- **Brand Names:** Daptacel and Infanrix
- **What it's for:** Prevents the bacterial infections diphtheria, tetanus (lockjaw), and pertussis (whooping cough). This combination vaccine is given as a series in infants and children 6 weeks through 6 years of age, prior to their 7th birthday. Diphtheria can infect the throat, causing a thick covering that can lead to problems with breathing, paralysis, or heart failure. Tetanus can cause painful tightening (spasms) of the muscles, seizures, paralysis, and death. Pertussis, also known as whooping cough,

has the initial symptoms of runny nose, sneezing, and a mild cough, which may seem like a typical cold. Usually, the cough slowly becomes more severe. Eventually the patient may experience bouts of rapid coughing followed by the "whooping" sound that gives the disease its common name as they try to inhale. While the coughing fit is occurring, the patient may vomit or turn blue from lack of air. Patients gradually recover over weeks to months.

- **Common side effects may include:** Fever, drowsiness, fussiness/irritability, and redness, soreness, or swelling at the injection site.
- **Tell your healthcare provider beforehand if:** The child is moderately or severely ill, has had swelling of the brain within 7 days after a previous dose of vaccine, has a neurologic disorder such as epilepsy, or has had a severe allergic reaction to a previous shot.

Tetanus Toxoid, Reduced Diphtheria Toxoid and Acellular Pertussis Vaccine Adsorbed (Tdap)

- **Brand Names:** Adacel and Boostrix
- **What it's for:** Booster shot for kids at 10 or 11 years of age to prevent the bacterial infections diphtheria, tetanus (lockjaw), and pertussis (whooping cough). In addition, Boostrix is approved for all individuals 10 years of age and older, (including the elderly). Adacel is approved for use in people ages 10 through 64 years.
- **Common side effects may include:** Pain, redness and swelling at the injection site, headache, and tiredness.
- **Tell your healthcare provider beforehand if:** The child is moderately or severely ill, has had swelling of the brain within 7 days after a previous dose of pertussis vaccine, or any allergic reaction to any vaccine that protects against diphtheria, tetanus or pertussis diseases.

Haemophilus B Conjugate Vaccine (Hib)

- **Brand Names:** ActHIB, Hiberix, PedvaxHIB
- **What it's for:** Prevents *Haemophilus influenzae* type b (Hib) invasive disease. Before the availability of Hib vaccines, Hib

disease was the leading cause of bacterial meningitis among children under 5 years of age in the United States. Meningitis is an infection of the tissue covering the brain and spinal cord, which can lead to lasting brain damage and deafness. Hib disease can also cause pneumonia, severe swelling in the throat, infections of the blood, joints, bones, and tissue covering of the heart, as well as death. Both ActHIB and PedvaxHIB are approved for routine administration for infants and children beginning at 2 months and through 18 months and 71 months of age respectively; Hiberix is approved as a booster shot in children 15 months through the age of before their 5th birthday.

- **Common side effects may include:** Fussiness, sleepiness, and soreness, swelling and redness at the injection site.
- **Tell your healthcare provider beforehand if:** The child is moderately or severely ill, or has ever had an allergic reaction to a previous dose of Hib vaccine.

Hepatitis A Vaccine

- **Brand Names:** Havrix and Vaqta
- **What it's for:** Prevents disease caused by hepatitis A virus. People infected with hepatitis A may not have any symptoms; and if they do have symptoms, they may feel like that they have a mild "flu-like" illness; or they may have jaundice (yellow skin or eyes), tiredness, stomachache, nausea and diarrhea. Young children may not have any symptoms, so when a child's caregiver becomes sick, that is when it is recognized that the child is infected. Hepatitis A is most often spread by an object contaminated with the feces of a person with hepatitis A, such as when a parent or caregiver does not properly wash his or her hands after changing diapers or cleaning up the stool of an infected person. Both vaccines are approved for use in people 12 months of age and older.
- **Common side effects may include:** Soreness and redness at the injection site, and loss of appetite.
- **Tell your healthcare provider beforehand if:** The child is moderately to severely ill, or has ever had an allergic reaction to a previous dose of the vaccine.

Hepatitis B Vaccine

- **Brand Names:** Engerix-B and Recombivax HB
- **What it's for:** Prevents infection caused by hepatitis B virus. Hepatitis B is spread when body fluid infected with hepatitis B enters the body of a person who is not infected. Hepatitis B can lead to chronic hepatitis (liver inflammation), liver cancer, and death. The vaccines are approved for individuals of all ages, including newborns. It is particularly important for those at increased risk of exposure to hepatitis B virus such as a baby born to mom who is infected with the virus.
- **Common side effects may include:** Soreness, redness, swelling at injection site, irritability, fever, diarrhea, fatigue/weakness, loss of appetite and headache.
- **Tell your healthcare provider beforehand if:** The child is moderately or severely ill, or has ever had a life-threatening allergic reaction to yeast or to a previous dose of the vaccine.

Human Papillomavirus Vaccine

- **Brand Names:** Cervarix, Gardasil and Gardasil 9
- **What it's for:** Gardasil prevents anal cancer and associated precancerous lesions caused by human papillomavirus (HPV) types 6, 11, 16, and 18 in people ages 9 through 26 years. In this same age group for females, it is also approved for prevention of cervical, vulvar, and vaginal cancer and the associated precancerous lesions caused by HPV types 6, 11, 16, and 18. Gardasil 9 is for use in females ages 9 through 26 and males ages 9 through 15. Gardasil 9 covers five more HPV types than Gardasil, preventing cervical, vulvar, vaginal and anal cancers caused by any of the following HPV Types 16, 18, 31, 33, 45, 52 and 58. Overall, Gardasil 9 has the potential to prevent approximately 90% of cervical, vulvar, vaginal and anal cancers. Gardasil and Gardasil 9 are also approved for the prevention of genital warts caused by types 6 and 11 in both males and females. Cervarix prevents cervical and associated precancerous lesions caused by HPV types 16 and 18 in females ages 9 through 25 years of age.
- **Common side effects may include:** Headache, fever, nausea, dizziness, fainting, and pain, swelling, redness, itchiness or bruising at the injection site.

- **Tell your healthcare provider beforehand if:** For Gardasil and Gardasil 9—the child has had an allergic reaction to yeast or to a previous dose of the vaccine. For Cervarix—the child has had an allergic reaction to a component of the vaccine, or to a previous dose of the vaccine.

Influenza Vaccine (Administered with a Needle)

- **Brand Names (for children):** Afluria, Fluarix, FluLaval, Fluvirin, Fluzone, Fluarix Quadrivalent, FluLaval Quadrivalent, and Fluzone Quadrivalent
- **What it's for:** Different vaccines are approved for different age groups to prevent influenza disease, caused by the strains of influenza virus that are included in the vaccine. Influenza, commonly called "flu," is a contagious respiratory virus that can cause mild to severe illness. The elderly, young children and people with certain health conditions (such as asthma, diabetes, or heart disease) are at high risk for serious influenza-related complications. Complications may include pneumonia, ear infections, sinus infections, dehydration, and worsening of certain medical conditions such as congestive heart failure, asthma or diabetes. The strains of influenza virus that cause disease in people frequently change, so yearly vaccination is needed to provide protection against the influenza viruses likely to cause illness each winter.
- **Common side effects may include:** Pain, redness and swelling at the injection site, low grade fever, and muscle aches, headache, fatigue and general feeling of being unwell.
- **Tell your healthcare provider beforehand if:** The child is moderately or severely ill, has immune system problems, or has had Guillain-Barre Syndrome (GBS), a neurological disorder that causes severe muscle weakness. Also, tell your healthcare provider about any allergies, including severe allergies to eggs and any allergic reaction to a previous dose of any influenza vaccine.

Influenza Vaccine, Intranasal (Nasal Spray)

- **Brand Names (for children):** FluMist Quadrivalent
- **What it's for:** Protects against four different strains of influenza virus included in the vaccine; for children and adults ages 2 through 49 years of age.

- **Common side effects may include:** Runny or stuffy nose and cough.
- **Tell your healthcare provider beforehand if:** The child is moderately or severely ill, has a weakened immune system, has asthma or recurrent wheezing, or has a history of Guillain-Barre Syndrome (GBS), a neurological disorder that causes severe muscle weakness. Also, tell your healthcare provider about any allergies, including severe allergies to eggs and any allergic reaction to a previous dose of any influenza vaccine. In addition, because of the association of Reye syndrome with aspirin and wild-type influenza infection, the healthcare provider should be made aware if the child is currently receiving aspirin or aspirin-containing therapy.

Measles, Mumps and Rubella Vaccine

- **Brand Name:** M-M-R II
- **What it's for:** Prevents measles, mumps, and rubella in those 12 months of age and older. Measles is a respiratory disease that causes a skin rash all over the body, and fever, cough and runny nose. Measles can be severe, causing ear infections, pneumonia, seizures, and swelling of the brain. Mumps causes fever, headache, loss of appetite and the well-known sign of swollen cheeks and jaw which is from the swelling of the salivary glands. Rare complications include deafness, meningitis (infection of the lining that surrounds the brain and spinal cord), and painful swelling of the testicles or ovaries. Rubella, also called German Measles, causes fever, a rash, and—mainly in women—can also cause arthritis. Rubella infection during pregnancy can lead to birth defects.
- **Common side effects may include:** Fever, mild rash, fainting, headache, dizziness, irritability and burning/stinging, redness, swelling, and tenderness at the injection site.
- **Tell your healthcare provider beforehand if:** The child is ill and has a fever or has ever had an allergic reaction to gelatin, the antibiotic neomycin, or a previous dose of the vaccine, has immune system problems, or cancer, or problems with the blood or lymph system.

Meningococcal Vaccine

- **Brand Names:** Bexsero, Menactra, Menveo and Trumenba

- **What it's for:** Prevents certain types of meningococcal disease, a life-threatening illness caused by the bacteria *Neisseria meningitidis* that infects the bloodstream and the lining that surrounds the brain and spinal cord (meningitis). *Neisseria meningitidis* is a leading cause of meningitis in young children. Even with appropriate antibiotics and intensive care, between 10 and 15 percent of people who develop meningococcal disease die from the infection. Another 10 to 20 percent suffer complications such as brain damage or loss of limb or hearing. Bexsero is approved for use in those 10 through 25 years of age to prevent invasive meningococcal disease caused by N. meningitidis serogroup B. Menactra is approved for use in infants and children beginning at 9 months of age, as well as for adults through 55 years of age. Menveo is approved for use in those 2 months through 55 years of age. Both Menactra and Menveo prevent meningococcal disease caused by N. meningitidis serogroups A, C, Y and W. Trumenba is approved for use in those 10 through 25 years of age to prevent invasive meningococcal disease caused by N. meningitidis serogroup B.
- **Common side effects may include:** Tenderness, pain, redness and swelling at the injection site, irritability, headache, fever, tiredness, chills, diarrhea and loss of appetite for a short while.
- **Tell your healthcare provider beforehand if:** The child is moderately or severely ill, has had a severe allergic reaction to a previous dose of meningococcal vaccine or diphtheria toxoid, has a known sensitivity to vaccine components, or a history of Guillain-Barre Syndrome (GBS).

Pneumococcal 13-Valent Conjugate Vaccine

- **Brand Name:** Prevnar 13
- **What it's for:** Prevents invasive disease caused by 13 different types of the bacterium Streptococcus pneumoniae in infants, children and adolescents ages 6 weeks through 17 years. In infants and children 6 weeks through 5 years of age, it is also approved for the prevention of otitis media (ear infection) caused by 7 different types of the bacterium. Streptococcus pneumoniae can cause infections of the blood, middle ear, and the covering of the brain and spinal cord, as well as pneumonia. Prevnar 13 is also approved for adults 50 years of age and older.

- **Common side effects may include:** Pain, redness and swelling at the injection site, irritability, decreased appetite and fever.
- **Tell your healthcare provider beforehand if:** The child is moderately or severely ill, has ever had an allergic reaction to a previous dose or component of the vaccine, including diphtheria toxoid (for example, DTaP vaccine).

Poliovirus Vaccine

- **Brand Name:** Ipol
- **What it's for:** Prevents polio in infants as young as 6 weeks of age. Polio is a disease that can cause paralysis or death.
- **Common side effects may include:** Redness, hardening and pain at the injection site, fever, irritability, sleepiness, fussiness, and crying.
- **Tell your healthcare provider beforehand if:** The child is moderately or severely ill, including illness with a fever, has ever had a severe allergic reaction to a previous dose of polio vaccine, any component of the vaccine, or an allergic reaction to the antibiotics neomycin, streptomycin, or polymyxin B.

Rotavirus Vaccine

- **Brand Names:** Rotarix and RotaTeq
- **What it's for:** Prevents gastroenteritis caused by rotavirus infection in infants as young as 6 weeks of age. Rotavirus disease is the leading cause of severe diarrhea and dehydration in infants worldwide. In the United States, the disease occurs more often during the winter. Before rotavirus vaccines were available, most children in the United States were infected with rotavirus before the age of two. In addition, rotavirus resulted in about 55,000–70,000 hospitalizations and 20–60 infant deaths in the United States each year.
- **Common side effects may include:** Fussiness/irritability, cough/runny nose, fever, and loss of appetite.
- **Tell your healthcare provider beforehand if:** The child has illness with a fever, a weakened immune system because of a disease, has a blood disorder, any type of cancer, has

gastrointestinal problems, has had stomach surgery or ever had intussusception, which is a form of blockage of the intestines, is allergic to any of the ingredients of the vaccine, or has ever had an allergic reaction to a previous dose of the vaccine, or has regular close contact with a member of a family or household who has a weak immune system.

Varicella Virus Vaccine

- **Brand Name:** Varivax
- **What it's for:** Prevents varicella (chickenpox) in children 12 months of age and older. Chickenpox usually causes a blister-like itchy rash, tiredness, headache and fever. It can be serious, particularly in babies, adolescents, adults and people with weak immune systems, causing less common, but more serious complications such as skin infection, scarring, pneumonia, brain swelling, Reye syndrome, (which affects the liver and brain) and death.
- **Common side effects may include:** Soreness, pain, redness or swelling at the injection site, fever, irritability, and chickenpox like rash on the body or at the site of the shot.
- **Tell your healthcare provider beforehand if:** The child is moderately or severely ill, including a fever, has a weak immune system, has received a blood or plasma transfusion or immune globulin within the last 5 months, takes any medicines, has allergies including any life-threatening allergic reaction to gelatin, the antibiotic neomycin, or a previous dose of chickenpox or any other vaccine.

Chapter 5

Promoting Wellness

Chapter Contents

Section 5.1

Nutrition for Children

This section includes text excerpted from "Health and Nutrition Information," ChooseMyPlate.gov, U.S. Department of Agriculture (USDA), July 31, 2015.

Health and Nutrition Information for Pre-Schoolers

Help your preschooler eat well, be active, and grow up healthy. Young children need your help to develop healthy eating and physical activity habits for life. During their early years, you and your preschooler's doctor are partners in maintaining your child's health.

The preschool years are an important time for developing healthy habits for life. From the ages of 2 to 5, children grow and develop in ways that affect behavior in all areas, including eating. As preschoolers grow, they change physically, mentally, and socially. Every child develops eating habits at a different pace.

My Plate Daily Checklist

The MyPlate Daily Checklist (formerly Daily Food Plan) shows what and how much your child should eat to meet his or her needs. Checklists are based on average needs by age and activity level, so you should use the Checklist as a general guide. Your preschooler's food needs also depend on how fast he or she is growing and other factors. So, do not be concerned if your preschooler does not eat the exact amounts suggested. Each child's needs may differ from the average, and appetites can vary from day to day. Try to balance the amounts over a few days or a week.

- Put the MyPlate Daily Checklist into action with meal and snack ideas.
- Offer different foods from day to day. Encourage your child to choose from a variety of foods.
- Serve foods in small portions at scheduled meals and snacks.
- Choose healthy snacks for your preschooler.

- Beverages count too. Make smart beverage choices.

Use the table below to access the right MyPlate Daily Checklist for your child. Be a healthy role model for your child!

Table 5.1. MyPlate Daily Checklist

<table>
<tr><th>Age</th><th>Sex</th><th>Daily Physical Activity</th><th>Calorie level of Food Plan</th></tr>
<tr><td>2 yrs</td><td>Boys and Girls</td><td>Any level</td><td>1000 calories</td></tr>
<tr><td rowspan="5">3 yrs</td><td rowspan="2">Boys</td><td>Less than 30 minutes</td><td>1200 calories</td></tr>
<tr><td>30–60 minutes, More than 60 minutes</td><td>1400 calories</td></tr>
<tr><td rowspan="3">Girls</td><td>Less than 30 minutes</td><td>1000 calories</td></tr>
<tr><td>30–60 minutes</td><td>1200 calories</td></tr>
<tr><td>More than 60 minutes</td><td>1400 calories</td></tr>
<tr><td rowspan="4">4-5 yrs</td><td rowspan="2">Boys and Girls</td><td>Less than 30 minutes</td><td>1200 calories</td></tr>
<tr><td>30–60 minutes</td><td>1400 calories</td></tr>
<tr><td>Boys</td><td>More than 60 minutes</td><td>1600 calories</td></tr>
<tr><td>Girls</td><td>More than 60 minutes</td><td>1400 calories</td></tr>
</table>

Food Groups

The kinds of food your preschooler eats and drinks are important for his or her health. Fruits, vegetables, grains, protein foods, and dairy provide the nutrients that their bodies need. Keep an eye on the amount of added sugars, sodium, and saturated (solid) fat.

- **Fruits:** Let your preschooler enjoy a variety of whole or bite-sized fruits such as apples, sliced bananas, and mandarin orange pieces. Serve 100% fruit juice in small amounts and less often.
- **Vegetables:** Prepare red, orange, and dark-green vegetables like tomatoes, sweet potatoes, and broccoli as part of your child's meals and snacks.
- **Grains:** Make at least half their grains whole grains by offering 100% whole-grain cereals, breads, and pasta.
- **Protein Foods:** Choose a variety of protein foods such as seafood, beans, and small portions of meat or poultry.
- **Dairy:** Give them low-fat milk, yogurt, and cheese to provide much needed calcium.

- **Encourage water instead of fruit juice or sugary drinks:** Too much 100% juice or sugar-sweetened beverages, such as soda, juice drinks, or sport drinks, can add more calories than your child needs.
- **Check out the sodium (salt) in canned foods, bread, and frozen meals:** Read the Nutrition Facts label to find foods with lower numbers.
- **Watch the amount of saturated fats in foods:** Cakes, cookies, ice cream, pizza, cheese, sausages, and hot dogs are okay sometimes but not every day.

Other Dietary Components

Added Sugars and Saturated Fats: Know Your Limits

In addition to the food groups, there are other components to consider when building a healthy eating pattern, including the amounts of added sugars, saturated fats, and sodium your child consumes. Added sugars and saturated fats add to total calories, but provide no vitamins or minerals. Allowing too many can fill your child up without supplying the nutrients they need. They can also add more calories than your child needs in a day.

Some examples of added sugars and saturated fats are:

- The sugars or sweeteners in soft drinks, fruit punch, candies, cakes, cookies, pies, and ice cream.
- The saturated fats in cookies, cakes, pizza, cheese, sausages, fatty meats, butter, and stick margarine.
- Some foods: such as milk, yogurt, and cereals—provide important nutrients, but they can also contain some added sugars or saturated fats. For example, sweetened yogurt and sweetened breakfast cereals contain added sugars. Whole milk and cheese contain saturated fat. Look for food choices that are low in saturated fats, unsweetened, or with no-added sugars.

There is room for foods with some added sugars or saturated fats now and then. But most daily food choices for preschoolers should be low in these dietary components.

Here are some ideas to help you choose foods lower in added sugars and saturated fat for your preschooler:

Table 5.2. Foods lower in added sugars and saturated fat

Instead of...	Choose
Regular cheese	Low-fat cheese
Sweetened yogurt	Plain yogurt plus fruit
Whole milk	Fat-free or low-fat milk
Sweetened breakfast cereals	Cereals with little or no added sugar
Cookies	Graham crackers
Fried chicken or fried fish	Baked chicken or fish
French fries	Oven-baked fries
Ice cream or frozen yogurt	Frozen fruits or frozen 100% fruit bars
Soft drinks or fruit punch	Water
Potato chips	Baked chips or whole grain crackers
Butter or margarine	Trans fat-free tub margarine, low in saturated fat
Jam or jelly	100% fruit spread

Sodium

Nearly all of us eat too much sodium, which is found in salt. This includes most children. Most salt that Americans eat comes from processed foods and foods eaten away from home. The taste for salt is learned. Adding less or no salt and choosing foods lower in salt can help your preschooler learn to like foods with a less salty taste.

Eating less salt is an important way to help your preschooler stay healthy as they grow. This may reduce their risk for high blood pressure and some chronic diseases when they are adults. The recommended daily limit for sodium is less than 1,500 milligrams for children 1 to 3 years old, and less than 1,900 milligrams for children 4 to 8 years old.

To eat less salt:

- Compare sodium content for similar foods, using the Nutrition Facts label to select brands lower in sodium. For example, a cup of tomato soup may have from 700 to 1260 milligrams of sodium.
- Look for "no salt added" or "low sodium" food products.
- Prepare foods with little or no added salt.
- Rinse canned foods such as beans with water before use to reduce the amount of salt.

Also look for foods that are good sources of potassium, which counteracts some of sodium's effects on blood pressure. Vegetables like sweet potatoes, beet greens, white beans, potatoes, tomato puree and paste, and soybeans and fruits like bananas, dried plums (prunes), cantaloupe, honeydew, and orange juice are examples of foods to choose for potassium.

Meals and Snacks

Your preschooler's food needs depend on how fast he or she is growing. A child's height and weight differ depending on family history, gender, nutrition, hours of sleep, and whether a child is sick or has special needs.

Table 5.3. Meals and snacks table for boys and girls

Boys				Girls			
Physical Activity				Physical Activity			
	< 30 min/ day	30–60 min/ day	> 60 min/ day		< 30 min/ day	30–60 min/ day	> 60 min/ day
2 yrs	1000 cals	1000 cals	1000 cals	2 yrs	1000 cals	1000 cals	1000 cals
3 yrs	1200 cals	1400 cals	1400 cals	3 yrs	1000 cals	1200 cals	1400 cals
4 yrs	1200 cals	1400 cals	1600 cals	4 yrs	1200 cals	1400 cals	1400 cals
5 yrs	1200 cals	1400 cals	1600 cals	5 yrs	1200 cals	1400 cals	1600 cals

Encourage your child to choose from a variety of foods and offer different types of foods during meals and snacks. Don't be too concerned if your child doesn't eat or drink the exact amounts offered at every meal. If you offer a variety of foods from each food group, his or her needs can be met over a few days or a week.

Picky Eating

Do you have a picky eater in your home? Do any of these statements remind you of your preschooler?

- "Michael won't eat anything green, just because of the color."
- "Ebony will only eat peanut butter sandwiches!"

- "Maria doesn't sit still at the table. She can't seem to pay attention long enough to eat a meal!"

You're not alone. Picky eating is a typical behavior for many preschoolers. It's simply another step in the process of growing up and becoming independent. As long as your preschooler is healthy, growing normally, and has plenty of energy, he or she is most likely getting needed nutrients.

- Many children will show one or more of the following behaviors during the preschool years. In most cases, these will go away with time.
- Your child may refuse a food based on a certain color or texture. For example, he or she could refuse foods that are red or green, contain seeds, or are squishy.
- For a period of time, your preschooler may only eat a certain type of food. Your child may choose 1 or 2 foods he or she likes and refuse to eat anything else.
- Sometimes your child may waste time at the table and seem interested in doing anything but eating.
- Your child may be unwilling to try new foods, especially fruits and vegetables. It is normal for your preschooler to prefer familiar foods and be afraid to try new things.

Having your preschooler help you in the kitchen is a good way to get your child to try new foods. Kids feel good about doing something "grown-up." Give them small jobs to do. Praise their efforts. Children are much less likely to reject foods that they helped make.

Section 5.2

Physical Fitness and Health

This section contains text excerpted from the following sources: Text beginning with the heading "Encourage Your Child to Participate in Activities" is excerpted from "How Much Physical Activity Do Children Need?" Centers for Disease Control and Prevention (CDC), June 4, 2015; text beginning with the heading "Healthy Tips for Active Play" is excerpted from "Physical Activity," ChooseMyPlate.gov, U.S. Department of Agriculture (USDA), June 16, 2015.

Encourage Your Child to Participate in Activities

This may sound like a lot, but don't worry! Your child may already be meeting the *Physical Activity Guidelines for Americans*. And, you'll soon discover all the easy and enjoyable ways to help your child meet the recommendations. Encourage your child to participate in activities that are age-appropriate, enjoyable and offer variety! Just make sure your child or adolescent is doing three types of physical activity:

- **Aerobic Activity**

  Aerobic activity should make up most of your child's 60 or more minutes of physical activity each day. This can include either moderate-intensity aerobic activity, such as brisk walking, or vigorous-intensity activity, such as running. Be sure to include vigorous-intensity aerobic activity on at least 3 days per week.

- **Muscle Strengthening**

  Include muscle strengthening activities, such as gymnastics or push-ups, at least 3 days per week as part of your child's 60 or more minutes.

- **Bone Strengthening**

  Include bone strengthening activities, such as jumping rope or running, at least 3 days per week as part of your child's 60 or more minutes.

  1. On a scale of 0 to 10, where sitting is a 0 and the highest level of activity is a 10, moderate-intensity activity is a 5 or 6.

When your son does moderate-intensity activity, his heart will beat faster than normal and he will breathe harder than normal. Vigorous-intensity activity is a level 7 or 8. When your son does vigorous-intensity activity, his heart will beat much faster than normal and he will breathe much harder than normal.

2. Another way to judge intensity is to think about the activity your child is doing and compare it to the average child. What amount of intensity would the average child use? For example, when your daughter walks to school with friends each morning, she's probably doing moderate-intensity aerobic activity. But while she is at school, when she runs, or chases others by playing tag during recess, she's probably doing vigorous-intensity activity.

What Do You Mean By "Age-Appropriate" Activities?

Some physical activity is better-suited for children than adolescents. For example, children do not usually need formal muscle-strengthening programs, such as lifting weights. Younger children usually strengthen their muscles when they do gymnastics, play on a jungle gym or climb trees. As children grow older and become adolescents, they may start structured weight programs. For example, they may do these types of programs along with their football or basketball team practice.

How Is It Possible for My Child to Meet the Guidelines?

Many physical activities fall under more than one type of activity. This makes it possible for your child to do two or even three types of physical activity in one day! For example, if your daughter is on a basketball team and practices with her teammates everyday, she is not only doing vigorous-intensity aerobic activity but also bone-strengthening. Or, if your daughter takes gymnastics lessons, she is not only doing vigorous-intensity aerobic activity but also muscle- and bone-strengthening! It's easy to fit each type of activity into your child's schedule—all it takes is being familiar with the Guidelines and finding activities that your child enjoys.

What Can I Do to Get—and Keep—My Child Active?

As a parent, you can help shape your child's attitudes and behaviors toward physical activity, and knowing these guidelines is a great place to start. Throughout their lives, encourage young people to be physically active for one hour or more each day, with activities ranging from informal, active play to organized sports. Here are some ways you can do this:

- Set a positive example by leading an active lifestyle yourself.
- Make physical activity part of your family's daily routine by taking family walks or playing active games together.
- Give your children equipment that encourages physical activity.
- Take young people to places where they can be active, such as public parks, community baseball fields or basketball courts.
- Be positive about the physical activities in which your child participates and encourage them to be interested in new activities.
- Make physical activity fun. Fun activities can be anything your child enjoys, either structured or non-structured. Activities can range from team sports or individual sports to recreational activities such as walking, running, skating, bicycling, swimming, playground activities or free-time play.
- Instead of watching television after dinner, encourage your child to find fun activities to do on their own or with friends and family, such as walking, playing chase or riding bikes.
- Be safe! Always provide protective equipment such as helmets, wrist pads or knee pads and ensure that activity is age-appropriate.

What If My Child Has a Disability?

Physical activity is important for all children. It's best to talk with a healthcare provider before your child begins a physical activity routine. Try to get advice from a professional with experience in physical activity and disability. They can tell you more about the amounts and types of physical activity that are appropriate for your child's abilities.

Healthy Tips for Active Play

Why Is Active Play Important?

Active play helps your child learn healthy habits. There are many health benefits of active play, such as:

- Active children are less likely to weigh too much.

- Keeping your child active now helps lower the chance of developing chronic diseases like Type 2 diabetes.
- Activities, like running and jumping rope, help your child learn movement skills to develop muscles and strong bones.
- Active play can also help the mind develop. Playing "pretend" lets kids be creative.
- Active children are more likely to be happy and feel good about themselves. Children feel proud after learning how to
- bounce a ball or ride a bike.

Your child loves to move!

Encourage your child to play actively several times each day. Active play for children can happen in short bursts of time and can be led by you or your child. Active play can include playing on the playground, playing tag with friends, or throwing a ball.

How Can You Raise an Active Child?

- **Make active play fun for the whole family.** Let your child help plan the fun.
- **Focus on fun, not performance.** All children like to play. They will win when they move, have fun, and are active daily.
- **Set limits on TV and computer time.** Limit TV and other screen time to less than 2 hours a day, as advised by many doctors. Try reading during inactive time rather than watching TV.
- **Be active yourself.** Active parents tend to raise active children. You influence your child's behavior, attitudes, and future habits. Be more active and limit your own time watching TV. Set the example by using safety gear, like bike helmets.

As children grow, they may be ready for new activities.

- By **age 2**, they can run, walk, gallop, jump, and swim with adult help.
- By **age 3,** they can hop, climb, ride a tricycle or bicycle with training wheels and a safety helmet, and catch, throw, bounce, and kick a ball.
- By **age 4,** they can skip, swim, and complete an obstacle course.

There are many activities you can do with your child.

Here are some ideas of how to be active with your child. Write down your own ideas, too!

Indoor play

- Act out a story
- Turn up the music and dance
- Walk inside a shopping mall
- Play games, such as duck-duck-goose, hide and seek, follow the leader, Simon says

Outdoor play

- Family walks after dinner
- Play catch
- Take a nature hike
- Games in the yard or park
- Kick a ball

Be an Active Family

Physical activity is important for children and adults of all ages. Being active as a family can benefit everyone.Adults need 2½ hours a week of physical activity, and children need 60 minutes a day.

Follow these tips to add more activity to your family's busy schedule:

1. **Set specific activity times.** Determine time slots throughout the week when the whole family is available. Devote a few of these times to physical activity. Try doing something active after dinner or begin the weekend with a Saturday morning walk.
2. **Plan ahead and track your progress.** Write your activity plans on a family calendar. Let the kids help in planning the activities. Allow them to check it off after completing each activity.
3. **Include work around the house.** Involve the kids in yard work and other active chores around the house. Have them help you with raking, weeding, planting, or vacuuming.

4. **Use what is available.** Plan activities that require little or no equipment or facilities. Examples include walking, jogging, jumping rope, playing tag, and dancing. Find out what programs your community recreation center offers for free or minimal charge.

5. **Build new skills.** Enroll the kids in classes they might enjoy such as gymnastics, dance, or tennis. Help them practice. This will keep things fun and interesting, and introduce new skills!

6. **Plan for all weather conditions.** Choose some activities that do not depend on the weather conditions. Try mall walking, indoor swimming, or active video games. Enjoy outdoor activities as a bonus whenever the weather is nice.

7. **Turn off the TV.** Set a rule that no one can spend longer than 2 hours per day playing video games, watching TV, and using the computer (except for school work). Instead of a TV show, play an active family game, dance to favorite music, or go for a walk.

8. **Start small.** Begin by introducing one new family activity and add more when you feel everyone is ready. Take the dog for a longer walk, play another ball game, or go to an additional exercise class.

9. **Include other families.** Invite others to join your family activities. This is a great way for you and your kids to spend time with friends while being physically active. Plan parties with active games such as bowling or an obstacle course, sign up for family programs at the YMCA, or join a recreational club.

10. **Treat the family with fun physical activity.** When it is time to celebrate as a family, do something active as a reward. Plan a trip to the zoo, park, or lake to treat the family.

Section 5.3

Healthy Sleep Habits

Text in this section is excerpted from "All about Sleep," © 1995–2016. The Nemours Foundation/KidsHealth®. Reprinted with permission.

Sleep—or lack of it—is probably the most-discussed aspect of baby care. As new parents quickly discover, the quality and quantity of their baby's sleep affects the well-being of everyone in the household. And sleep struggles rarely end when child moves from a crib to a bed. Instead of cries, it's pleas or refusals; instead of a 3 a.m. feeding, it's a nightmare or request for water.

So how do you get kids to bed through the cries, screams, and avoidance tactics? How should you respond when you're awakened in the middle of the night? And how much sleep is enough for your kids?

How Much Is Enough?

Sleep quantity needs vary based on age. But common "rules" about how many hours of sleep an infant or a 2-year-old need might not be helpful when it comes to your own child. These numbers are simply averages reported for large groups of kids of particular ages.

There's no magical number of hours all kids need in a certain age group. Two-year-old Lilly might sleep for 12 hours, while 2-year-old Marcus is just as alert the next day after sleeping for only 9 hours.

Still, sleep is very important to kids' well-being. The link between a lack of sleep and a child's behavior isn't always obvious. When adults are tired, they can be grumpy or lack energy, but kids can become hyper, disagreeable, and have extreme changes in behavior.

Here are some approximate numbers based on age, with age-appropriate tips to help you get your child to sleep.

Babies (Up to 6 Months)

Newborns' internal clocks aren't fully developed. They sleep up to 18 hours a day, divided about equally between night and day. Newborns should be wakened every 3 to 4 hours until they have good weight gain, usually within the first few weeks. After that, it's OK if a baby sleeps for longer periods.

After those first weeks, infants may sleep for as long as 4 or 5 hours at a time—this is about how long their small bellies can go between feedings. If babies do sleep a good stretch at night, they may want to nurse or get the bottle more often during the day.

Just when parents feel that sleeping through the night is a far-off dream, their baby usually begins to sleep longer stretches at night. At 3 months, a baby averages about 14 hours of sleep total, with 8 to 9 hours at night (usually with an interruption or two) and two or three daytime naps.

It's important to know that babies can cry and make all sorts of other noises during light sleep. Even if they do wake up in the night, they may only be awake for a few minutes before falling asleep again on their own.

But if a baby under 6 months old continues to cry, it's time to respond. Your baby may be truly uncomfortable: hungry, wet, cold, or even sick. But routine nighttime awakenings for changing and feeding should be as quick and quiet as possible. Don't provide any unnecessary stimulation, such as talking, playing, turning on the lights, or using a bright mobile device while waiting for your child to sleep. Encourage the idea that nighttime is for sleeping. You have to teach this because your baby doesn't care what time it is as long as his or her needs are met.

Ideally, place your baby in the crib before he or she falls asleep. It's not too early to establish a simple bedtime routine. Any soothing activities (bathing, reading, singing) done consistently and in the same order each night can be part of the routine. Your baby will associate them with sleeping and they'll help him or her wind down.

The goal is for babies to fall asleep by themselves and learn to soothe themselves and go back to sleep if they should wake up in the middle of the night.

6 to 12 Months

At 6 months, babies still need an average of 14 hours of sleep a day, with 2 to 3 daytime naps, lasting anywhere from 2 hours to 30 minutes each. Some babies, particularly those who are breastfed, may still wake at night. But most no longer need a middle-of-the-night feeding.

If your baby wakes in the middle of the night, but you don't think it's due to hunger, wait a few minutes before going to your baby.

Sometimes, babies just need a few minutes to settle down on their down. Those who don't settle should be comforted without being picked up (talk softly to your baby, rub the back), then left to settle down again—unless they are sick. Sick babies need to be picked up and cared for. If your baby doesn't seem sick and continues to cry, you can wait a little longer, then repeat the short crib-side visit.

Between 6 and 12 months, separation anxiety, a normal part of development, comes into play. But the rules at night are the same through a baby's first birthday: Try not to pick up your baby, turn on the lights, sing, talk, play, or feed your child. All of these activities do not allow your baby to learn to fall asleep on his or her own and encourage more awakenings.

Toddlers

From ages 1 to 3, most toddlers sleep about 12 to 14 hours over a 24-hour period. Separation anxiety, or just wanting to be up with mom and dad (and not miss anything), can motivate a child to stay awake. So can the simple toddler style of always saying "No!"

It's important to set regular bedtimes and naptimes, and to stick to them. Parents sometimes make the mistake of thinking that keeping kids up will make them sleepier at bedtime. But the truth is that kids can have a harder time sleeping if they're overtired. Though most toddlers take 1- to 3-hour naps during the day, you don't have to force your child to nap. But it's important to schedule some quiet time, even if your toddler chooses not to sleep.

Establish a bedtime routine to help kids relax and get ready for sleep. For a toddler, the routine might be 5-30 minutes long and include calming activities such as reading a story, bathing, and listening to soft music.

Whatever the nightly ritual is, your toddler will probably insist that it be the same every night. Just don't allow rituals to become too long or complicated. Whenever possible, let your toddler make bedtime choices within the routine: which pajamas to wear, which stuffed animal to take to bed, what music to play. This gives your little one a sense of control.

Even the best sleepers give parents an occasional wake-up call. Teething can awaken a toddler and so can dreams. Active dreaming begins at this age, and for very young children dreams can be pretty alarming. Nightmares are particularly frightening to a toddler, who can't distinguish imagination from reality. (So carefully select what TV programs, if any, your toddler sees before bedtime.)

Comfort and hold your child at these times. Let your toddler talk about the dream if he or she wants to, and stay until your child is calm. Then encourage your child to go back to sleep as soon as possible.

Pre-Schoolers

Preschoolers sleep about 11 to 12 hours per night. Those who get enough rest at night may no longer need a daytime nap. Instead, they may benefit from some quiet time in the afternoon.

Most nursery schools and kindergartens have quiet periods when the kids lie on mats or just rest. As kids give up their naps, they may go to bed at night earlier than they did as toddlers.

School-Age Kids and Preteens

School-age kids need 10 to 11 hours of sleep a night. Bedtime problems can start at this age for a variety of reasons. Homework, sports and after-school activities, computers, TVs, mobile devices, and hectic family schedules all can contribute to kids not getting the sleep they need. Sleep-deprived kids can become hyper or irritable, and may have a hard time paying attention in school.

It's still important to have a consistent bedtime, especially on school nights. Leave enough technology-free time before bed to allow your child to unwind before lights-out. A good rule of thumb is switching off the electronics at least an hour before bed and keeping TVs, computers, and mobile devices out of kids' bedrooms.

Teens

Teens need about 9 hours of sleep per night, but many don't get it. Early school start times on top of schedules packed with school, homework, friends, and activities mean that many are chronically sleep deprived.

Sleep deprivation adds up over time, so an hour less per night is like a full night without sleep by the end of the week. Among other things, a lack of sleep can lead to:

- being less attentive
- inconsistent performance
- short-term memory loss
- delayed response time

This can lead to anger problems, trouble in school (academically and with teachers and peers), the use of stimulants like caffeine or energy drinks to feel more awake, and car crashes due to delayed response times or falling asleep at the wheel.

Teens also undergo a change in their sleep patterns—their bodies want to stay up late and wake up later, which often leads to them trying to catch up on sleep during the weekend. But this irregularity can make getting to sleep at a reasonable hour during the week even harder.

Ideally, a teen should try to go to bed at the same time every night and wake up at the same time every morning, allowing for at least 9 hours of sleep.

Bedtime Routines

No matter what your child's age, establish a bedtime routine that encourages good sleep habits. These tips can help kids ease into a good night's sleep:

- Stick to a bedtime, and give your kids a heads-up 30 minutes and then 10 minutes beforehand.
- Include a winding-down period in the routine.
- Encourage older kids and teens to set and maintain a bedtime that allows for the full hours of sleep needed at their age.

Section 5.4

The Importance of Handwashing

This section includes text excerpted from "When and How to Wash Your Hands," Centers for Disease Control and Prevention (CDC), September 4, 2015.

Keeping hands clean through improved hand hygiene is one of the most important steps we can take to avoid getting sick and spreading germs to others. Many diseases and conditions are spread by not washing hands with soap and clean, running water. If clean, running water is not accessible, as is common in many parts of the world, use soap and available water. If soap and water are unavailable, use an alcohol-based hand sanitizer that contains at least 60% alcohol to clean hands.

When Should You Wash Your Hands?

- Before, during, and after preparing food
- Before eating food
- Before and after caring for someone who is sick
- Before and after treating a cut or wound
- After using the toilet
- After changing diapers or cleaning up a child who has used the toilet
- After blowing your nose, coughing, or sneezing
- After touching an animal, animal feed, or animal waste
- After handling pet food or pet treats
- After touching garbage

How Should You Wash Your Hands?

- **Wet** your hands with clean, running water (warm or cold), turn off the tap, and apply soap.
- **Lather** your hands by rubbing them together with the soap. Be sure to lather the backs of your hands, between your fingers, and under your nails.
- **Scrub** your hands for at least 20 seconds. Need a timer? Hum the "Happy Birthday" song from beginning to end twice.
- **Rinse** your hands well under clean, running water.
- **Dry** your hands using a clean towel or air dry them.

What Should You Do If You Don't Have Soap and Clean, Running Water?

Washing hands with soap and water is the best way to reduce the number of germs on them in most situations. If soap and water are not available, use an alcohol-based hand sanitizer that contains at least 60% alcohol. Alcohol-based hand sanitizers can quickly reduce the number of germs on hands in some situations, but sanitizers do not eliminate all types of germs and might not remove harmful chemicals.

Hand sanitizers are not as effective when hands are visibly dirty or greasy.

How Do You Use Hand Sanitizers?

Apply the product to the palm of one hand (read the label to learn the correct amount).

- Rub your hands together.
- Rub the product over all surfaces of your hands and fingers until your hands are dry.

Why Wash Your Hands?

Keeping hands clean is one of the most important steps we can take to avoid getting sick and spreading germs to others. Many diseases and conditions are spread by not washing hands with soap and clean, running water.

How Germs Get onto Hands and Make People Sick

Feces (poop) from people or animals is an important source of germs like *Salmonella, E. coli* O157, and norovirus that cause diarrhea, and it can spread some respiratory infections like adenovirus and hand-foot-mouth disease. These kinds of germs can get onto hands after people use the toilet or change a diaper, but also in less obvious ways, like after handling raw meats that have invisible amounts of animal poop on them. A single gram of human feces—which is about the weight of a paper clip—can contain one trillion germs. Germs can also get onto hands if people touch any object that has germs on it because someone coughed or sneezed on it or was touched by some other contaminated object. When these germs get onto hands and are not washed off, they can be passed from person to person and make people sick.

Washing Hands Prevents Illnesses and Spread of Infections to Others

Handwashing with soap removes germs from hands. This helps prevent infections because:

- People frequently touch their eyes, nose, and mouth without even realizing it. Germs can get into the body through the eyes, nose and mouth and make us sick.
- Germs from unwashed hands can get into foods and drinks while people prepare or consume them. Germs can multiply in some types of foods or drinks, under certain conditions, and make people sick.
- Germs from unwashed hands can be transferred to other objects, like handrails, table tops, or toys, and then transferred to another person's hands.
- Removing germs through handwashing therefore helps prevent diarrhea and respiratory infections and may even help prevent skin and eye infections.

Teaching people about handwashing helps them and their communities stay healthy. Handwashing education in the community:

- Reduces the number of people who get sick with diarrhea by 31%
- Reduces diarrheal illness in people with weakened immune systems by 58%
- Reduces respiratory illnesses, like colds, in the general population by 16–21%

Not Washing Hands Harms Children around the World

- About 1.8 million children under the age of 5 die each year from diarrheal diseases and pneumonia, the top two killers of young children around the world.
- Handwashing with soap could protect about 1 out of every 3 young children who get sick with diarrhea and almost 1 out of 5 young children with respiratory infections like pneumonia.
- Although people around the world clean their hands with water, very few use soap to wash their hands. Washing hands with soap removes germs much more effectively.
- Handwashing education and access to soap in schools can help improve attendance.
- Good handwashing early in life may help improve child development in some settings.

Handwashing Helps Battle the Rise in Antibiotic Resistance

- Preventing sickness reduces the amount of antibiotics people use and the likelihood that antibiotic resistance will develop. Handwashing can prevent about 30% of diarrhea-related sicknesses and about 20% of respiratory infections (e.g., colds). Antibiotics often are prescribed unnecessarily for these health issues. Reducing the number of these infections by washing hands frequently helps prevent the overuse of antibiotics—the single most important factor leading to antibiotic resistance around the world. Handwashing can also prevent people from getting sick with germs that are already resistant to antibiotics and that can be difficult to treat.

Chapter 6

Preventing Childhood Injuries

Chapter Contents

Section 6.1

Preventing Burns

This section contains text excerpted from the following sources: Text in this section begins with excerpts from "Burn Prevention," Centers for Disease Control and Prevention (CDC), April 28, 2016; Text under the heading "Key Prevention Tips" is excerpted from "Smoke Alarms," U.S. Fire Administration (USFA), Federal Emergency Management Agency (FEMA), September 24, 2013.

We all want to keep our children safe and secure and help them live to their full potential. Knowing how to prevent leading causes of child injury, like burns, is a step toward this goal.

Every day, over 300 children ages 0 to 19 are treated in emergency rooms for burn-related injuries and two children die as a result of being burned.

Younger children are more likely to sustain injuries from scald burns that are caused by hot liquids or steam, while older children are more likely to sustain injuries from flame burns that are caused by direct contact with fire.

Thankfully, there are ways you can help protect the children you love from burns.

Key Prevention Tips

Put Smoke Alarms in Your Home to Keep Your Family Safe

Almost 2,500 people die in home fires every year in the United States. Most of these people live in homes that do not have working smoke alarms. Smoke alarms save lives. Keep your family safe. Put working smoke alarms in your home.

- Smoke is poison. It can kill you.
- Smoke alarms make a loud noise when there is smoke in your home.
- Smoke alarms wake you up if you are sleeping.
- Put a smoke alarm on every level of your home and outside each sleeping area. Put a smoke alarm inside every bedroom.

- Smoke goes up. Put smoke alarms on the ceiling or high on the wall.

Make Sure Your Smoke Alarms Work

Smoke alarms save lives. Keep your family safe. Put working smoke alarms in your home.

- Your family is not safe if they can't hear the smoke alarms.
- Test your smoke alarms. Push the test button. You will hear a loud noise. If you don't hear the noise, you need a new battery or a new alarm. Fix this immediately.
- Make sure the smoke alarm always has a good battery. Put a new battery in the alarm every year.
- Smoke alarms with long-life batteries will work for up to 10 years. You do not change the battery.
- Smoke alarms do not last forever. Get new smoke alarms every 10 years.

Be Ready, Make an Escape Plan

When you hear a smoke alarm, you only have about three minutes to get everyone outside and safe.

- Tell your family what to do if they hear the smoke alarm.
- Make an escape plan so everyone knows how to get out fast.
- Pick a meeting place outside of your home where everyone will meet.
- Some children and older adults cannot hear the smoke alarm when they are sleeping. Make a plan for how to wake them up.
- Practice your escape plan with everyone in your family two times each year.

Use Your Escape Plan If There Is a Fire

When you hear a smoke alarm, you only have about three minutes to get everyone outside and safe.

- Go to your outside meeting place immediately.
- Call 911 or the fire department from outside.
- Never go back inside a burning building.

Section 6.2

Preventing Drowning

This section contains text excerpted from the following sources: Text in this section begins with excerpts from "Drowning Prevention," Centers for Disease Control and Prevention (CDC), April 30, 2016; Text beginning with the heading "Unintentional Drowning: Get the Facts" is excerpted from from "Unintentional Drowning: Get the Facts," Centers for Disease Control and Prevention (CDC), April 28, 2016.

We all want to keep our children safe and secure and help them live to their full potential. Knowing how to prevent leading causes of child injury, like drowning, is a step toward this goal. When most of us are enjoying time at the pool or beach, injuries aren't the first thing on our minds. Yet, drownings are a leading cause of injury death for young children ages 1 to 14, and three children die every day as a result of drowning. In fact, drowning kills more children 1—4 than anything else except birth defects.

Thankfully, parents can play a key role in protecting the children they love from drowning.

Unintentional Drowning: Get the Facts

Every day, about ten people die from unintentional drowning. Of these, two are children aged 14 or younger. Drowning ranks fifth among the leading causes of unintentional injury death in the United States.

What Factors Influence Drowning Risk?

The main factors that affect drowning risk are lack of swimming ability, lack of barriers to prevent unsupervised water access, lack of close supervision while swimming, location, failure to wear life jackets, alcohol use, and seizure disorders.

- **Lack of Swimming Ability:** Many adults and children report that they can't swim. Research has shown that participation in formal swimming lessons can reduce the risk of drowning among children aged 1 to 4 years.

- **Lack of Barriers:** Barriers, such as pool fencing, prevent young children from gaining access to the pool area without caregivers' awareness. A four-sided isolation fence (separating the pool area from the house and yard) reduces a child's risk of drowning 83% compared to three-sided property-line fencing.
- **Lack of Close Supervision:** Drowning can happen quickly and quietly anywhere there is water (such as bathtubs, swimming pools, buckets), and even in the presence of lifeguards.
- **Location:** People of different ages drown in different locations. For example, most children ages 1–4 drown in home swimming pools. The percentage of drownings in natural water settings, including lakes, rivers and oceans, increases with age. More than half of fatal and nonfatal drownings among those 15 years and older (57% and 57% respectively) occurred in natural water settings.
- **Failure to Wear Life Jackets:** In 2010, the U.S. Coast Guard received reports for 4,604 boating incidents; 3,153 boaters were reported injured, and 672 died. Most (72%) boating deaths that occurred during 2010 were caused by drowning, with 88% of victims not wearing life jackets.

Key Prevention Tips

Learn life-saving skills.

Everyone should know the basics of swimming (floating, moving through the water) and cardiopulmonary resuscitation (CPR).

Fence it off.

Install a four-sided isolation fence, with self-closing and self-latching gates, around backyard swimming pools. This can help keep children away from the area when they aren't supposed to be swimming. Pool fences should completely separate the house and play area from the pool.

Make life jackets a must.

Make sure kids wear life jackets in and around natural bodies of water, such as lakes or the ocean, even if they know how to swim. Life jackets can be used in and around pools for weaker swimmers too.

Be on the look out.

When kids are in or near water (including bathtubs), closely supervise them at all times. Because drowning happens quickly and quietly, adults watching kids in or near water should avoid distracting activities like playing cards, reading books, talking on the phone, and using alcohol or drugs.

Section 6.3

Preventing Falls

This section includes text excerpted from "Fall Prevention," Centers for Disease Control and Prevention (CDC), April 28, 2016.

We all want to keep our children safe and secure and help them live to their full potential. Knowing how to prevent leading causes of child injury, like falls, is a step toward this goal.

Falls are the leading cause of non-fatal injuries for all children ages 0 to 19. Every day, approximately 8,000 children are treated in the U.S. emergency rooms for fall-related injuries. This adds up to almost 2.8 million children each year.

Thankfully, many falls can be prevented, and parents and caregivers can play a key role in protecting children.

Key Prevention Tips

Play safely.

Falls on the playground are a common cause of injury. Check to make sure that the surfaces under playground equipment are safe, soft, and consist of appropriate materials (such as wood chips or sand, not dirt or grass). The surface materials should be an appropriate depth and well-maintained.

Make your home safer.

Use home safety devices, such as guards on windows that are above ground level, stair gates, and guard rails. These devices can help keep a busy, active child from taking a dangerous tumble.

Keep sports safe.

Make sure your child wears protective gear during sports and recreation. For example, when in-line skating, use wrist guards, knee and elbow pads, and a helmet.

Supervision is key.

Supervise young children at all times around fall hazards, such as stairs and playground equipment, whether you're at home or out to play.

Section 6.4

Preventing Poisoning

This section contains text excerpted from the following sources: Text in this section begins with excerpts from "Poisoning Prevention," Centers for Disease Control and Prevention (CDC), April 28, 2016; Text beginning with the heading "Keep Young Children Safe from Poisoning" is excerpted from "Tips to Prevent Poisonings," Centers for Disease Control and Prevention (CDC), November 24, 2015.

Every day, over 300 children in the United States ages 0 to 19 are treated in an emergency department, and two children die, as a result of being poisoned. It's not just chemicals in your home marked with clear warning labels that can be dangerous to children.

Everyday items in your home, such as household cleaners and medicines, can be poisonous to children as well. Medication dosing mistakes and unsupervised ingestions are common ways that children are poisoned. Active, curious children will often investigate—and sometimes try to eat or drink—anything that they can get into.

Thankfully, there are ways you can help poison-proof your home and protect the children you love.

Key Prevention Tips

Lock them up and away.

Keep medicines and toxic products, such cleaning solutions and detergent pods, in their original packaging where children can't see or get them.

Know the number.

Put the nationwide poison control center phone number, 1-800-222-1222, on or near every telephone in your home and program it into your cell phone. Call the poison control center if you think a child has been poisoned but they are awake and alert; they can be reached 24 hours a day, seven days a week. Call 911 if you have a poison emergency and your child has collapsed or is not breathing.

Read the label.

Follow label directions carefully and read all warnings when giving medicines to children.

Don't keep it if you don't need it.

Safely dispose of unused, unneeded, or expired prescription drugs and over the counter drugs, vitamins, and supplements. To dispose of medicines, mix them with coffee grounds or kitty litter and throw them away. You can also turn them in at a local take-back program or during National Drug Take-Back events.

Keep Young Children Safe from Poisoning

Be Prepared

- Put the poison help number, 1-800-222-1222, on or near every home telephone and save it on your cell phone. The line is open 24 hours a day, 7 days a week.

Be Smart about Storage

- Store all medicines and household products up and away and out of sight in a cabinet where a child cannot reach them.
- When you are taking or giving medicines or are using household products:
- Do not put your next dose on the counter or table where children can reach them—it only takes seconds for a child to get them.
- If you have to do something else while taking medicine, such as answer the phone, take any young children with you.
- Secure the child safety cap completely every time you use a medicine.
- After using them, do not leave medicines or household products out. As soon as you are done with them, put them away and out of sight in a cabinet where a child cannot reach them.

- Be aware of any legal or illegal drugs that guests may bring into your home. Ask guests to store drugs where children cannot find them. Children can easily get into pillboxes, purses, backpacks, or coat pockets.

What to Do if a Poisoning Occurs

- Remain calm.
- Call 911 if you have a poison emergency and the victim has collapsed or is not breathing. If the victim is awake and alert, dial 1-800-222-1222. Try to have this information ready:
- the victim's age and weight
- the container or bottle of the poison if available
- the time of the poison exposure
- the address where the poisoning occurred
- Stay on the phone and follow the instructions from the emergency operator or poison control center.

Section 6.5

Preventing Motor Vehicle Injuries

This section includes text excerpted from "Road Traffic Safety," Centers for Disease Control and Prevention (CDC), April 28, 2016.

We all want to keep our children safe and secure and help them live to their full potential. Knowing how to prevent leading causes of child injury, like road traffic injuries, is a step toward this goal.

Every hour, nearly 150 children between ages 0 and 19 are treated in emergency departments for injuries sustained in motor vehicle crashes. More children ages 5 to 19 die from crash-related injuries than from any other type of injury.

Thankfully, parents can play a key role in protecting the children they love from road traffic injuries.

Key Prevention Tips

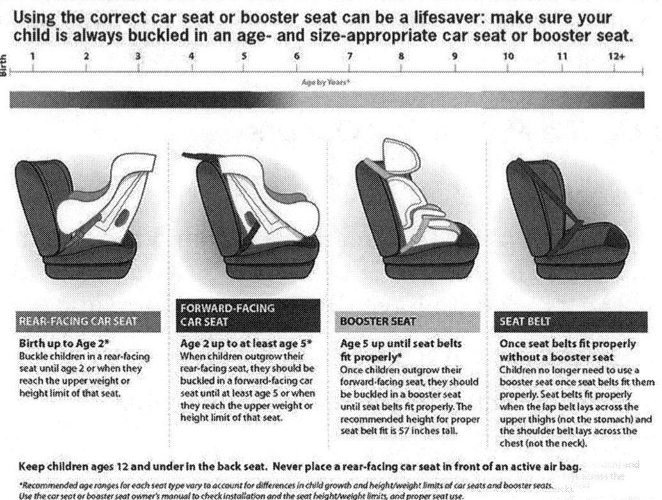

Figure 6.1. *Car Seat or Booster Seat*

Know the stages

Make sure children are properly buckled up in a car seat, booster seat, or seat belt, whichever is appropriate for their age, height and weight.

Birth up to Age 2: Rear-facing car seat.

For the best possible protection, infants and children should be buckled in a rear-facing car seat, in the back seat, until age 2 or when they reach the upper weight or height limits of their particular seat. Check the seat's owner's manual and/or labels on the seat for weight and height limits.

Age 2 up to at least Age 5: Forward-facing car seat.

When children outgrow their rear-facing seats they should be buckled in a forward-facing car seat, in the back seat, until at least age 5 or when they reach the upper weight or height limit of their particular seat. Check the seat's owner's manual and/or labels on the seat for weight and height limits.

Age 5 up until seat belts fit properly: Booster seat.

Once children outgrow their forward-facing seat, (by reaching the upper height or weight limit of their seat), they should be buckled in a belt positioning booster seat until seat belts fit properly. Seat belts fit properly when the lap belt lays across the upper thighs (not the stomach) and the shoulder belt lays across the chest (not the neck). Remember to keep children properly buckled in the back seat for the best possible protection.

Once Seat Belts Fit Properly without a Booster Seat: Seat Belt

Children no longer need to use a booster seat once seat belts fit them properly. Seat belts fit properly when the lap belt lays across the upper thighs (not the stomach) and the shoulder belt lays across the chest (not the neck). For the best possible protection keep children properly buckled in the back seat.

Install and Use Car and Booster Seats Properly

Install and use car seats and booster seats according to the seat's owner's manual or get help installing them from a certified Child Passenger Safety Technician.

Don't Seat Children in Front of an Airbag

Buckle all children aged 12 and under in the back seat. Airbags can kill young children riding in the front seat. Never place a rear-facing car seat in front of an air bag.

Seat Children in the Middle of the Back Seat

Buckle children in the middle of the back seat when possible, because it is the safest spot in the vehicle.

Use Proper Restraints Every Trip

Buckle children in car seats, booster seats, or seat belts on every trip, no matter how short.

Parents and Caregivers: Always Wear a Seat Belt

Set a good example by always using a seat belt themselves.

Additional Tips

Sign a Driving Agreement.

If you're a parent of a teen who is learning to drive, sign a Parent-Teen Driving Agreement with your teen to limit risky driving situations, such as having multiple teen passengers and driving at night.

Helmets can Help.

Children should wear an appropriate helmet any time they are on a motorcycle, bicycle, skateboard, scooter, or skates.

Section 6.6

Preventing Sports Injuries

This section contains text excerpted from the following sources: Text in this section begins with excerpts from "Playground Safety," Centers for Disease Control and Prevention (CDC), May 2, 2016; Text beginning with the heading "Sports Safety" is excerpted from "Sports Safety," Centers for Disease Control and Prevention (CDC), April 30, 2016.

Each year in the United States, emergency departments (EDs) treat more than 200,000 children ages 14 and younger for playground-related injuries. More than 20,000 of these children are treated for a traumatic brain injury (TBI), including concussion. Overall, more research is needed to better understand what specific activities are putting kids at risk of injury and what changes in playground equipment and surfaces might help prevent injuries.

Occurrence and Consequences of Playground-Related Injuries

All Emergency Department-Treated, Playground-Related Injuries

- About 56% of playground-related injuries that are treated in EDs are fractures and contusions/abrasions.
- About 75% of injuries related to playground equipment occur on public playgrounds. Most occur at a place of recreation or school.

Playground-Related TBIs

- The overall rate of ED visits for playground-related TBI has significantly increased in recent years (2005–2013).
- About two-thirds of playground-related TBIs occurred at school and places or recreation or sports and often involved monkey bars, climbing equipment, or swings.

- Most ED visits for playground-related TBIs occur during weekdays, Monday through Friday.
- Playground-related TBI ED visits occurred frequently during the months of April, May, and September.

Deaths

Between 2001 and 2008, the Consumer Product Safety Commission investigated 40 deaths associated with playground equipment. The average age of children who died was six years old. Of these, 27 (68%) died from strangulation and six (15%) died from falls to the playground surface. Most strangulation involved the combination of slides or swings and jump ropes, other ropes, dog leashes or clothes drawstrings.

Injury Risk Factors

All Emergency Department-Treated, Playground-Related Injuries

- While all children who use playgrounds are at risk for injury, boys sustain ED-treated injuries (55%) slightly more often than girls (45%).
- Children ages 5 to 9 have higher rates of ED visits for playground injuries than any other age group. Most of these injuries occur at school. On public playgrounds, more injuries occur on monkey bars and climbing equipment than on any other equipment.
- Playgrounds that are well maintained have fewer risks to children such as rusty or broken equipment.

Playground-Related TBIs

- Boys more often sustain playground-related TBIs compared to girls.
- Most children who are treated for playground-related TBIs are 5 to 9 years of age.
- Playground-related TBIs varied by age group and equipment type:
    - 0–4 year olds are often injured on swings and slides.

- 5–9 year olds are often injured on swings, monkey bars, and climbing equipment.
- 10–14 year olds are often injured on swings, monkey bars, and climbing equipment.
- 5 to 14 year olds sustain TBIs more frequently at school.

What Can Be Done?

Take steps to keep kids safe by:

- Checking that playgrounds have soft material under them such as wood chips, sand, or mulch.
- Reading playground signs and using playground equipment that is right for your child's age.
- Making sure there are guardrails in good condition to help prevent falls.
- Looking out for things in the play area that can trip your child, like tree stumps or rocks.

Sports Safety

Taking part in sports and recreation activities is an important part of a healthy, physically active lifestyle for kids. But injuries can, and do, occur. More than 2.6 million children 0–19 years old are treated in the emergency department each year for sports and recreation-related injuries.

Thankfully, there are steps that parents can take to help make sure kids stay safe on the field, the court, or wherever they play or participate in sports and recreation activities.

Key Prevention Tips

Gear up. When children are active in sports and recreation, make sure they use the right protective gear for their activity, such as helmets, wrist guards, knee or elbow pads.

Use the right stuff. Be sure that sports protective equipment is in good condition, fits appropriately and is worn correctly all the time—for example, avoid missing or broken buckles or compressed or worn padding. Poorly fitting equipment may be uncomfortable and may not offer the best protection.

Practice makes perfect. Have children learn and practice skills they need in their activity. For example, knowing how to tackle safely is important in preventing injuries in football and soccer. Have children practice proper form—this can prevent injuries during baseball, softball, and many other activities. Also, be sure to safely and slowly increase activities to improve physical fitness; being in good condition can protect kids from injury.

Pay attention to temperature. Allow time for child athletes to gradually adjust to hot or humid environments to prevent heat-related injuries or illness. Parents and coaches should pay close attention to make sure that players are hydrated and appropriately dressed.

Be a good model. Communicate positive safety messages and serve as a model of safe behavior, including wearing a helmet and following the rules.

Chapter 7

Fevers and Febrile Seizures in Children

Chapter Contents

Section 7.1

Fevers in Children

Text in this section is excerpted from "Fever and Taking Your Child's Temperature," © 1995–2016. The Nemours Foundation/KidsHealth®. Reprinted with permission.

You've probably experienced waking in the middle of the night to find your child flushed, hot, and sweaty. Your little one's forehead feels warm. You immediately suspect a fever, but are unsure of what to do next. Should you get out the thermometer? Call the doctor?

In healthy kids, fevers usually don't indicate anything serious. Although it can be frightening when your child's temperature rises, fever itself causes no harm and can actually be a good thing—it's often the body's way of fighting infections. And not all fevers need to be treated. High fever, however, can make a child uncomfortable and make problems (such as dehydration) worse.

Here's more about fevers, how to measure and treat them, and when to call your doctor.

Fever Facts

Fever happens when the body's internal "thermostat" raises the body temperature above its normal level. This thermostat is found in a part of the brain called the hypothalamus. The hypothalamus knows what temperature your body should be (usually around 98.6°F/37°C) and will send messages to your body to keep it that way.

Most people's body temperatures even change a little bit during the course of the day: It's usually a little lower in the morning and a little higher in the evening and can vary as kids run around, play, and exercise.

Sometimes, though, the hypothalamus will "reset" the body to a higher temperature in response to an infection, illness, or some other cause. Why? Researchers believe turning up the heat is the body's way of fighting the germs that cause infections and making the body a less comfortable place for them.

Causes of Fever

It's important to remember that fever by itself is not an illness—it's usually a symptom of another problem.

Fevers have a few potential causes:

Infection: Most fevers are caused by infection or other illness. A fever helps the body fight infections by stimulating natural defense mechanisms.

Overdressing: Infants, especially newborns, may get fevers if they're over bundled or in a hot environment because they don't regulate their body temperature as well as older kids. However, because fevers in newborns can indicate a serious infection, even infants who are overdressed must be checked by a doctor if they have a fever.

Immunizations: Babies and kids sometimes get a low-grade fever after getting vaccinated.

Although teething may cause a slight rise in body temperature, it's probably not the cause if a child's temperature is higher than 100°F (37.8°C).

When Fever Is a Sign of Something Serious

In the past, doctors advised treating a fever on the basis of temperature alone. But now they recommend considering both the temperature and a child's overall condition.

Kids whose temperatures are lower than 102°F (38.9°C) often don't need medicine unless they're uncomfortable. There's one important exception to this rule: If you have an infant 3 months or younger with a rectal temperature of 100.4°F (38°C) or higher, call your doctor or go to the emergency department immediately. Even a slight fever can be a sign of a potentially serious infection in very young infants.

If your child is between 3 months and 3 years old and has a fever of 102.2°F (39°C) or higher, call your doctor to see if he or she needs to see your child. For older kids, take behavior and activity level into account. Watching how your child behaves will give you a pretty good idea of whether a minor illness is the cause or if your child should be seen by a doctor.

The illness is probably not serious if your child:

- is still interested in playing
- is eating and drinking well

- is alert and smiling at you
- has a normal skin color
- looks well when his or her temperature comes downAnd don't worry too much about a child with a fever who doesn't want to eat. This is very common with infections that cause fever. For kids who still drink and urinate (pee) normally, not eating as much as usual is OK.

Is it a Fever?

A gentle kiss on the forehead or a hand placed lightly on the skin is often enough to give you a hint that your child has a fever. However, this method of taking a temperature (called tactile temperature) doesn't give an accurate measurement.

Use a reliable thermometer to confirm a fever, which is when a child's temperature is at or above one of these levels:

- measured orally (in the mouth): 99.5°F (37.5°C)
- measured rectally (in the bottom): 100.4°F (38°C)
- measured in an axillary position (under the arm): 99°F (37.2°C)

But how high a fever is doesn't tell you much about how sick your child is. A simple cold or other viral infection can sometimes cause a rather high fever (in the 102°–104°F/38.9°–40°C range), but this doesn't usually indicate a serious problem. And serious infections, especially those in infants, might cause no fever or even an abnormally low body temperature (below 97°F or 36.1°C).

Because fevers can rise and fall, a child might have chills as the body's temperature begins to rise. The child may sweat to release extra heat as the temperature starts to drop.

Sometimes kids with a fever breathe faster than usual and may have a faster heart rate. Call the doctor if your child is having trouble breathing, is breathing faster than normal, or continues to breathe fast after the fever comes down.

Fever: A Common Part of Childhood

All kids get fevers, and in most cases they're completely back to normal within a few days. For older babies and kids (but not necessarily for infants younger than 3 months), the way they act is more important than the reading on your thermometer. Everyone gets cranky when they have a fever. This is normal and should be expected.

But if you're ever in doubt about what to do or what a fever might mean, or if your child is acting ill in a way that concerns you even if there's no fever, always call your doctor for advice.

Section 7.2

Febrile Seizures

This section includes text excerpted from "Febrile Seizures Fact Sheet," National Institute of Neurological Disorders and Stroke (NINDS), November 3, 2015.

What Are Febrile Seizures?

Febrile seizures are seizures or convulsions that occur in young children and are triggered by fever. Young children between the ages of about 6 months and 5 years old are the most likely to experience febrile seizures; this risk peaks during the second year of life. The fever may accompany common childhood illnesses such as a cold, the flu, or an ear infection. In some cases, a child may not have a fever at the time of the seizure but will develop one a few hours later.

The vast majority of febrile seizures are convulsions. Most often during a febrile seizure, a child will lose consciousness and both arms and legs will shake uncontrollably. Less common symptoms include eye rolling, rigid (stiff) limbs, or twitching on only one side or a portion of the body, such as an arm or a leg. Sometimes during a febrile seizure, a child may lose consciousness but will not noticeably shake or move.

Most febrile seizures last only a few minutes and are accompanied by a fever above 101°F (38.3°C). Although they can be frightening for parents, brief febrile seizures (less than 15 minutes) do not cause any long-term health problems. Having a febrile seizure does not mean a child has epilepsy, since that disorder is characterized by reoccurring seizures that are not triggered by fever. Even prolonged seizures (lasting more 15 minutes) generally have a good outcome but carry an increased risk of developing epilepsy.

How Common Are Febrile Seizures?

Febrile seizures are the most common type of convulsions in infants and young children and occur in 2 to 5 percent of American children before age 5. Approximately 40 percent of children who experience one febrile seizure will have a recurrence. Children at highest risk for recurrence are those who have:

- their first febrile seizure at a young age (younger than 18 months)
- a family history of febrile seizures
- a febrile seizure as the first sign of an illness
- a relatively low temperature increases with their first febrile seizure.

A prolonged initial febrile seizure does not substantially boost the risk of reoccurring febrile seizures. However, if another does occur, it is more likely to be prolonged.

What Should Be Done for a Child Having a Febrile Seizure?

It is important that parents and caretakers remain calm, take first aid measures, and carefully observe the child. If a child is having a febrile seizure, parents and caregivers should do the following:

- Note the start time of the seizure. If the seizure lasts longer than 5 minutes, call an ambulance. The child should be taken immediately to the nearest medical facility for diagnosis and treatment.
- Call an ambulance if the seizure is less than 5 minutes but the child does not seem to be recovering quickly.
- Gradually place the child on a protected surface such as the floor or ground to prevent accidental injury. Do not restrain or hold a child during a convulsion.
- Position the child on his or her side or stomach to prevent choking. When possible, gently remove any objects from the child's mouth. Nothing should ever be placed in the child's mouth during a convulsion. These objects can obstruct the child's airway and make breathing difficult.

- Seek immediate medical attention if this is the child's first febrile seizure and take the child to the doctor once the seizure has ended to check for the cause of the fever. This is especially urgent if the child shows symptoms of stiff neck, extreme lethargy, or abundant vomiting, which may be signs of meningitis, an infection over the brain surface.

Are Febrile Seizures Harmful?

The vast majority of febrile seizures are short and do not cause any long-term damage. During a seizure, there is a small chance that the child may be injured by falling or may choke on food or saliva in the mouth. Using proper first aid for seizures can help avoid these hazards.

There is no evidence that short febrile seizures cause brain damage. Large studies have found that even children with prolonged febrile seizures have normal school achievement and perform as well on intellectual tests as their siblings who do not have seizures. Even when the seizures last a long time, most children recover completely.

Multiple or prolonged seizures are a risk factor for epilepsy but most children who experience febrile seizures do not go on to develop the reoccurring seizures that are characteristic of epilepsy. Some children, including those with cerebral palsy, delayed development, or other neurological abnormalities as well as those with a family history of epilepsy are at increased risk of developing epilepsy whether or not they have febrile seizures. Febrile seizures may be more common in these children but do not contribute much to the overall risk of developing epilepsy.

Children who experience a brief, full body febrile seizure are slightly more likely to develop epilepsy than the general population. Children who have a febrile seizure that lasts longer than 10 minutes; a focal seizure (a seizure that starts on one side of the brain); or seizures that reoccur within 24 hours, have a moderately increased risk (about 10 percent) of developing epilepsy as compared to children who do not have febrile seizures.

Of greatest concern is the small group of children with very prolonged febrile seizures lasting longer than 30 minutes. In these children, the risk of epilepsy is as high as 30 to 40 percent though the condition may not occur for many years. Recent studies suggest that prolonged febrile seizures can injure the hippocampus, a brain structure involved with temporal lobe epilepsy (TLE).

How Are Febrile Seizures Evaluated?

Before diagnosing febrile seizures in infants and children, doctors sometimes perform tests to be sure that the seizures are not caused by an underlying or more serious health condition. For example, meningitis, an infection of the membranes surrounding the brain, can cause both fever and seizures that can look like febrile seizures but are much more serious. If a doctor suspects a child has meningitis a spinal tap may be needed to check for signs of the infection in the cerebrospinal fluid (fluid surrounding the brain and spinal cord). If there has been severe diarrhea or vomiting, dehydration could be responsible for seizures. Also, doctors often perform other tests such as examining the blood and urine to pinpoint the cause of the child's fever.

If the seizure is either very prolonged or is accompanied by a serious infection, or if the child is younger than 6 months of age, the clinician may recommend hospitalization. In most cases, however, a child who has a febrile seizure usually will not need to be hospitalized.

Can Subsequent Febrile Seizures Be Prevented?

Experts recommend that children who have experienced a febrile seizure not take any anti-seizure medication to prevent future seizures, as the side effects of these daily medications outweigh any benefits. This is especially true since most febrile seizures are brief and harmless.

If a child has a fever, most parents will use fever-lowering drugs such as acetaminophen or ibuprofen to make the child more comfortable. However, available studies show this does not reduce the risk of having another febrile seizure.

Although the majority of children with febrile seizures do not need medication, children especially prone to febrile seizures may be treated with medication, such as diazepam, when they have a fever. This medication may lower the risk of having another febrile seizure. It is usually well tolerated, although it occasionally can cause drowsiness, a lack of coordination, or hyperactivity. Children vary widely in their susceptibility to such side effects.

A child whose first febrile seizure is a prolonged one does not necessarily have a higher risk of having reoccurring prolonged seizures. But if the child has another seizure, it is likely to be prolonged. Because very long febrile seizures are associated with the potential for injury and an increased risk of developing epilepsy, some doctors may prescribe medication to these children to prevent prolonged seizures. The parents of children who have experienced a long febrile may wish to talk to their doctor about this treatment option.

Chapter 8

Responding to Medical Emergencies

Handling Medical Emergencies

Even healthy kids get hurt or sick sometimes. In some cases, you will know that you need to head straight to the emergency room (ER) at the nearest hospital. In other cases, it's harder to determine whether an injury or illness needs the attention of a medical professional or can be treated at home.

Different problems require different levels of care. When your child needs some sort of medical help, you have many options:

- **Handle the problem at home.** Many minor injuries and illnesses, including some cuts, certain types of rashes, coughs, colds, scrapes, and bruises, can be handled with home care and over-the-counter (OTC) treatments.
- **Call your doctor.** If you're unsure of the level of medical care your child needs, your doctor—or a nurse who works in the office—can help you decide what steps to take and how.
- **Visit an urgent care center.** An urgent care center can be a good option for non-emergencies at night and on weekends when your doctor may not be in the office. At these centers, you can

---

Text in this chapter is excerpted from "Is it a Medical Emergency?" © 1995–2016. The Nemours Foundation/KidsHealth®. Reprinted with permission.

usually get things like X-rays, stitches, and care for minor injuries that aren't life threatening yet require medical attention on the same day.

- **Visit a hospital emergency room.** An ER—also called an emergency department (ED)—can handle a wide variety of serious problems, such as severe bleeding, head trauma, seizures, meningitis, breathing difficulties, dehydration, and serious bacterial infections.
- **Call 911 for an ambulance.** Some situations are so serious that you need the help of trained medical personnel on the way to the hospital. These might include if your child: has been in a car accident, has a head or neck injury, has ingested too much medication and is now hard to rouse, or is not breathing or is turning blue. In these cases, dial 911 for an ambulance.

As a parent, it can be hard to make these judgment calls. You don't want to rush to the ER if it isn't really an emergency and can wait until a doctor's appointment. On the other hand, you don't want to hesitate to get medical attention if your child needs treatment right away. As your kids grow, you'll learn to trust yourself to decide when it's an emergency.

Remember that in cases when you know the problem is minor, it's best to contact your child's doctor, go to an urgent care center, or handle it at home. ERs can be crowded and it can take a long time for minor problems to be treated.

Should I Go to The ER?

Here are some reasons to go to the ER:

- if your child has difficulty breathing or shortness of breath
- if your child has had a change in mental status, such as suddenly becoming unusually sleepy or difficult to wake, disoriented, or confused
- if your child has a cut in the skin that is bleeding and won't stop
- if your child has a stiff neck along with a fever
- if your child has a rapid heartbeat that doesn't slow down
- if your child accidentally ingests a poisonous substance or too much medication
- if your child has had more than minor head trauma

Other situations may seem alarming, but don't require a trip to the ER. The list below includes some of the symptoms that may require calling your doctor:

- high fever
- ear pain
- pain in the abdomen
- headache that doesn't go away
- rash
- mild wheezing
- persistent cough

When in doubt, call your doctor. Even if the doctor isn't available, the office nurse can talk with you and determine whether you should go to the ER. On weekends and at night, doctors have answering services that allow them to get in touch with you if you leave a message.

Urgent Care Centers

Sometimes an injury or an illness isn't life threatening but needs medical attention on the same day. If that's the case, and your doctor doesn't have office hours at the time, consider going to an urgent care center.

Urgent care centers usually allow you to walk in without an appointment, just as you would in an ER. But they're equipped and staffed to treat minor, non-critical issues. Patients usually will be seen by a doctor and also might be able to get X-rays or blood drawn.

Most of these clinics offer extended hours on evenings and on weekends for patients to receive treatment when the family doctor is not available. Some are open 24 hours a day every day. In addition to accepting walk-in patients, some allow you to call ahead to be seen.

Some cases where you might take your child to an urgent care center include:

- cuts
- minor injuries
- vomiting or diarrhea
- ear pain
- sore throat

- infected bug bites
- mild allergic reactions
- suspected sprain or broken bone
- minor animal bites

The doctors who work at freestanding urgent care centers often are ER doctors or family physicians who focus on treating adult and pediatric diseases. Some centers are also staffed by nurse practitioners and physician assistants. The ERs in many children's hospitals have special sections similar to an urgent care center for treatment of minor injuries and illnesses.

Find out about the urgent care centers near you—before a situation comes up where you need to go to one. Ask your doctor about local facilities. In general, you should find a clinic that meets the state licensing requirements and is staffed by doctors who are board certified in their specialties, such as pediatrics, family medicine, or emergency medicine. It's also a good idea to find out if the center accepts your insurance plan.

Talk with your doctor before your child gets sick about how to handle emergencies and ask about the doctor's policy on addressing medical needs outside of office hours. Having that information ahead of time will mean one less thing to worry about when your child is sick!

Chapter 9

Helping Children Avoid Potential Health Problems

Chapter Contents

Section 9.1

Obesity in Children

This section contains text excerpted from the following sources: Text under the heading "BMI for Children and Teens" is excerpted from "Defining Childhood Obesity," Centers for Disease Control and Prevention (CDC), June 16, 2015; Text beginning with the heading "Help Children Maintain a Healthy Weight" is excerpted from "Tips for Parents—Ideas to Help Children Maintain a Healthy Weight," Centers for Disease Control and Prevention (CDC), May 15, 2015.

BMI for Children and Teens

Body mass index (BMI) is a measure used to determine childhood overweight and obesity. Overweight is defined as a BMI at or above the 85th percentile and below the 95th percentile for children and teens of the same age and sex. Obesity is defined as a BMI at or above the 95th percentile for children and teens of the same age and sex.

BMI is calculated by dividing a person's weight in kilograms by the square of height in meters. For children and teens, BMI is age- and sex-specific and is often referred to as BMI-for-age. A child's weight status is determined using an age- and sex-specific percentile for BMI rather than the BMI categories used for adults. This is because children's body composition varies as they age and varies between boys and girls. Therefore, BMI levels among children and teens need to be expressed relative to other children of the same age and sex.

For example, a 10-year-old boy of average height (56 inches) who weighs 102 pounds would have a BMI of 22.9 kg/m. This would place the boy in the 95th percentile for BMI, and he would be considered as obese. This means that the child's BMI is greater than the BMI of 95% of 10-year-old boys in the reference population.

The CDC Growth Charts are the most commonly used indicator to measure the size and growth patterns of children and teens in the United States. BMI-for-age weight status categories and the corresponding percentiles were based on expert committee recommendations and are shown in the following table.

Table 9.1. Weight Status Category and Percentile Range

Weight Status Category	Percentile Range
Underweight	Less than the 5th percentile
Normal or Healthy Weight	5th percentile to less than the 85th percentile
Overweight	85th to less than the 95th percentile
Obese	95th percentile or greater

BMI does not measure body fat directly, but research has shown that BMI is correlated with more direct measures of body fat, such as skinfold thickness measurements, bioelectrical impedance, densitometry (underwater weighing), dual energy X-ray absorptiometry (DXA) and other methods. BMI can be considered an alternative to direct measures of body fat. A trained healthcare provider should perform appropriate health assessments in order to evaluate an individual's health status and risks.

Help Children Maintain a Healthy Weight

You've probably read about it in newspapers and seen it on the news: in the United States, the number of obese children and teens has continued to rise over the past two decades. You may wonder: Why are doctors and scientists troubled by this trend? And as parents or other concerned adults, you may also ask: What steps can we take to help prevent obesity in our children? This page provides answers to some of the questions you may have and provides you with resources to help you keep your family healthy.

Why is Childhood Obesity Considered a Health Problem?

Doctors and scientists are concerned about the rise of obesity in children and youth because obesity may lead to the following health problems:

- Heart disease, caused by:
    - high cholesterol and/or
    - high blood pressure
- Type 2 diabetes
- Asthma

- Sleep apnea
- Social discrimination

Childhood obesity is associated with various health-related consequences. Obese children and adolescents may experience immediate health consequences and may be at risk for weight-related health problems in adulthood.

Psychosocial Risks

Some consequences of childhood and adolescent overweight are psychosocial. Obese children and adolescents are targets of early and systematic social discrimination. The psychological stress of social stigmatization can cause low self-esteem which, in turn, can hinder academic and social functioning, and persist into adulthood.

Cardiovascular Disease Risks

Obese children and teens have been found to have risk factors for cardiovascular disease (CVD), including high cholesterol levels, high blood pressure, and abnormal glucose tolerance. In a population-based sample of 5- to 17-year-olds, almost 60% of overweight children had at least one CVD risk factor while 25 percent of overweight children had two or more CVD risk factors.

Additional Health Risks

Less common health conditions associated with increased weight include asthma, hepatic steatosis, sleep apnea and Type 2 diabetes.

- Asthma is a disease of the lungs in which the airways become blocked or narrowed causing breathing difficulty. Studies have identified an association between childhood overweight and asthma.
- Hepatic steatosis is the fatty degeneration of the liver caused by a high concentration of liver enzymes. Weight reduction causes liver enzymes to normalize.
- Sleep apnea is a less common complication of overweight for children and adolescents. Sleep apnea is a sleep-associated breathing disorder defined as the cessation of breathing during sleep that lasts for at least 10 seconds. Sleep apnea is characterized by loud snoring and labored breathing. During sleep apnea,

oxygen levels in the blood can fall dramatically. One study estimated that sleep apnea occurs in about 7% of overweight children.

- Type 2 diabetes is increasingly being reported among children and adolescents who are overweight. While diabetes and glucose intolerance, a precursor of diabetes, are common health effects of adult obesity, only in recent years has Type 2 diabetes begun to emerge as a health-related problem among children and adolescents. Onset of diabetes in children and adolescents can result in advanced complications such as CVD and kidney failure.

In addition, studies have shown that obese children and teens are more likely to become obese as adults.

What Can I Do As a Parent or Guardian to Help Prevent Childhood Overweight and Obesity?

To help your child maintain a healthy weight, balance the calories your child consumes from foods and beverages with the calories your child uses through physical activity and normal growth.

Remember that the goal for overweight and obese children and teens is to reduce the rate of weight gain while allowing normal growth and development. Children and teens should not be placed on a weight reduction diet without the consultation of a healthcare provider.

Balancing Calories: Help Kids Develop Healthy Eating Habits

One part of balancing calories is to eat foods that provide adequate nutrition and an appropriate number of calories. You can help children learn to be aware of what they eat by developing healthy eating habits, looking for ways to make favorite dishes healthier, and reducing calorie-rich temptations.

Encourage Healthy Eating Habits

There's no great secret to healthy eating. To help your children and family develop healthy eating habits:

- Provide plenty of vegetables, fruits, and whole-grain products.
- Include low-fat or non-fat milk or dairy products.
- Choose lean meats, poultry, fish, lentils, and beans for protein.

- Serve reasonably-sized portions.
- Encourage your family to drink lots of water.
- Limit sugar-sweetened beverages.
- Limit consumption of sugar and saturated fat.

Remember that small changes every day can lead to a recipe for success!

Look for Ways to Make Favorite Dishes Healthier

The recipes that you may prepare regularly, and that your family enjoys, with just a few changes can be healthier and just as satisfying.

Remove Calorie-Rich Temptations

Although everything can be enjoyed in moderation, reducing the calorie-rich temptations of high-fat and high-sugar, or salty snacks can also help your children develop healthy eating habits. Instead only allow your children to eat them sometimes, so that they truly will be treats! Here are examples of easy-to-prepare, low-fat and low-sugar treats that are 100 calories or less:

- A medium-size apple
- A medium-size banana
- 1 cup blueberries
- 1 cup grapes
- 1 cup carrots, broccoli, or bell peppers with 2 tbsp. hummus

Balancing Calories: Help Kids Stay Active

Another part of balancing calories is to engage in an appropriate amount of physical activity and avoid too much sedentary time. In addition to being fun for children and teens, regular physical activity has many health benefits, including:

- Strengthening bones
- Decreasing blood pressure
- Reducing stress and anxiety
- Increasing self-esteem
- Helping with weight management

Help Kids Stay Active

Children and teens should participate in at least 60 minutes of moderate intensity physical activity most days of the week, preferably daily. Remember that children imitate adults. Start adding physical activity to your own daily routine and encourage your child to join you.

Some examples of moderate intensity physical activity include:

- Brisk walking
- Playing tag
- Jumping rope
- Playing soccer
- Swimming
- Dancing

Reduce Sedentary Time

In addition to encouraging physical activity, help children avoid too much sedentary time. Although quiet time for reading and homework is fine, limit the time your children watch television, play video games, or surf the web to no more than 2 hours per day. Additionally, the American Academy of Pediatrics (AAP) does not recommend television viewing for children age 2 or younger. Instead, encourage your children to find fun activities to do with family members or on their own that simply involve more activity.

Section 9.2

The Effects of Secondhand Smoke on Children

This section includes text excerpted from "Children in the Home," Centers for Disease Control and Prevention (CDC), September 15, 2016.

Children and Secondhand Smoke Exposure

Tobacco smoke hurts babies and children. Children who are exposed to secondhand tobacco smoke breathe the same dangerous chemicals that smokers inhale.The main place where young children are exposed to secondhand smoke is at home. Smoke-free home and vehicle rules help protect children and adults:

- The home is the place where children are most exposed to secondhand smoke, and it's a major place for secondhand smoke exposure for adults.
- Children who live in homes where smoking is allowed have higher levels of cotinine (a biological marker of secondhand smoke exposure) than children who live in homes where smoking is not allowed.
- Although secondhand smoke exposure among children has fallen over the past 15 years, children are still more heavily exposed to secondhand smoke than adults.
- About two in five U.S. children aged 3–11 years (40.6%) are exposed to secondhand smoke.
- In the United States., the percentage of children and teens living with at least one smoker is about three times the percentage of nonsmoking adults who live with a smoker.

Making your home and vehicles smoke free can reduce secondhand smoke exposure among children and nonsmoking adults. Some studies indicate that these rules can also help smokers quit and can reduce adolescents' risk of becoming smokers.

Health Effects of Smoking and Secondhand Smoke on Children

- Because their bodies are developing, infants and young children are especially vulnerable to the poisons in secondhand smoke.
- Both babies whose mothers smoke while pregnant and babies who are exposed to secondhand smoke after birth are more likely to die from sudden infant death syndrome (SIDS) than babies who are not exposed to cigarette smoke.
- Mothers who are exposed to secondhand smoke while pregnant are more likely to have lower birth weight babies, which makes babies weaker and increases the risk for many health problems.
- Babies whose mothers smoke while pregnant or who are exposed to secondhand smoke after birth have weaker lungs than other babies, which increases the risk for many health problems.
- Secondhand smoke exposure causes acute lower respiratory infections such as bronchitis and pneumonia in infants and young children.
- Secondhand smoke exposure causes children who already have asthma to experience more frequent and severe attacks.
- Secondhand smoke exposure causes respiratory symptoms, including cough, phlegm, wheezing, and breathlessness, among school-aged children.
- Children exposed to secondhand smoke are at increased risk for ear infections and are more likely to need an operation to insert ear tubes for drainage.

Quit Tips

Are you one of the more than 70% of smokers who want to quit? Then try following this advice:

1. **Don't smoke any cigarettes.** Each cigarette you smoke damages your lungs, your blood vessels, and cells throughout your body. Even occasional smoking is harmful.
2. **Write down why you want to quit.** Do you want to:

   Be around for your loved ones?

   Have better health?

Set a good example for your children?

Protect your family from breathing other people's smoke?

Really wanting to quit smoking is very important to how much success you will have in quitting.

3. **Know that it will take commitment and effort to quit smoking.** Nearly all smokers have some feelings of nicotine withdrawal when they try to quit. Nicotine is addictive.a Knowing this will help you deal with withdrawal symptoms that can occur, such as bad moods and really wanting to smoke.

   There are many ways smokers quit, including using nicotine replacement products (gum and patches) or U.S. Food and Drug Administration (FDA)-approved, non-nicotine cessation medications. Some people do not experience any withdrawal symptoms. For most people, symptoms only last a few days to a couple of weeks.a Take quitting one day at a time, even one minute at a time—whatever you need to succeed.

4. **Get help if you want it.** Smokers can receive free resources and assistance to help them quit by calling the 1-800-QUIT-NOW quitline (1-800-784-8669). Your healthcare providers are also a good source for help and support.

5. **Remember this good news!** More than half of all adult smokers have quit, and you can, too. Millions of people have learned to face life without a cigarette. Quitting smoking is the single most important step you can take to protect your health and the health of your family.

Section 9.3

Protecting Children from the Sun

This section includes text excerpted from "How Can I Protect My Children from the Sun?" Centers for Disease Control and Prevention (CDC), December 12, 2013.

How Can I Protect My Children from the Sun?

Just a few serious sunburns can increase your child's risk of skin cancer later in life. Kids don't have to be at the pool, beach, or on vacation to get too much sun. Their skin needs protection from the sun's harmful ultraviolet (UV) rays whenever they're outdoors.

Seek shade. UV rays are strongest and most harmful during midday, so it's best to plan indoor activities then. If this is not possible, seek shade under a tree, an umbrella, or a pop-up tent. Use these options to prevent sunburn, not to seek relief after it's happened.

Cover up. When possible, long-sleeved shirts and long pants and skirts can provide protection from UV rays. Clothes made from tightly woven fabric offer the best protection. A wet T-shirt offers much less UV protection than a dry one, and darker colors may offer more protection than lighter colors. Some clothing certified under international standards comes with information on its ultraviolet protection factor.

Get a hat. Hats that shade the face, scalp, ears, and neck are easy to use and give great protection. Baseball caps are popular among kids, but they don't protect their ears and neck. If your child chooses a cap, be sure to protect exposed areas with sunscreen.

Wear sunglasses. They protect your child's eyes from UV rays, which can lead to cataracts later in life. Look for sunglasses that wrap around and block as close to 100% of both UVA and UVB rays as possible.

Apply sunscreen. Use sunscreen with at least Sun Protection Factor (SPF) 15 and Ultra Violet A (UVA) and Ultra Violet B (UVB) protection every time your child goes outside. For the best protection, apply sunscreen generously 30 minutes before going outdoors. Don't forget to protect ears, noses, lips, and the tops of feet.

Take sunscreen with you to reapply during the day, especially after your child swims or exercises. This applies to waterproof and water-resistant products as well.

Follow the directions on the package for using a sunscreen product on babies less than 6 months old. All products do not have the same ingredients; if your or your child's skin reacts badly to one product, try another one or call a doctor. Your baby's best defense against sunburn is avoiding the sun or staying in the shade.

Keep in mind, sunscreen is not meant to allow kids to spend more time in the sun than they would otherwise. Try combining sunscreen with other options to prevent UV damage.

Too Much Sun Hurts

Turning pink? Unprotected skin can be damaged by the sun's UV rays in as little as 15 minutes. Yet it can take up to 12 hours for skin to show the full effect of sun exposure. So, if your child's skin looks "a little pink" today, it may be burned tomorrow morning. To prevent further burning, get your child out of the sun.

Tan? There's no other way to say it—tanned skin is damaged skin. Any change in the color of your child's skin after time outside—whether sunburn or suntan—indicates damage from UV rays.

Cool and cloudy? Children still need protection. UV rays, not the temperature, do the damage. Clouds do not block UV rays, they filter them—and sometimes only slightly.

Oops! Kids often get sunburned when they are outdoors unprotected for longer than expected. Remember to plan ahead, and keep sun protection handy—in your car, bag, or child's backpack.

Sun Safety at School: What You Can Do

Parents and Guardians

- Urge your school's parent—teacher association to advocate for sun safety policies and practices such as ensuring that the dress code allows students to wear hats when outdoors.
- Develop partnerships to help support environmental improvements such as adding trees to schools property. Reach out to

local businesses, the media and recreational programs, as well as nonprofit and civic organizations.

- Participate on your school's health team.
- Be a good role model by practicing sun safety yourself.
- Encourage your children to make sun safety a habit.
- Make sure your children wear hats, coverup clothing and sunglasses and apply sunscreen when they participate in outdoor activities.

Part Two

Childhood Infections and Related Concerns

Chapter 10

Foodborne Illness

Chapter Contents

Section 10.1

Understanding Foodborne Illness

This section contains text excerpted from the following sources: Text under the heading "What Are Foodborne Illnesses?" is excerpted from "Foodborne Illnesses," National Institute of Diabetes and Digestive and Kidney Diseases (NIDDK), June 2014; Text under the heading "Foods to Avoid" is excerpted from "Food Safety: It's Especially Important for At-Risk Groups," U.S. Food and Drug Administration (FDA), April 6, 2016.

What Are Foodborne Illnesses?

Foodborne illnesses are infections or irritations of the gastrointestinal (GI) tract caused by food or beverages that contain harmful bacteria, parasites, viruses, or chemicals. The GI tract is a series of hollow organs joined in a long, twisting tube from the mouth to the anus. Common symptoms of foodborne illnesses include vomiting, diarrhea, abdominal pain, fever, and chills.

Most foodborne illnesses are acute, meaning they happen suddenly and last a short time, and most people recover on their own without treatment. Rarely, foodborne illnesses may lead to more serious complications. Each year, an estimated 48 million people in the United States experience a foodborne illness. Foodborne illnesses cause about 3,000 deaths in the United States annually.

What Causes Foodborne Illnesses?

The majority of foodborne illnesses are caused by harmful bacteria and viruses. Some parasites and chemicals also cause foodborne illnesses.

Bacteria

Bacteria are tiny organisms that can cause infections of the GI tract. Not all bacteria are harmful to humans.

Some harmful bacteria may already be present in foods when they are purchased. Raw foods including meat, poultry, fish and shellfish, eggs, unpasteurized milk and dairy products, and fresh produce often contain bacteria that cause foodborne illnesses. Bacteria can contaminate food—making it harmful to eat—at any time during growth, harvesting or slaughter, processing, storage, and shipping.

Foods may also be contaminated with bacteria during food preparation in a restaurant or home kitchen. If food preparers do not thoroughly wash their hands, kitchen utensils, cutting boards, and other kitchen surfaces that come into contact with raw foods, cross-contamination—the spread of bacteria from contaminated food to uncontaminated food—may occur.

If hot food is not kept hot enough or cold food is not kept cold enough, bacteria may multiply. Bacteria multiply quickly when the temperature of food is between 40 and 140 degrees. Cold food should be kept below 40 degrees and hot food should be kept above 140 degrees. Bacteria multiply more slowly when food is refrigerated, and freezing food can further slow or even stop the spread of bacteria. However, bacteria in refrigerated or frozen foods become active again when food is brought to room temperature. Thoroughly cooking food kills bacteria.

Many types of bacteria cause foodborne illnesses. Examples include

- *Salmonella,* a bacterium found in many foods, including raw and undercooked meat, poultry, dairy products, and seafood. *Salmonella* may also be present on egg shells and inside eggs.
- *Campylobacter jejuni* (*C. jejuni*), found in raw or undercooked chicken and unpasteurized milk.
- *Shigella*, a bacterium spread from person to person. These bacteria are present in the stools of people who are infected. If people who are infected do not wash their hands thoroughly after using the bathroom, they can contaminate food that they handle or prepare. Water contaminated with infected stools can also contaminate produce in the field.
- *Escherichia coli* (*E. coli*), which includes several different strains, only a few of which cause illness in humans. *E. coli O157:H7* is the strain that causes the most severe illness. Common sources of *E. coli* include raw or undercooked hamburger, unpasteurized fruit juices and milk, and fresh produce.
- *Listeria monocytogenes* (*L. monocytogenes*), which has been found in raw and undercooked meats, unpasteurized milk, soft cheeses, and ready-to-eat deli meats and hot dogs.
- *Vibrio*, a bacterium that may contaminate fish or shellfish.

- *Clostridium botulinum* (*C. botulinum*), a bacterium that may contaminate improperly canned foods and smoked and salted fish.

Viruses

Viruses are tiny capsules, much smaller than bacteria, that contain genetic material. Viruses cause infections that can lead to sickness. People can pass viruses to each other. Viruses are present in the stool or vomit of people who are infected. People who are infected with a virus may contaminate food and drinks, especially if they do not wash their hands thoroughly after using the bathroom.

Common sources of foodborne viruses include:

- food prepared by a person infected with a virus
- shellfish from contaminated water
- produce irrigated with contaminated water

Common foodborne viruses include

- norovirus, which causes inflammation of the stomach and intestines
- hepatitis A, which causes inflammation of the liver

Parasites

Parasites are tiny organisms that live inside another organism. In developed countries such as the United States, parasitic infections are relatively rare.

Cryptosporidium parvum and *Giardia intestinalis* are parasites that are spread through water contaminated with the stools of people or animals who are infected. Foods that come into contact with contaminated water during growth or preparation can become contaminated with these parasites. Food preparers who are infected with these parasites can also contaminate foods if they do not thoroughly wash their hands after using the bathroom and before handling food.

Trichinella spiralis is a type of roundworm parasite. People may be infected with this parasite by consuming raw or undercooked pork or wild game.

Chemicals

Harmful chemicals that cause illness may contaminate foods such as

- fish or shellfish, which may feed on algae that produce toxins, leading to high concentrations of toxins in their bodies. Some types of fish, including tuna and mahi mahi, may be contaminated with bacteria that produce toxins if the fish are not properly refrigerated before they are cooked or served.
- certain types of wild mushrooms.
- unwashed fruits and vegetables that contain high concentrations of pesticides.

What Are the Symptoms of Foodborne Illnesses?

Symptoms of foodborne illnesses depend on the cause. Common symptoms of many foodborne illnesses include:

- vomiting
- diarrhea or bloody diarrhea
- abdominal pain
- fever
- chills

Symptoms can range from mild to serious and can last from a few hours to several days.

C. botulinum and some chemicals affect the nervous system, causing symptoms such as:

- headache
- tingling or numbness of the skin
- blurred vision
- weakness
- dizziness
- paralysis

What Are the Complications of Foodborne Illnesses?

Foodborne illnesses may lead to dehydration, hemolytic uremic syndrome (HUS), and other complications. Acute foodborne illnesses may also lead to chronic—or long lasting—health problems.

Dehydration

When someone does not drink enough fluids to replace those that are lost through vomiting and diarrhea, dehydration can result. When dehydrated, the body lacks enough fluid and electrolytes—minerals in salts, including sodium, potassium, and chloride—to function properly. Infants, children, older adults, and people with weak immune systems have the greatest risk of becoming dehydrated.

Signs of dehydration are:

- excessive thirst
- infrequent urination
- dark-colored urine
- lethargy, dizziness, or faintness

Signs of dehydration in infants and young children are

- dry mouth and tongue
- lack of tears when crying
- no wet diapers for 3 hours or more
- high fever
- unusually cranky or drowsy behavior
- sunken eyes, cheeks, or soft spot in the skull

Also, when people are dehydrated, their skin does not flatten back to normal right away after being gently pinched and released.

Severe dehydration may require intravenous fluids and hospitalization. Untreated severe dehydration can cause serious health problems such as organ damage, shock, or coma—a sleep like state in which a person is not conscious.

Hemolytic Uremic Syndrome (HUS)

Hemolytic uremic syndrome is a rare disease that mostly affects children younger than 10 years of age. HUS develops when *E. coli* bacteria lodged in the digestive tract make toxins that enter the bloodstream. The toxins start to destroy red blood cells, which help the blood to clot, and the lining of the blood vessels.

In the United States, *E. coli O157:H7* infection is the most common cause of HUS, but infection with other strains of *E. coli,* other bacteria, and viruses may also cause HUS. A recent study found that about

6 percent of people with *E. coli O157:H7* infections developed HUS. Children younger than age 5 have the highest risk, but females and people age 60 and older also have increased risk.

Symptoms of *E. coli O157:H7* infection include diarrhea, which may be bloody, and abdominal pain, often accompanied by nausea, vomiting, and fever. Up to a week after *E. coli* symptoms appear, symptoms of HUS may develop, including irritability, paleness, and decreased urination. HUS may lead to acute renal failure, which is a sudden and temporary loss of kidney function. HUS may also affect other organs and the central nervous system. Most people who develop HUS recover with treatment. Research shows that in the United States between 2000 and 2006, fewer than 5 percent of people who developed HUS died of the disorder. Older adults had the highest mortality rate—about one-third of people age 60 and older who developed HUS died.

Studies have shown that some children who recover from HUS develop chronic complications, including kidney problems, high blood pressure, and diabetes.

When Should People with Foodborne Illnesses See a Healthcare Provider?

People with any of the following symptoms should see a healthcare provider immediately:

- signs of dehydration
- prolonged vomiting that prevents keeping liquids down
- diarrhea for more than 2 days in adults or for more than 24 hours in children
- severe pain in the abdomen or rectum
- a fever higher than 101 degrees
- stools containing blood or pus
- stools that are black and tarry
- nervous system symptoms
- signs of HUS

If a child has a foodborne illness, parents or guardians should not hesitate to call a healthcare provider for advice.

Eating, Diet, And Nutrition

The following steps may help relieve the symptoms of foodborne illnesses and prevent dehydration in adults:

- drinking plenty of liquids such as fruit juices, sports drinks, caffeine-free soft drinks, and broths to replace fluids and electrolytes
- sipping small amounts of clear liquids or sucking on ice chips if vomiting is still a problem
- gradually reintroducing food, starting with bland, easy-to-digest foods such as rice, potatoes, toast or bread, cereal, lean meat, applesauce, and bananas
- avoiding fatty foods, sugary foods, dairy products, caffeine, and alcohol until recovery is complete

Infants and children present special concerns. Infants and children are likely to become dehydrated more quickly from diarrhea and vomiting because of their smaller body size. The following steps may help relieve symptoms and prevent dehydration in infants and children:

- giving oral rehydration solutions such as Pedialyte, Naturalyte, Infalyte, and CeraLyte to prevent dehydration
- giving food as soon as the child is hungry
- giving infants breast milk or full strength formula, as usual, along with oral rehydration solutions

Older adults and adults with weak immune systems should also drink oral rehydration solutions to prevent dehydration.

Foods to Avoid

If you are at greater risk of foodborne illness, you are advised not to eat:

- Raw or undercooked meat or poultry.
- Raw fish, partially cooked seafood (such as shrimp and crab), and refrigerated smoked seafood.
- Raw shellfish (including oysters, clams, mussels, and scallops) and their juices.
- Unpasteurized (raw) milk and products made with raw milk, like yogurt and cheese

- Soft cheeses made from unpasteurized milk, such as Feta, Brie, Camembert, blue-veined, and Mexican-style cheeses (such as such as Queso Fresco, Panela, Asadero, and Queso Blanco).
- Raw or undercooked eggs or foods containing raw or undercooked eggs, including certain homemade salad dressings (such as Caesar salad dressing), homemade cookie dough and cake batters, and homemade eggnog.
- Unwashed fresh vegetables, including lettuce/salads.
- Unpasteurized fruit or vegetable juices (these juices will carry a warning label).
- Hot dogs, luncheon meats (cold cuts), fermented and dry sausage, and other deli-style meats, poultry products, and smoked fish—unless they are reheated until steaming hot.
- Salads (without added preservatives) prepared on site in a deli-type establishment, such as ham salad, chicken salad, or seafood salad.
- Unpasteurized, refrigerated pâtés or meat spreads.
- Raw sprouts (alfalfa, bean, or any other sprout).

Section 10.2

Raw Milk Risks

This section includes text excerpted from "Raw Milk Questions and Answers," Centers for Disease Control and Prevention (CDC), February 20, 2015.

Raw milk is milk from cows, goats, sheep, or other animals that has not been pasteurized. Although precise data are not available, it is thought that less than 1% of milk sold to consumers in the United States has not been pasteurized.

What Are the Risks Associated with Drinking Raw Milk?

Raw milk can carry harmful bacteria and other germs that can make you very sick or kill you. While it is possible to get foodborne illnesses from many different foods, raw milk is one of the riskiest of all.

Getting sick from raw milk can mean many days of diarrhea, stomach cramping, and vomiting. Less commonly, it can mean kidney failure, paralysis, chronic disorders, and even death.

Many people who chose raw milk thinking they would improve their health instead found themselves (or their loved ones) sick in a hospital for several weeks fighting for their lives from infections caused by germs in raw milk. For example, a person can develop severe or even life-threatening diseases, such as Guillain-Barré syndrome, which can cause paralysis, and hemolytic uremic syndrome, which can result in kidney failure and stroke.

- Illness can occur from the same brand and source of raw milk that people had been drinking for a long time without becoming ill.
- A wide variety of germs that are sometimes found in raw milk, can make people sick, including bacteria (e.g., *Brucella, Campylobacter, Listeria, Mycobacterium bovis* (a cause of tuberculosis), *Salmonella*, Shiga toxin-producing *Escherichia coli* [e.g., *E. coli O157*], *Shigella, Yersinia*), parasites (e.g., Giardia), and viruses (e.g., norovirus).
- Each ill person's symptoms can differ, depending on the type of germ, the amount of contamination, and the person's immune defenses.

Who Is at Greatest Risk of Getting Sick from Drinking Raw Milk?

The risk of getting sick from drinking raw milk is greater for infants and young children, the elderly, pregnant women, and people with weakened immune systems, such as people with cancer, an organ transplant, or human immunodeficiency virus (HIV) / Acquired Immune Deficiency Syndrome (AIDS), than it is for healthy school-aged children and adults. But, it is important to remember that healthy people of any age can get very sick or even die if they drink raw milk contaminated with harmful germs.

Can Drinking Raw Milk Hurt Me or My Family?

Yes. Raw milk can cause serious infections. Raw milk and raw milk products (such as cheeses and yogurts made with raw milk) can be contaminated with bacteria that can cause serious illness, hospitalization, or death. These harmful bacteria include *Brucella, Campylobacter, Listeria, Mycobacterium bovis, Salmonella*, Shiga toxin-producing *E. coli, Shigella, Streptococcus pyogenes*, and *Yersinia enterocolitica*. From 1998 through 2011, 148 outbreaks due to consumption of raw milk or raw milk products were reported to CDC. These resulted in 2,384 illnesses, 284 hospitalizations, and 2 deaths. Most of these illnesses were caused by *Escherichia coli, Campylobacter, Salmonella,* or *Listeria*. It is important to note that a substantial proportion of the raw milk-associated disease burden falls on children; among the 104 outbreaks from 1998–2011 with information on the patients' ages available, 82% involved at least one person younger than 20 years old.

Because not all cases of foodborne illness are recognized and reported, the actual number of illnesses associated with raw milk likely is greater.

Aren't Raw or Natural Foods Better than Processed Foods?

Many people believe that foods with no or minimal processing are better for their health. Many people also believe that small, local farms are better sources of healthy food. However, some types of processing are needed to protect health. For example, consumers process raw meat, poultry, and fish for safety by cooking. Similarly, when milk is pasteurized, it is heated just long enough to kill disease-causing germs. Most nutrients remain after milk is pasteurized. There are many local, small farms that offer pasteurized organic milk and cheese products.

Does Drinking Raw Milk Prevent or Cure Any Diseases, Such as Asthma, Allergies, Heart Disease, or Cancer?

No. There are no health benefits from drinking raw milk that cannot be obtained from drinking pasteurized milk that is free of disease-causing bacteria. The process of pasteurization of milk has never been found to be the cause of chronic diseases, allergies, or developmental or behavioral problems.

I Know People Who Have Been Drinking Raw Milk for Years, and They Never Got Sick. Why Is That?

The presence of germs in raw milk is unpredictable. The number of disease-causing germs in the raw milk may be too low to make a person sick for a long time, and later high enough to make the same person seriously ill. For some people, drinking contaminated raw milk just once could make them really sick. Even if you trust the farmer and your store, raw milk is never a guaranteed safe product. Drinking raw milk means taking a real risk of getting very sick.

Chapter 11

Streptococcal Bacterial Infections

Chapter Contents

Section 11.1

Group A Streptococcal Infections

This section includes text excerpted from "Group A Streptococcus Frequently Asked Questions," Centers for Disease Control and Prevention (CDC), May 1, 2014.

What Is Group A Streptococcus?

Group A *Streptococcus* (group A strep) are bacteria that can cause a wide range of infections. People may also carry group A strep in the throat or on the skin and have no symptoms of illness. Most group A strep infections are relatively mild illnesses, such as "strep throat" or impetigo (a skin infection). Occasionally these bacteria can cause serious and even life-threatening diseases. These diseases can sometimes lead to sepsis, the body's overwhelming and life-threatening response to infection that can cause tissue damage, organ failure, and death.

How Are Group A Strep Spread?

These bacteria are spread through direct contact with mucus from the nose or throat of people who are sick with a group A strep infection or through contact with infected wounds or sores on the skin. The bacteria may also be spread through contact with people without symptoms but who carry the bacteria in their throat or on their skin. Ill people, such as those who have strep throat or skin infections, are most likely to spread the infection. People who carry the bacteria but have no symptoms are much less contagious. Treating an infected person with an antibiotic for 24 hours or longer generally prevents the spread of the bacteria to others. However, it is important to complete the entire course of antibiotics as prescribed. It is not likely that household items, like toys, spread these bacteria. However, it is possible to spread these bacteria by drinking from the same glass or eating from the same plate as someone who is ill with a group A strep infection like strep throat.

What Kind of Illnesses Are Caused by Group A Strep?

Infection with group A strep can result in a range of illnesses:

- Mild illness such as strep throat or impetigo
- Serious illness such as pneumonia (lung infection), necrotizing fasciitis, or streptococcal toxic shock syndrome (STSS)

Serious, sometimes life-threatening group A strep disease may occur when these bacteria get into parts of the body where bacteria usually are not found, such as the blood, muscle, or the lungs. These infections are called "invasive group A strep disease." Two of the most serious, but least common, forms of invasive group A strep disease are necrotizing fasciitis and STSS. Necrotizing fasciitis (occasionally described by the media as "the flesh-eating bacteria") rapidly destroys muscles, fat, and skin tissue. STSS causes blood pressure to drop rapidly and organs (e.g., kidney, liver, lungs) to fail. STSS is not the same as the staphylococcal toxic shock syndrome that has been associated with tampon usage. Less serious invasive illnesses caused by group A strep include cellulitis and pneumonia. In the United States, about 1 out of 4 patients with necrotizing fasciitis due to group A strep and approximately 4 out of 10 with STSS die. About 10 to 15 out of 100 patients with any form of invasive group A strep disease die.

How Common Is Invasive Group A Strep Disease?

Approximately 9,000 to 11,500 cases of invasive group A strep disease occur each year in the United States, resulting in 1,000 to 1,800 deaths annually. Most of these cases are less serious invasive infections, like cellulitis. STSS and necrotizing fasciitis are each responsible for an average of about 6 to 7 out of 100 of these invasive cases. In contrast, there are several million cases of non-invasive group A strep infections, like strep throat and impetigo, each year.

Who Is Most at Risk of Getting Invasive Group A Strep Disease?

Few people who come in contact with group A strep will develop invasive group A strep disease. Most people will have a throat or skin infection, and some may have no symptoms at all. Although healthy people can get invasive group A strep disease, people with chronic illnesses like cancer, diabetes, and chronic heart or lung disease, and those who use medicines, such as steroids, have an increased risk. People with skin lesions (such as cuts, chickenpox, or surgical wounds), the elderly, and adults with a history of alcohol abuse or injection drug use also have an increased risk for disease.

What Are the Early Signs and Symptoms of Necrotizing Fasciitis and Streptococcal Toxic Shock Syndrome?

Early signs and symptoms of necrotizing fasciitis include:

- Severe pain and swelling, often rapidly increasing
- Fever
- Redness at a wound site

Early signs and symptoms of STSS include:

- Sudden onset of generalized or localized severe pain, often in an arm or leg
- Dizziness
- Flu-like symptoms such as fever, chills, muscle aches, nausea, vomiting
- Confusion
- A flat red rash over large areas of the body (only occurs in 1 out of 10 cases)

How Is Invasive Group A Strep Disease Treated?

Group A strep infections can be treated with many different antibiotics (medicines that kill bacteria in the body). For STSS and necrotizing fasciitis, high dose penicillin and clindamycin are recommended. For those with very serious illness, supportive care in an intensive care unit may also be needed. For people with necrotizing fasciitis, early and aggressive surgery is often needed to remove damaged tissue and stop disease spread. Early treatment may reduce the risk of death from invasive group A strep disease. However, even the best medical care does not prevent death in every case.

What Can Be Done to Help Prevent Group A Strep Infections?

The spread of all types of group A strep infection can be reduced by good hand washing, especially after coughing and sneezing and before preparing foods or eating. People with sore throats should be seen by a doctor who can perform tests to find out whether the illness is strep throat. If the test result shows strep throat, the person should stay home from work, school, or daycare until 24 hours after taking an antibiotic. All wounds should be kept clean and watched for possible signs of infection such as redness, swelling, drainage, and pain at the wound site. A person with signs of an infected wound, especially if fever occurs, should immediately seek medical care. It is not necessary for all people exposed to someone with an invasive group A strep infection (i.e., necrotizing fasciitis or STSS) to receive antibiotic therapy to prevent infection. However, in some situations, antibiotic therapy may be recommended. That decision should be made after talking with your doctor.

Section 11.2

Pneumococcal Disease

This section includes text excerpted from "Pneumococcal Disease and the Vaccine (Shot) to Prevent It," Centers for Disease Control and Prevention (CDC), November 10, 2014.

What Is Pneumococcal Disease?

Pneumococcal disease is an illness caused by bacteria called pneumococcus. It is often mild but can cause serious symptoms, lifelong disability, or death. Children younger than 2 years of age are among those most at risk for the disease.

What Are the Symptoms of Pneumococcal Disease?

There are many types of pneumococcal disease. Symptoms depend on the part of the body that is infected.

Pneumococcal pneumonia (lung infection) is the most common serious form. It causes the following:

- Fever and chills
- Cough

- Rapid breathing or difficulty breathing
- Chest pain

Pneumococcal meningitis is an infection of the covering of the brain and spinal cord. It causes the following:

- Stiff neck
- Fever and headache
- Increased pain from bright lights
- Confusion

In babies, meningitis may cause poor eating and drinking, low alertness, and vomiting.

Blood infection (bacteremia and sepsis) causes fever, chills, and low alertness.

Pneumococcal disease causes up to half of middle ear infections (otitis media). Symptoms are ear pain, a red, swollen eardrum, and sometimes, fever and sleepiness.

How Serious Is It?

Pneumococcal disease ranges from mild to very dangerous. About 2,000 cases of serious disease (bacteremia, pneumonia with bacteremia, and meningitis) occur each year in children under 5 in the United States. These illnesses can lead to disabilities like deafness, brain damage, or loss of arms or legs. About 1 out of 15 children who get pneumococcal meningitis dies.

How Does Pneumococcal Disease Spread?

Pneumococcal disease spreads when an infected person coughs or sneezes. Some children may not even feel sick, but they could have the bacteria in their noses and throats. These children can still spread pneumococcal disease.

Do Children in the United States Still Get Pneumococcal Disease?

Yes. Each year in the United States, pneumococcus causes thousands of cases of pneumonia and ear infections. Babies younger than 2 years of age are most likely to have a serious case of pneumococcal disease.

Why Should My Child Get the Pneumococcal Shot?

The pneumococcal shot:

- Protects your child from pneumococcal disease, a potentially serious, and even deadly infection
- Prevents your child from developing pneumococcal meningitis and pneumonia
- Keeps your child from missing school or childcare (and keeps you from missing work to care for your sick child)

Is The Pneumococcal Shot Safe?

The pneumococcal vaccine is very safe, and it is effective at preventing pneumococcal disease. Vaccines, like any medicine, can have side effects. Most children who get the PCV13 shot have no side effects.

What Are the Side Effects?

The most common side effects are usually mild and include the following:

- Fussiness
- Sleepiness
- Loss of appetite (not wanting to eat)
- Soreness, redness, and swelling where the child got the shot
- Fever

Section 11.3

Rheumatic Fever

This section includes text excerpted from "Rheumatic Fever," Genetic and Rare Diseases (GARD) Information Center, National Institutes of Health (NIH), January 12, 2015.

Rheumatic fever is an inflammatory condition that may develop after infection with group A *Streptococcus* bacteria, such as strep throat or scarlet fever. It is primarily diagnosed in children between the ages of 6 and 16 and can affect the heart, joints, nervous system and/or skin. Early signs and symptoms include sore throat; swollen red tonsils; fever; headache; and/or muscle and joint aches. Some affected people develop rheumatic heart disease, which can lead to serious inflammation and scarring of the heart valves. It is not clear why some people who are infected with group A *Streptococcus* bacteria go on to develop rheumatic fever, while others do not; however, it appears that some families may have a genetic susceptibility to develop the condition. Treatment usually includes antibiotics and/or anti-inflammatory medications.

Symptoms of Rheumatic Fever

Rheumatic fever is primarily diagnosed in children between the ages of 6 and 16 and can affect many different systems of the body, including the heart, joints, nervous system and/or skin. The condition usually develops approximately 14-28 days after infection with group A *Streptococcus* bacteria, such as strep throat or scarlet fever. Early signs and symptoms may include sore throat; swollen red tonsils; fever; headache; and/or muscle aches. Affected people may also experience:

- Abdominal pain
- Rheumatic heart disease
- Joint pain and/or swelling
- Nosebleeds
- Skin nodules (painless, firm, round lumps underneath the skin)

- Skin rash
- Sydenham chorea (abrupt, non-repetitive limb movements and grimaces)

People with a history of rheumatic fever have a high risk of developing recurrent episodes of the condition. This can cause progressive (worsening over time) heart damage.

Cause of Rheumatic Fever

Rheumatic fever is an inflammatory condition that may develop approximately 14-28 days after infection with group A *Streptococcus* bacteria, such as strep throat or scarlet fever. About 5% of those with untreated strep infection will develop rheumatic fever. Although group A *Streptococcus* bacterial infections are highly contagious, rheumatic fever is not spread from person to person. The exact underlying cause of the condition is not well understood and it is unclear why some people with strep infections go on to develop rheumatic fever, while others do not. However, some scientists suspect that an exaggerated immune response in genetically susceptible people may play a role in the development of the condition.

Inheritance

Rheumatic fever is likely inherited in a multifactorial manner, which means it is caused by multiple genes interacting with each other and with environmental factors. The condition is thought to occur in genetically susceptible children who are infected with group A *Streptococcus* bacteria and live in poor social conditions. Some studies suggest that differences in the expression of various genes involved in the immune response may contribute to rheumatic fever susceptibility.

Diagnosis of Rheumatic Fever

A diagnosis of rheumatic fever is usually based on the following:

- Characteristic signs and symptoms identified by physical examination and/or specialized testing such as a blood test, chest X-ray and echocardiogram
- Confirmation of group A *Streptococcus* bacterial infection with a throat culture or blood tests

The diagnosis can also be supported by blood tests that confirm the presence of certain proteins that increase in response to inflammation (called acute-phase reactants) and tend to be elevated in rheumatic fever. Additional tests may be recommended to rule out other conditions that cause similar features.

Treatment for Rheumatic Fever

Treatment of rheumatic fever usually consists of antibiotics to treat the underlying group A *Streptococcus* bacterial infection and anti-inflammatory medications such as aspirin or corticosteroids. Because people with a history of rheumatic fever have a high risk of developing recurrent episodes of the condition, low dose antibiotics are often continued over a long period of time to prevent recurrence.

Prognosis of Rheumatic Fever

The long-term outlook (prognosis) for people with rheumatic fever depends on the severity of the heart involvement at the initial diagnosis. Severe carditis (inflammation of the heart) is associated with a poor prognosis and generally leads to rheumatic heart disease. People with a history of rheumatic fever have a high risk of developing recurrent episodes of the condition, which can cause progressive (worsening over time) heart damage. Prophylactic low dose antibiotics can significantly improve prognosis in many cases by preventing these recurrences.

Section 11.4

Scarlet Fever

This section includes text excerpted from "Scarlet Fever: A Group A Streptococcal Infection," Centers for Disease Control and Prevention (CDC), January 19, 2016.

Scarlet fever results from group A strep infection. If your child has a sore throat and rash, their doctor can test for strep. Quick treatment with antibiotics can protect your child from possible long-term health problems.

Scarlet fever—or scarlatina—is a bacterial infection caused by group A *Streptococcus* or "group A strep." This illness affects a small percentage of people who have strep throat or, less commonly, streptococcal skin infections. Scarlet fever is treatable with antibiotics and usually is a mild illness, but it needs to be treated to prevent rare but serious long-term health problems. Treatment with antibiotics also helps clear up symptoms faster and reduces spread to other people.

Although anyone can get scarlet fever, it usually affects children between 5 and 15 years old. The classic symptom of the disease is a certain type of red rash that feels rough, like sandpaper.

How Do You Get Scarlet Fever?

Group A strep bacteria can live in a person's nose and throat. The bacteria are spread through contact with droplets from an infected person's cough or sneeze. If you touch your mouth, nose, or eyes after touching something that has these droplets on it, you may become ill. If you drink from the same glass or eat from the same plate as the sick person, you could also become ill. It is possible to get scarlet fever from contact with sores from group A strep skin infections.

Common Symptoms of Scarlet Fever

- A very red, sore throat
- A fever (101° F or above)
- A red rash with a sandpaper feel
- Bright red skin in underarm, elbow, and groin creases
- A whitish coating on the tongue or back of the throat
- A "strawberry" tongue
- Headache or body aches
- Nausea, vomiting, or abdominal pain
- Swollen glands

Scarlet Fever: What to Expect

Illness usually begins with a fever and sore throat. There also may be chills, vomiting, and abdominal pain. The tongue may have a whitish coating and appear swollen. It may also have a "strawberry"-like (red and bumpy) appearance. The throat and tonsils may be very red and sore, and swallowing may be painful.

One or two days after the illness begins, the characteristic red rash appears (although the rash can appear before illness or up to 7 days later). Certain strep bacteria produce a toxin (poison) which causes some people to break out in the rash—the "scarlet" of scarlet fever. The rash may first appear on the neck, underarm, and groin (the area where your stomach meets your thighs), then spread over the body. Typically, the rash begins as small, flat red blotches which gradually become fine bumps and feel like sandpaper.

Although the cheeks might have a flushed appearance, there may be a pale area around the mouth. Underarm, elbow, and groin skin creases may become brighter red than the rest of the rash. These are called Pastia's lines. The scarlet fever rash generally fades in about 7 days. As the rash fades, the skin may peel around the fingertips, toes, and groin area. This peeling can last up to several weeks.

Scarlet fever is treatable with antibiotics. Since either viruses or other bacteria can also cause sore throats, it's important to ask the doctor about getting a strep test (a simple swab of the throat) if your child complains of having a sore throat. If the test is positive, meaning your child is infected with group A strep bacteria, your child's doctor will prescribe antibiotics to avoid possible, although rare, long-term health problems, reduce symptoms, and prevent further spread of the disease.

Long-Term Health Problems from Scarlet Fever

Long-term health problems from scarlet fever may include:

- Rheumatic fever (an inflammatory disease that can affect the heart, joints, skin, and brain)
- Kidney disease (inflammation of the kidneys, called poststreptococcal glomerulonephritis)
- Otitis media (ear infections)
- Skin infections
- Abscesses of the throat
- Pneumonia (lung infection)
- Arthritis (joint inflammation)

Most of these health problems can be prevented by treatment with antibiotics.

Preventing Infection: Wash Those Hands

The best way to keep from getting infected is to wash your hands often and avoid sharing eating utensils, linens, towels or other personal items. It is especially important for anyone with a sore throat to wash his or her hands often. There is no vaccine to prevent strep throat or scarlet fever. Children with scarlet fever or strep throat should stay home from school or daycare for at least 24 hours after starting antibiotics.

Section 11.5

Strep Throat

This section includes text excerpted from "Is It Strep Throat?" Centers for Disease Control and Prevention (CDC), October 19, 2015.

Is It Strep Throat?

Strep throat is a common type of sore throat in children, but it's not very common in adults. Healthcare professionals can do a quick test to determine if a sore throat is strep throat and decide if antibiotics are needed. Proper treatment can help you feel better faster and prevent spreading it to others!

Many things can cause that unpleasant, scratchy, and sometimes painful condition known as a sore throat. Viruses, bacteria, allergens, environmental irritants (such as cigarette smoke), chronic postnasal drip, and fungi can all cause a sore throat. While many sore throats will get better without treatment, some throat infections—including strep throat—may need antibiotic treatment.

How You Get Strep Throat

Strep throat is an infection in the throat and tonsils caused by group A *Streptococcus* bacteria (called "group A strep"). Group A strep bacteria can also live in a person's nose and throat without causing illness. The bacteria are spread through contact with droplets after an infected person coughs or sneezes. If you touch your mouth, nose, or eyes after touching something that has these droplets on it, you may become ill. If you drink from the same glass or eat from the same plate as the infected person, you could also become ill. It is also possible to get strep throat from contact with sores from group A strep skin infections.

Common Symptoms of Strep Throat

The most common symptoms of strep throat include:

- Sore throat, usually starts quickly and can cause severe pain when swallowing
- A fever (101°F or above)
- Red and swollen tonsils, sometimes with white patches or streaks of pus
- Tiny, red spots (petechiae) on the roof of the mouth (the soft or hard palate)
- Headache, nausea, or vomiting
- Swollen lymph nodes in the front of the neck
- Sandpaper-like rash

A Simple Test Gives Fast Results

Healthcare professionals can test for strep by swabbing the throat to quickly see if group A strep bacteria are causing a sore throat. A strep test is needed to tell if you have strep throat; just looking at your throat is not enough to make a diagnosis. If the test is positive, your healthcare professional can prescribe antibiotics. If the strep test is negative, but your clinician still strongly suspects you have this infection, then they can take a throat culture swab to test for the bacteria, but those results will take a little longer to come back.

Antibiotics Get You Well Fast

The strep test results will help your healthcare professional decide if you need antibiotics, which can:

- Decrease the length of time you're sick
- Reduce your symptoms

- Help prevent the spread of infection to friends and family members
- Prevent more serious complications, such as tonsil and sinus infections, and acute rheumatic fever (a rare inflammatory disease that can affect the heart, joints, skin, and brain)

You should start feeling better in just a day or two after starting antibiotics. Call your healthcare professional if you don't feel better after taking antibiotics for 48 hours. People with strep throat should stay home from work, school, or daycare until they have taken antibiotics for at least 24 hours so they don't spread the infection to others.

Be sure to finish the entire prescription, even when you start feeling better, unless your healthcare professional tells you to stop taking the medicine. When you stop taking antibiotics early, you risk getting an infection later that is resistant to antibiotic treatment.

More Prevention Tips: Wash Those Hands

The best way to keep from getting strep throat is to wash your hands often and avoid sharing eating utensils, like forks or cups. It is especially important for anyone with a sore throat to wash their hands often and cover their mouth when coughing and sneezing. There is no vaccine to prevent strep throat.

Section 11.6

Impetigo

This section includes text excerpted from "Impetigo," National Institute of Allergy and Infectious Diseases (NIAID), October 22, 2013.

What Is Impetigo?

Impetigo is an infection of the top layers of the skin and is most common among children ages 2 to 6 years. It usually starts when bacteria get into a cut, scratch, or insect bite.

Cause of Impetigo

Impetigo is usually caused by staphylococcus (staph) bacteria, but it also can be caused by group A *Streptococcus* bacteria. Skin infections are usually caused by different types (strains) of strep bacteria than those that cause strep throat. Therefore, the types of strep germs that cause impetigo are usually different from those that cause strep throat.

Transmission of Impetigo

The infection is spread by direct contact with lesions (wounds or sores) or nasal discharge from an infected person. Scratching may spread the lesions. It usually takes 1 to 3 days from the time of infection until you show symptoms. If your skin doesn't have breaks in it, you can't be infected by dried strep bacteria in the air.

Symptoms of Impetigo

Symptoms start with red or pimple-like lesions surrounded by reddened skin. These sores can be anywhere on your body, but mostly on your face, arms, and legs. The sores fill with pus, then break open after a few days and form a thick crust. Itching is common.

Diagnosis of Impetigo

Your healthcare provider can diagnose the infection by looking at the skin lesions.

Treatment for Impetigo

If your impetigo is caused by strep bacteria, your healthcare provider will prescribe oral antibiotics, as with strep throat. This treatment may also include an antibiotic ointment to be used on your skin.

Chapter 12

Other Bacterial Infections

Chapter Contents

Section 12.1

Cat Scratch Disease

This section includes text excerpted from "Cat-Scratch Disease," Centers for Disease Control and Prevention (CDC), April 30, 2014.

Overview

Cat-scratch disease (CSD) is a bacterial infection spread by cats. The disease spreads when an infected cat licks a person's open wound, or bites or scratches a person hard enough to break the surface of the skin. About three to 14 days after the skin is broken, a mild infection can occur at the site of the scratch or bite. The infected area may appear swollen and red with round, raised lesions and can have pus. The infection can feel warm or painful. A person with CSD may also have a fever, headache, poor appetite, and exhaustion. Later, the person's lymph nodes closest to the original scratch or bite can become swollen, tender, or painful.

Wash cat bites and scratches well with soap and running water. Do not allow cats to lick your wounds. Contact your doctor if you develop any symptoms of cat-scratch disease or infection.

CSD is caused by a bacterium called *Bartonella henselae*. About 40% of cats carry *B. henselae* at some time in their lives, although most cats with this infection show NO signs of illness. Kittens younger than 1 year are more likely to have B. henselae infection and to spread the germ to people. Kittens are also more likely to scratch and bite while they play and learn how to attack prey.

How Cats and People Become Infected

Cats can get infected with *B. henselae* from flea bites and flea dirt (droppings) getting into their wounds. By scratching and biting at the fleas, cats pick up the infected flea dirt under their nails and between their teeth. Cats can also become infected by fighting with other cats that are infected. The germ spreads to people when infected cats bite or scratch a person hard enough to break their skin. The germ can also spread when infected cats lick at wounds or scabs that you may have.

Serious but Rare Complications

People

Although rare, CSD can cause people to have serious complications. CSD can affect the brain, eyes, heart, or other internal organs. These rare complications, which may require intensive treatment, are more likely to occur in children younger than 5 years and people with weakened immune systems.

Cats

Most cats with *B. henselae* infection show NO signs of illness, but on rare occasions this disease can cause inflammation of the heart—making cats very sick with labored breathing. *B. henselae* infection may also develop in the mouth, urinary system, or eyes. Your veterinarian may find that some of your cat's other organs may be inflamed.

Prevention

People

Do:

- Wash cat bites and scratches right away with soap and running water.
- Wash your hands with soap and running water after playing with your cat, especially if you live with young children or people with weakened immune systems.
- Since cats less than one year of age are more likely to have CSD and spread it to people, persons with a weakened immune system should adopt cats older than one year of age.

Do not:

- Play rough with your pets because they may scratch and bite.
- Allow cats to lick your open wounds.
- Pet or touch stray or feral cats.

Cats

Control fleas

- Keep your cat's nails trimmed.
- Apply a flea product (topical or oral medication) approved by your veterinarian once a month.

- Beware: Over-the-counter flea products may not be safe for cats. Check with your veterinarian before applying ANY flea product to make sure it is safe for your cat and your family.
- Check for fleas by using a flea comb on your cat to inspect for flea dirt.
- Control fleas in your home by
- Vacuuming frequently
- Contacting a pest-control agent if necessary

Protect your cat's health

- Schedule routine veterinary health check-ups.
- Keep cats indoors to
- Decrease their contact with fleas
- Prevent them from fighting with stray or potentially infected animals

Available Tests and Treatments

People

Talk to your doctor about testing and treatments for CSD. People are only tested for CSD when the disease is severe and the doctor suspects CSD based on the patient's symptoms. CSD is typically not treated in otherwise healthy people.

Cats

Talk to your veterinarian about testing and treatments for your cat. Your veterinarian can tell you whether your cat requires testing or treatment.

Section 12.2

Diphtheria

This section contains text excerpted from the following sources: Text beginning with the heading "About Diphtheria" is excerpted from "About Diphtheria," Centers for Disease Control and Prevention (CDC), January 15, 2016; Text beginning with the heading "Diphtheria Vaccine for Baby" is excerpted from "Diphtheria," Centers for Disease Control and Prevention (CDC), February 2013.

About Diphtheria

Diphtheria once was a major cause of illness and death among children. The United States recorded 206,000 cases of diphtheria in 1921 and 15,520 deaths. Before there was treatment for diphtheria, up to half of the people who got the disease died from it.

Starting in the 1920s, diphtheria rates dropped quickly in the United States and other countries with the widespread use of vaccines. In the past decade, there were less than five cases of diphtheria in the United States reported to Centers for Disease Control and Prevention (CDC). However, the disease continues to cause illness globally. In 2014, 7,321 cases of diphtheria were reported to the World Health Organization (WHO), but there are likely many more cases.

Causes and Transmission

Diphtheria is an infection caused by the *Corynebacterium diphtheriae* bacterium.

Diphtheria is spread (transmitted) from person to person, usually through respiratory droplets, like from coughing or sneezing. Rarely, people can get sick from touching open sores (skin lesions) or clothes that touched open sores of someone sick with diphtheria. A person also can get diphtheria by coming in contact with an object, like a toy, that has the bacteria that cause diphtheria on it.

Symptoms

When the bacteria that cause diphtheria get into and attach to the lining of the respiratory system, which includes parts of the body that help you breathe, they produce a poison (toxin) that can cause:

- Weakness
- Sore throat
- Fever
- Swollen glands in the neck

The poison destroys healthy tissues in the respiratory system. Within two to three days, the dead tissue forms a thick, gray coating that can build up in the throat or nose. This thick gray coating is called a "pseudomembrane." It can cover tissues in the nose, tonsils, voice box, and throat, making it very hard to breathe and swallow.

The poison may also get into the bloodstream and cause damage to the heart, kidneys, and nerves.

Complications

Complications from diphtheria may include:

- Blocking of the airway
- Damage to the heart muscle (myocarditis)
- Nerve damage (polyneuropathy)
- Loss of the ability to move (paralysis)
- Lung infection (respiratory failure or pneumonia)

For some people, diphtheria can lead to death. Even with treatment, about 1 out of 10 diphtheria patients die. Without treatment, as many as 1 out of 2 patients can die from the disease.

Diagnosis and Treatment

Doctors usually decide if a person has diphtheria by looking for common signs and symptoms. They can use a swab from the back of the throat and test it for the bacteria that cause diphtheria. A doctor can also take a sample from a skin lesion (like a sore) and try and grow the bacteria to be sure a patient has diphtheria.

It is important to start treatment right away if a doctor suspects diphtheria and not to wait for laboratory confirmation. In the United States, before there was treatment for diphtheria, up to half of the people who got the disease died from it.

Diphtheria treatment today involves:

- Using diphtheria antitoxin to stop the poison (toxin) produced by the bacteria from damaging the body
- Using medicines (called antibiotics) to kill and get rid of the bacteria

Diphtheria patients are usually kept in isolation, until they are no longer contagious—this usually takes about 48 hours after starting antibiotics. After the patient finishes taking the antibiotic, the doctor will run tests to make sure the bacteria are not in the patient's body anymore.

Prevention

The best way to prevent diphtheria is to get vaccinated. In the United States, there are four vaccines used to prevent diphtheria:

1. DTaP
2. Tdap
3. DT
4. Td

Each of these vaccines prevents diphtheria and tetanus; DTaP and Tdap also help prevent pertussis (whooping cough). DTaP and DT are given to children younger than seven years old, while Tdap and Td are given to older children, teens, and adults.

Babies and Children

The current childhood immunization schedule for diphtheria includes five doses of DTaP for children younger than seven years old.

Preteens and Teens

The adolescent immunization schedule recommends that preteens get a booster dose of Tdap at 11 or 12 years old. Teens who did not get Tdap when they were 11 or 12 years old should get a dose the next time they see their doctor.

Section 12.3

H. pylori *Bacteria and Peptic Ulcers*

This section includes text excerpted from "Definition and Facts for Peptic Ulcer Disease," National Institute of Diabetes and Digestive and Kidney Diseases (NIDDK), November 13, 2014.

What Is a Peptic Ulcer?

A peptic ulcer is a sore on the lining of your stomach or duodenum. Rarely, a peptic ulcer may develop just above your stomach in your esophagus. Doctors call this type of peptic ulcer an esophageal ulcer.

Who Is More Likely to Develop Peptic Ulcers Caused by H. pylori*?*

About 30 to 40 percent of people in the United States get an *Helicobacter pylori* (*H. pylori*) infection. In most cases, the infection remains dormant, or quiet without signs or symptoms, for years. Most people get an *H. pylori* infection as a child.

Adults who have an *H. pylori* infection may get a peptic ulcer, also called an H. pylori-induced peptic ulcer. However, most people with an *H. pylori* infection never develop a peptic ulcer. Peptic ulcers caused by *H. pylori* are uncommon in children.

H. pylori are spiral-shaped bacteria that can damage the lining of your stomach and duodenum and cause peptic ulcer disease. Researchers are not certain how *H. pylori* spread. They think the bacteria may spread through:

- unclean food
- unclean water
- unclean eating utensils
- contact with an infected person's saliva and other bodily fluids, including kissing

Researchers have found *H. pylori* in the saliva of some infected people, which means an *H. pylori* infection could spread through direct contact with saliva or other bodily fluids.

What Other Problems Can a Peptic Ulcer Cause?

A peptic ulcer can cause other problems, including:

- bleeding from a broken blood vessel in your stomach or small intestine
- perforation of your stomach or small intestine
- a blockage that can stop food from moving from your stomach into your duodenum
- peritonitis

You may need surgery to treat these problems.

What Are the Symptoms of a Peptic Ulcer?

A dull or burning pain in your stomach is the most common symptom of a peptic ulcer. You may feel the pain anywhere between your belly button and breastbone. The pain most often:

- happens when your stomach is empty—such as between meals or during the night
- stops briefly if you eat or if you take antacids
- lasts for minutes to hours
- comes and goes for several days, weeks, or months

Less common symptoms may include:

- bloating
- burping
- feeling sick to your stomach
- poor appetite
- vomiting
- weight loss

Even if your symptoms are mild, you may have a peptic ulcer. You should see your doctor to talk about your symptoms. Without treatment, your peptic ulcer can get worse.

What Causes a Peptic Ulcer?

Causes of peptic ulcers include:

- long-term use of nonsteroidal anti-inflammatory drugs (NSAIDs), such as aspirin and ibuprofen
- an infection with the bacteria *Helicobacter pylori* (*H. pylori*)
- rare cancerous and noncancerous tumors in the stomach, duodenum, or pancreas—known as Zollinger-Ellison syndrome

Sometimes peptic ulcers are caused by both NSAIDs and *H. pylori*.

How Do H. pylori *Cause a Peptic Ulcer and Peptic Ulcer Disease?*

H. pylori are spiral-shaped bacteria that can cause peptic ulcer disease by damaging the mucous coating that protects the lining of the stomach and duodenum. Once *H. pylori* have damaged the mucous coating, powerful stomach acid can get through to the sensitive lining. Together, the stomach acid and *H. pylori* irritate the lining of the stomach or duodenum and cause a peptic ulcer.

When Should You Call or See a Doctor?

You should call or see your doctor right away if you:

- feel weak or faint
- have difficulty breathing
- have red blood in your vomit or vomit that looks like coffee grounds
- have red blood in your stool or black stools
- have sudden, sharp stomach pain that doesn't go away

These symptoms could be signs that a peptic ulcer has caused a more serious problem.

How Can I Prevent a Peptic Ulcer?

To help prevent a peptic ulcer caused by NSAIDs, ask your doctor if you should:

- stop using NSAIDs

- take NSAIDs with a meal if you still need NSAIDs
- take a lower dose of NSAIDs
- take medicines to protect your stomach and duodenum while taking NSAIDs
- switch to a medicine that won't cause ulcers

To help prevent a peptic ulcer caused by *H. pylori,* your doctor may recommend that you avoid drinking alcohol.

Section 12.4

Haemophilus influenza *Type B*

This section contains text excerpted from the following sources: Text beginning with the heading "About *Haemophilus influenzae* Disease" is excerpted from "About *Haemophilus influenzae* Disease," Centers for Disease Control and Prevention (CDC), July 25, 2016; Text beginning with the heading "Protect Your Child against Hib Disease" is excerpted from "Protect Your Child against Hib Disease," Centers for Disease Control and Prevention (CDC), March 14, 2016.

About Haemophilus influenzae *Disease*

H.influenzae is a type of bacteria that can cause infections in people of all ages ranging from mild, such as an ear infection, to severe, such as a bloodstream infection.

Types of Haemophilus influenzae *Infections*

H. influenzae, including Hib, can cause many different kinds of infections. These infections can range from mild ear infections to severe diseases, like bloodstream infections.

When the bacteria invade parts of the body that are normally free from germs, like spinal fluid or blood, this is known as "invasive disease." Invasive disease is usually severe and can sometimes result in death.

The most common types of invasive disease caused by *H. influenzae* are:

- Pneumonia (lung infection)
- Bacteremia (blood infection)
- Meningitis (infection of the covering of the brain and spinal cord)
- Epiglottitis (swelling of the windpipe that can cause breathing trouble)
- Cellulitis (skin infection)
- Infectious arthritis (inflammation of the joint)

H. influenzae can also be a common cause of ear infections in children and bronchitis in adults.

Causes, How It Spreads, and People at Increased Risk

Causes

Haemophilus influenzae disease is caused by the bacterium *Haemophilus influenzae*. There are six identifiable types of *H. influenzae* (a through f) and other non-identifiable types (called nontypeable). The one that people are most familiar with is *H. influenzae* type b, or Hib.

These bacteria live in the nose and throat, and usually cause no harm. However, the bacteria can sometimes move to other parts of the body and cause infection. Some of these infections are considered "invasive" and can be very serious and sometimes even deadly.

The incubation period (time between exposure and first symptoms) of *H. influenzae* disease is not certain, but could be as short as a few days.

How It Spreads

H. influenzae, including Hib, are spread person-to-person through respiratory droplets that occur when someone who has the bacteria in their nose or throat coughs or sneezes. Most of the time, *H. influenzae* are spread by people who have the bacteria in their noses and throats but who are not ill (asymptomatic).

Sometimes *H. influenzae* spread to other people who have had close or lengthy contact with a person sick with *H. influenzae* disease. In certain cases, people in close contact with that person should receive antibiotics (medicines that kill bacteria in the body) to prevent them from getting the disease.

People at Increased Risk

H. influenzae, including Hib, disease occurs mostly in babies and children younger than five years old. Adults 65 years or older, American Indians, and Alaska Natives are also at increased risk for getting sick with invasive *H. influenzae* disease.

People with certain medical conditions are also at increased risk for developing *H. influenzae* disease. Those medical conditions include:

- Sickle cell disease
- Asplenia (no spleen)
- HIV (human immunodeficiency virus) infection
- Antibody and complement deficiency syndromes
- Receipt of chemotherapy or radiation therapy for malignant neoplasms
- Receipt of hematopoietic stem cell

Signs and Symptoms

Haemophilus influenzae, including Hib, disease causes different symptoms depending on which part of the body is affected. The most common severe types of *H. influenzae* disease are:

- Pneumonia (lung infection)
- Bacteremia (bloodstream infection)
- Meningitis (infection of the covering of the brain and spinal cord)

Pneumonia

Pneumonia occurs when the lungs become infected, causing inflammation (swelling). *H. influenzae* pneumonia is considered non-invasive if there's not bacteremia or pleural fluid (fluid surrounding the lungs) infection occurring at the same time. When there is pneumonia with either bacteremia or pleural fluid infection occurring at the same time, it is considered invasive.

Symptoms of pneumonia usually include:

- Fever and chills
- Cough
- Shortness of breath or difficulty breathing

- Sweating
- Chest pain
- Headache
- Muscle pain or aches
- Excessive tiredness

Bacteremia

Bacteremia is an infection of the blood. It can cause symptoms such as:

- Fever and chills
- Excessive tiredness
- Pain in the belly
- Nausea with or without vomiting
- Diarrhea
- Anxiety
- Shortness of breath or difficulty breathing
- Altered mental status (confusion)Bacteremia from *H. influenzae* can occur with or without pneumonia.

Meningitis

Meningitis is an infection of the covering of the brain and spinal cord. Symptoms typically include sudden onset of:

- Fever
- Headache
- Stiff neck
- Nausea with or without vomiting
- Increased sensitivity to light (photophobia)
- Altered mental status (confusion)Babies may appear to be lethargic (limp, loss of alertness) or irritable, or may not eat well. In young children, doctors may also test the child's reflexes, which can be abnormal with meningitis.

Diagnosis, Treatment, and Complications

Diagnosis

Haemophilus influenzae, including Hib, disease is usually diagnosed with one or more laboratory tests using a sample of body fluid, such as blood or spinal fluid.

Treatment

H. influenzae, including Hib, disease is treated with antibiotics (medicines that kill bacteria in the body), usually for 10 days. Most cases of invasive disease (when bacteria invade parts of the body that are normally free from germs) require care in a hospital.

When *H. influenzae* cause a non-invasive infection, like bronchitis or an ear infection, antibiotics may be given to prevent complications.

Complications

Complications depend on the type of invasive infection caused the bacteria. For example, if *H. influenzae* cause meningitis (infection of the covering of the brain and spinal cord), a person can suffer from brain damage or hearing loss. Bacteremia (blood infection) can result in loss of limb(s). Invasive *H. influenzae* infections can sometimes result in death. Even with antibiotic treatment, about 3 to 6 out of every 100 children with meningitis caused by Hib die from the disease.

When *H. influenzae* cause a non-invasive infection, like bronchitis or an ear infection, complications are rare and typically not severe. If appropriate, antibiotics can be given to prevent complications.

Prevention

Vaccine

There's a vaccine that can prevent *Haemophilus influenzae* type b (Hib) disease, the most common type ("strain") of *Haemophilus influenzae* bacteria. However, this vaccine does not prevent disease caused by the other types of *H. influenzae*.

Hib vaccine is recommended for all children younger than 5 years old in the United States and is usually given to babies starting at 2 months old. In certain situations, people at increased risk for getting invasive Hib disease (when bacteria invade parts of the body that are normally free from germs) who are fully vaccinated may need additional doses of Hib vaccine. Unimmunized older children, teens, and adults with certain medical conditions should also receive Hib vaccine.

Re-Infection

A child with *H. influenzae*, including Hib, disease may not develop protective levels of antibodies (proteins produced by the body to fight off diseases). This means that someone could get *H. influenzae* disease again. Children younger than 2 years old who have recovered from invasive Hib disease are not be considered protected and should receive Hib vaccine as soon as possible.

Antibiotic Prophylaxis

Sometimes Hib is spread to people who have had close or lengthy contact with someone who has or had Hib disease. In certain cases, people in close contact with someone who is sick with Hib should receive antibiotics to prevent them from getting the disease. This is known as prophylaxis. A doctor or local health department will make recommendations for who should receive prophylaxis.

Section 12.5

Lyme Disease

This section includes text excerpted from "Lyme Disease," National Institute of Allergy and Infectious Diseases (NIAID), April 6, 2016.

What Is Lyme Disease?

Lyme disease, or borreliosis, is caused by the bacterium Borrelia burgdorferi and is transmitted to humans through the bite of an infected blacklegged deer tick. It is the most common tickborne infectious disease in the United States. State health departments reported

27,203 confirmed cases and 9,104 probable cases of Lyme disease to the Centers for Disease Control and Prevention in 2013.

Symptoms

Typically, the first symptom of Lyme disease is a rash known as erythema migrans, which starts as a small red spot at the site of the tick bite and gets larger over a period of days or weeks, forming a circular or oval-shaped red rash. The rash may look like a bull's eye, appearing as a red ring around a clear area with a red center. It appears within a few weeks of a tick bite and usually occurs at the place of the bite. The rash can range in size from that of a small coin to the width of a person's back. As infection spreads, rashes can appear at different sites on the body. The rash is often accompanied by other symptoms, such as fever, headache, stiff neck, body aches and fatigue. Although these symptoms may be like those of common viral infections, such as the flu, Lyme disease symptoms tend to last longer or may come and go over time.

Some people who have Lyme disease may develop arthritis or nervous system problems and more rarely, heart problems. Lyme disease may also cause eye inflammation, hepatitis (liver disease), and severe fatigue. However, these problems usually only appear in conjunction with other symptoms of the disease.

Diagnosis

Healthcare providers may have difficulty diagnosing Lyme disease because many of its symptoms are similar to those of other illnesses, such as the flu. The bull's eye rash is the only symptom that is unique to Lyme disease, but not everyone infected with Lyme bacteria develops the rash. Research supported by the National Institutes of Health (NIH) and the Centers for Disease Control and Prevention (CDC) suggest that a tick must be attached to the body for at least 36 hours to transmit Lyme disease. Although transmission cannot occur without the tick bite, many people may not remember being bitten because the deer tick is tiny and its bite is usually painless.

If a person has symptoms of Lyme disease but does not have the distinctive rash, healthcare providers will rely on a detailed medical history. The medical history includes whether symptoms first appeared during the summer months, if the person had been outdoors in an area where Lyme disease is common, and whether the person was bitten by a tick, along with a careful physical exam and laboratory tests to check for the presence of antibodies to *B. burgdorferi* to help provide a diagnosis.

Treatment

Antibiotics are prescribed to effectively treat Lyme disease. These medicines can help speed healing of the erythema migrans rash and keep symptoms, such as arthritis and nervous system problems, from developing. In general, the sooner treatment begins after infection, the quicker and more complete the recovery. Treatment for pregnant women is similar to treatment for others, but certain antibiotics are not used because they may affect the fetus.

After receiving treatment for Lyme disease, patients may still experience muscle or joint aches and nervous system symptoms, such as trouble with memory and concentration. To help combat these problems, researchers are trying to find out how long a person should take antibiotics for the various symptoms that may follow a bout with Lyme disease. Individuals who have previously had Lyme disease can be infected again if bitten by an infected tick.

The Ticks That Cause Lyme Disease

Two types of blacklegged ticks, which look quite similar, are largely responsible for transmitting Lyme disease in the United States:

- *Ixodes scapularis* is most commonly found in the U.S. Northeast and Midwest, and can also be found in the South and Southeast.
- *Ixodes pacificus* is found on the U.S. West Coast.

Prevention

The best way to prevent Lyme disease is to avoid contact with deer ticks, especially during the summer months when infections are most common. Other useful tips:

- Wear long pants, long sleeves and long socks to keep ticks off the skin. Tuck shirts into pants, and pant legs into socks or shoes, to keep ticks on the surface of your clothing. If outside for a long period of time, tape the area where pants and socks meet to prevent ticks from crawling under clothing.
- Wear light-colored clothing to make it easier to spot ticks.
- Spray clothing with the repellant permethrin, found in lawn and garden stores. Do not apply permethrin directly to the skin.
- Spray exposed clothing and skin with repellant containing 20 to 30 percent DEET to prevent tick bites. Carefully read and

understand manufacturer instructions when using repellant, especially when using the products on infants and children.

- Pregnant women in particular should avoid ticks in Lyme disease areas as infection may be transmitted to the fetus.
- Avoid wooded areas and nearby shady grasslands. Deer ticks are common in these areas, and particularly common where the two areas merge.
- Maintain a clear backyard by removing yard litter and excess brush that could attract deer and rodents.
- Once indoors after being outside, check for ticks, especially in the hairy areas of the body, and wash all clothing.
- Before letting pets indoors, check them for ticks. Ticks may fall off and then attach to humans. Pets can also develop Lyme disease.

Section 12.6

Methicillin-Resistant Staphylococcus aureus *(MRSA)*

This section includes text excerpted from "General Information about MRSA in the Community," Centers for Disease Control and Prevention (CDC), February 9, 2016.

Methicillin-resistant *Staphylococcus aureus* (MRSA) is a type of staph bacteria that is resistant to several antibiotics. In the general community, MRSA most often causes skin infections. In some cases, it causes pneumonia (lung infection) and other issues. If left untreated, MRSA infections can become severe and cause sepsis—a life-threatening reaction to severe infection in the body.

In a healthcare setting, such as a hospital or nursing home, MRSA can cause severe problems such as bloodstream infections, pneumonia and surgical site infections.

Who Is at Risk, and How Is MRSA Spread in The Community?

Anyone can get MRSA on their body from contact with an infected wound or by sharing personal items, such as towels or razors, that have touched infected skin. MRSA infection risk can be increased when a person is in activities or places that involve crowding, skin-to-skin contact, and shared equipment or supplies. People including athletes, daycare and school students, military personnel in barracks, and those who recently received inpatient medical care are at higher risk.

How Common Is MRSA?

Studies show that about one in three people carry staph in their nose, usually without any illness. Two in 100 people carry MRSA. There are no data showing the total number of people who get MRSA skin infections in the community.

Can I Prevent MRSA? How?

There are the steps you can take to reduce your risk of MRSA infection:

- Maintain good hand and body hygiene. Wash hands often, and clean your body regularly, especially after exercise.
- Keep cuts, scrapes and wounds clean and covered until healed.
- Avoid sharing personal items such as towels and razors.
- Get care early if you think you might have an infection.

What are MRSA Symptoms?

Sometimes, people with MRSA skin infections first think they have a spider bite. However, unless a spider is actually seen, the irritation is likely not a spider bite. Most staph skin infections, including MRSA, appear as a bump or infected area on the skin that might be:

- Red
- Swollen
- Painful
- Warm to the touch
- Full of pus or other drainage
- Accompanied by a fever

What Should I Do If I See These Symptoms?

If you or someone in your family experiences these signs and symptoms, cover the area with a bandage, wash your hands, and contact your doctor. It is especially important to contact your doctor if signs and symptoms of an MRSA skin infection are accompanied by a fever.

What Should I do if I Think I Have a Skin Infection?

- You can't tell by looking at the skin if it is a staph infection (including MRSA).
- Contact your doctor if you think you have an infection. Finding infections early and getting care make it less likely that the infection will become severe.
- Do not try to treat the infection yourself by picking or popping the sore.
- Cover possible infections with clean, dry bandages until you can be seen by a doctor, nurse, or other healthcare provider.

How to Prevent Spreading MRSA

- Cover your wounds. Keep wounds covered with clean, dry bandages until healed. Follow your doctor's instructions about proper care of the wound. Pus from infected wounds can contain MRSA so keeping the infection covered will help prevent the spread to others. Bandages and tape can be thrown away with the regular trash. Do not try to treat the infection yourself by picking or popping the sore.
- Clean your hands often. You, your family, and others in close contact should wash their hands often with soap and water or use an alcohol-based hand rub, especially after changing the bandage or touching the infected wound.
- Do not share personal items. Personal items include towels, washcloths, razors and clothing, including uniforms.
- Wash used sheets, towels, and clothes with water and laundry detergent. Use a dryer to dry them completely.
- Wash clothes according to manufacturer's instructions on the label. Clean your hands after touching dirty clothes.

Section 12.7

Mycoplasma Infection (Walking Pneumonia)

This section includes text excerpted from "*Mycoplasma pneumoniae* Infection," Centers for Disease Control and Prevention (CDC), March 15, 2016.

About the Disease

Mycoplasma pneumoniae is an "atypical" bacterium (the singular form of bacteria) that commonly causes infections of the respiratory system. The most common type of illness caused by these bacteria, especially in children, is tracheobronchitis, commonly called a chest cold. This illness is often seen with other upper respiratory tract symptoms, like a sore throat. Sometimes *Mycoplasma pneumoniae (M. pneumoniae)* infection can cause pneumonia, a more serious infection of the lungs, which may require treatment or care in a hospital.

M. pneumoniae infections are sometimes referred to as "walking pneumonia." Some experts estimate that between 1 and 10 out of every 50 cases of community-acquired pneumonia (lung infections developed outside of a hospital) in the United States is caused by *M. pneumoniae*. However, not everyone who is exposed to *M. pneumoniae* develops pneumonia.

In general, *M. pneumoniae* infection is a mild illness that is most common in young adults and school-aged children. Outbreaks of *M. pneumoniae* occur mostly in crowded environments, like schools, college dormitories, military barracks, and nursing homes, when small droplets of water that contain the bacteria get into the air by coughing and sneezing while in close contact with others, who then breathe in the bacteria. *M. pneumoniae* infections often spread within households.

Causes

Mycoplasma pneumoniae is a bacterium that causes illness by damaging the lining of the respiratory system (throat, lungs, windpipe).

Transmission

A person who is sick with *M. pneumoniae* infection has these bacteria in their nose, throat, windpipe, and lungs. *M. pneumoniae* is transmitted (spread) from person-to-person when small droplets of water that contain the bacteria get into the air and people breathe them in. People who are sick with *M. pneumoniae* infection usually spread the disease by coughing or sneezing while in close contact with others, who then breathe in the bacteria.

Most people who are exposed for a short amount of time to someone with *M. pneumoniae* infection do not become ill. *M. pneumoniae* infections are known to have long incubation periods (the time between first catching the bacteria from an ill person and development of symptoms). However, it is common for this illness to spread between family members who live together. The incubation period is usually between 1 to 4 weeks.

Outbreaks occur mostly in crowded settings like schools, college dormitories, military barracks, nursing homes, and hospitals. Transmission of *M. pneumoniae* to the community has been seen during school-based outbreaks, with most community cases thought to be family members of ill school children.

Signs and Symptoms

In general, *Mycoplasma pneumoniae* infection is a mild illness with symptoms that appear and get worse over a period of 1 to 4 weeks. This bacterium can cause several types of infections. Pneumonia (lung infection) may be the most serious type of *M. pneumoniae* infection, but not everyone will develop pneumonia. It is estimated that only 1 out of every 3 people who get ill from *M. pneumoniae* actually get pneumonia.

The most common type of illness, especially in children, is tracheobronchitis, commonly known as chest cold. This chest cold often comes with:

- Sore throat
- Fatigue (being tired)
- Fever
- Slowly worsening cough that can last for weeks or months
- Headache

Children younger than 5 years old often do not run a fever when they have *M. pneumoniae* infection. Instead they may have signs that appear more like a cold than pneumonia. They sometimes wheeze, vomit, or have diarrhea.

Prevention

Like many respiratory diseases, *Mycoplasma pneumoniae* infection is spread by coughing and sneezing. Some tips to prevent the spread of *M. pneumoniae* include:

- Cover your mouth and nose with a tissue when you cough or sneeze.
- Put your used tissue in the waste basket.
- If you don't have a tissue, cough or sneeze into your upper sleeve or elbow, not your hands.
- Wash your hands often with soap and water for at least 20 seconds.
- If soap and water are not available, use an alcohol-based hand rub.

There is no vaccine to prevent *M. pneumoniae* infection.

Treatment

Pneumonia (lung infection) caused by *Mycoplasma pneumoniae* is routinely treated with antibiotics, although most people will recover from the illness on their own without medicine. The illness will usually not last as long if antibiotics are started early.

There are several types of antibiotics available to treat pneumonia caused by *M. pneumoniae*. If you or your child is diagnosed with a *M. pneumoniae* infection, your doctor will explain how to treat it.

M. pneumoniae has increasingly been shown to be resistant to some antibiotics.

Complications

While *M. pneumoniae* infection usually causes mild disease, severe complications can occur that result in needing care or treatment in a hospital. Complications that have been reported include:

- Serious pneumonia
- Encephalitis (swelling of the brain)

- Hemolytic anemia (too few red blood cells, which means fewer cells to deliver oxygen in the body)
- Renal dysfunction (kidney problems)
- Skin disorders (Stevens-Johnson syndrome, erythema multiforme, toxic epidermal necrolysis)

People at Risk

People of all ages are at risk of infection from *Mycoplasma pneumoniae,* but it is most common in young adults and school-aged children. People at highest risk include those who live or work in crowded settings, such as:

- Schools
- College dormitories
- Military barracks
- Nursing homes
- Hospitals

People at risk for serious disease include people:

- Recovering from a respiratory illness
- With a weakened immune system
- With asthma

Section 12.8

Tetanus

This section includes text excerpted from "Tetanus and the Vaccine (Shot) to Prevent It," Centers for Disease Control and Prevention (CDC), November 10, 2014.

What Is Tetanus?

Tetanus is a serious disease caused by a toxin (poison) made by bacteria. It causes painful muscle stiffness and can be deadly.

Tetanus is very dangerous. It can cause breathing problems, muscle spasms, and paralysis (unable to move parts of the body). Muscle spasms can be strong enough to break a child's spine or other bones.

It can take months to recover fully from tetanus. A child might need weeks of hospital care. As many as 1 out of 5 people who get tetanus dies.

What Are the Symptoms of Tetanus?

Tetanus in children starts with headache, jaw cramping, and muscle spasms (sudden, involuntary muscle tightening).

It also causes the following:

- Painful muscle stiffness all over the body
- Trouble swallowing
- Seizures (jerking or staring)
- Fever and sweating
- High blood pressure and fast heart rate
- Tetanus is often called "lockjaw" because the jaw muscles tighten, and the person cannot open his mouth.

How Could My Child Get Tetanus?

The bacteria that cause tetanus are found in soil. They get into the body through a puncture, cut, or sore of the skin. A person can also be infected after a burn or an animal bite.

Tetanus does not spread from one person to another.

Why Should My Child Get the DTaP Shot?

The DTaP shot:

- Protects your child from tetanus, a potentially serious disease (and also protects against diphtheria and whooping cough)
- Protects your child from painful muscle stiffness from tetanus
- Keeps your child from missing school or childcare (and keeps you from missing work to care for your sick child)

Is The DTaP Shot Safe?

Yes. The DTaP shot is very safe, and it is effective at preventing tetanus. Vaccines, like any medicine, can have side effects. Most children who get the shot have no side effects.

What Are the Side Effects?

Most children don't have any side effects from the shot. When side effects do occur, they are usually mild and may include:

- Redness, swelling, and pain at the injection site
- Fever
- Vomiting

These types of side effects happen in about 1 child out of every 4 children who get the shot.

More serious side effects are very rare but can include:

- A fever over 105 degrees
- Nonstop crying for 3 hours or more
- Seizures (jerking or twitching of the muscles or staring)

Booster Vaccines Needed to Keep Up Protection from Tetanus

The DTaP does not offer lifetime protection. People need booster vaccines to keep up protection from tetanus.

Children should get a booster vaccine called Tdap (which protects against tetanus, diphtheria, and whooping cough) at 11 or 12 years of age.

Adults need a booster called the Td vaccine (for tetanus and diphtheria) every 10 years. Adults should also receive a one-time shot of the Tdap vaccine in place of one Td shot.

Section 12.9

Tuberculosis

This section includes text excerpted from "Tuberculosis (TB)," Centers for Disease Control and Prevention (CDC), October 10, 2014.

TB in Children in the United States

TB disease in children under 15 years of age (also called pediatric tuberculosis) is a public health problem of special significance because it is a marker for recent transmission of TB. Also of special significance, infants and young children are more likely than older children and adults to develop life-threatening forms of TB disease (e.g., disseminated TB, TB meningitis). Among children, the greatest numbers of TB cases are seen in children less than 5 years of age, and in adolescents older than 10 years of age.

Basic TB Facts

TB is caused by a bacterium called *Mycobacterium tuberculosis*. TB bacteria are spread from person to person through the air. The TB bacteria are put into the air when a person with TB disease of the lungs or throat coughs, sneezes, speaks, or sings. People nearby may breathe in these bacteria and become infected.

People with TB disease of the lungs or throat can spread bacteria to others with whom they spend time every day. However, children are less likely to spread TB bacteria to others. This is because the forms of TB disease most commonly seen in children are usually less infectious than the forms seen in adults.

Not everyone infected with TB bacteria becomes sick. As a result, two TB-related conditions exist: latent TB infection and TB disease.

Latent TB Infection

Persons with latent TB infection:

- Usually have a skin test or blood test indicating TB infection;
- Have TB bacteria in their bodies, but the bacteria are not active;

- Are not sick and do not have symptoms;
- Cannot spread bacteria to others; and
- Are often given medicine to prevent them from developing TB disease.

TB Disease

If TB bacteria become active in the body and multiply, the person will get sick with TB disease.

Persons with TB disease:

- Usually have a skin test or blood test indicating TB infection;
- Are sick from TB bacteria that are active (meaning that they are multiplying and destroying tissue in their body);
- Usually have symptoms of TB disease; and
- Must be given medicine to treat TB disease.

Once infected with TB bacteria, children are more likely to get sick with TB disease and to get sick more quickly than adults. In comparison to children, TB disease in adults is usually due to past TB infection that becomes active years later, when a person's immune system becomes weak for some reason (e.g., human immunodeficiency virus (HIV) infection, diabetes).

Confirming the diagnosis of TB disease in children with a laboratory test can be challenging. This is because:

- It is difficult to collect sputum specimens from infants and young children; and
- The laboratory tests used to find TB in sputum are less likely to have a positive result in children; this is due to the fact that children are more likely to have TB disease caused by a smaller number of bacteria (paucibacillary disease).

For these reasons, the diagnosis of TB disease in children is often made without laboratory confirmation and instead based on combination of the following factors:

- Clinical signs and symptoms typically associated with TB disease,
- Positive tuberculin skin test (TST) or positive TB blood test (IGRA),

- Chest X-ray that has patterns typically associated with TB disease, and
- History of contact with a person with infectious TB disease.

Testing for TB in Children

In the absence of symptoms, usually the only sign of TB infection is a positive reaction to the TB skin test or TB blood test. TB skin testing is considered safe in children, and is preferred over TB blood tests for children less than 5 years of age.

All children with a positive test for TB infection, symptoms of TB, or a history of contact with a person with infectious TB disease should undergo a medical evaluation. Medical evaluations for TB disease include a chest X-ray and physical examination to exclude TB disease, and must be done before beginning treatment for latent TB infection.

Signs and Symptoms of TB Disease in Children

Signs and symptoms of TB disease in children include:

- Cough;
- Feelings of sickness or weakness, lethargy, and/or reduced playfulness;
- Weight loss or failure to thrive;
- Fever; and/or
- Night sweats.

The most common form of TB disease occurs in the lungs, but TB disease can affect other parts of the body as well. Symptoms of TB disease in other parts of the body depend on the area affected. Infants, young children, and immunocompromised children (e.g., children with HIV) are at the highest risk of developing the most severe forms of TB such as TB meningitis or disseminated TB disease.

Treatment

A pediatric TB expert should be involved in the treatment of TB in children and in the management of infants, young children, and immunocompromised children who have been exposed to someone with infectious TB disease. It is very important that children or anyone being treated for latent TB infection or TB disease finish the medicine and take the drugs exactly as instructed.

Latent TB Infection

Treatment is recommended for children with latent TB infection to prevent them from developing TB disease. Infants, young children, and immunocompromised children with latent TB infection or children in close contact with someone with infectious TB disease, require special consideration because they are at increased risk for getting TB disease. Consultation with a pediatric TB expert is recommended before treatment begins. Isoniazid is the anti-TB medicine that is most commonly used for treatment of latent TB infection. In children, the recommended length of treatment with isoniazid is 9 months.

TB Disease

TB disease is treated by taking several anti-TB medicines for 6 to 9 months. It is important to note that if a child stops taking the drugs before completion, the child can become sick again. If drugs are not taken correctly, the bacteria that are still alive may become resistant to those drugs. TB that is resistant to drugs is harder and more expensive to treat, and treatment lasts much longer (up to 18 to 24 months).

Vaccines

BCG, or bacille Calmette-Guerin, is a vaccine to prevent TB disease. BCG is used in many countries to prevent childhood TB disease. However, the BCG vaccine is not generally used in the United States, because of the low risk of infection with TB bacteria and the variable effectiveness of the vaccine. The BCG vaccine should only be considered for very select persons who meet specific criteria and in consultation with a TB doctor.

Section 12.10

Whooping Cough (Pertussis)

This section contains text excerpted from the following sources: Text beginning with the heading "What Is Pertussis (Whooping Cough)?" is excerpted from "Pertussis (Whooping Cough) Vaccine," Vaccines.gov, U.S. Department of Health and Human Services (HHS), April 17, 2015; Text beginning with the heading "Can Pertussis Be Prevented with Vaccines?" is excerpted from "Pertussis Frequently Asked Questions," Centers for Disease Control and Prevention (CDC), August 31, 2015.

What Is Pertussis (Whooping Cough)?

Pertussis, a respiratory illness commonly known as whooping cough, is a very contagious disease caused by a type of bacteria. Pertussis is found only in humans and is spread from person-to-person. People with pertussis usually spread the disease by coughing or sneezing while in close contact with others, who then breathe in the pertussis bacteria.

Symptoms of pertussis usually develop within seven to ten days after being exposed, but sometimes not for as long as six weeks. Pertussis can cause severe coughing spells, vomiting, and disturbed sleep. It can lead to weight loss, incontinence, rib fractures, and passing out from violent coughing. Although you are often exhausted after a coughing fit, you usually appear fairly well in-between. Coughing fits generally become more common and severe as the illness continues, and can occur more often at night. The illness can be milder (less severe) and the typical "whoop" absent in children, teens, and adults who have been vaccinated. Since symptoms can vary and may look much like the common cold during the early stages of disease, children and adults may not know they have whooping cough and can end up spreading it to infants they are in close contact with.

Who Gets Pertussis (Whooping Cough)?

Everyone is at risk for pertussis, but it is most severe for babies, especially in the first months of life before pertussis immunizations begin; about half of infants younger than one year of age who get the disease are hospitalized. Of infants who are hospitalized with pertussis, one in four get pneumonia (lung infection), one or two in a hundred will have convulsions, and one or two in a hundred will die.

Up to five in 100 preteens, teens, and adults with pertussis are hospitalized. Of those patients, up to two in 100 are diagnosed with pneumonia. The most common complications in a study of adults with pertussis were:

- Weight loss (33%)
- Loss of bladder control (28%)
- Passing out (6%)
- Rib fractures from severe coughing (4%)

It is especially important for women to get Tdap in the third trimester of every pregnancy so that they can create antibodies and pass this protection to their babies before birth. These antibodies help protect newborns right after birth and until babies are old enough to get their own DTaP vaccine at two months of age.

Getting vaccinated with DTaP or Tdap (depending on your age) is also important for anyone who is around infants. Remember that even fully-vaccinated children and adults can get pertussis. If you are caring for infants, check with your healthcare provider about what's best for your situation.

Early symptoms can last for one to two weeks and usually include:

- Runny nose
- Low-grade fever (generally minimal throughout the course of the disease)
- Mild, occasional cough
- Apnea—a pause in breathing (in infants)

As the disease progresses, the traditional symptoms of pertussis may appear and include:

- Fits (paroxysms) of many, rapid coughs followed by a high-pitched "whoop"
- Vomiting (throwing up)
- Exhaustion (very tired) after coughing fits

The coughing fits can go on for up to ten weeks or more.

How Contagious Is Pertussis?

Pertussis spreads easily from person to person through coughing and sneezing. A person with pertussis can infect up to 12 to 15 other people. That's why being up-to-date with pertussis vaccines and practicing good cough and sneeze etiquette are so important.

Many babies who get pertussis are infected by older siblings, parents or caregivers who might not know they have the disease. If pertussis is circulating in the community, there's a chance that even a fully vaccinated person of any age can catch this very contagious disease. But if you've been vaccinated, your infection is usually less serious.

If you or your child develops a cold that includes a very bad cough or a cough that lasts a long time, it may be pertussis. The best way to know is to contact your doctor.

Can Pertussis Be Prevented with Vaccines?

Yes. Pertussis, or whooping cough, can be prevented with vaccines. Before pertussis vaccines became widely available in the 1940s, about 200,000 children got sick with it each year in the United States and about 9,000 died as a result of the infection. Now we see about 10,000 to 40,000 cases reported each year and unfortunately up to 20 deaths.

Pertussis vaccines are recommended for people of all ages. Babies and children should get 5 doses of DTaP for maximum protection. A dose is given at 2, 4 and 6 months, at 15 through 18 months, and again at 4 through 6 years. A booster dose of Tdap is given to preteens at 11 or 12 years old.

Teens or adults who didn't get Tdap as a preteen should get one dose. Getting Tdap is especially important for pregnant women during the third trimester of each pregnancy. It's also important that those who care for babies are up-to-date with pertussis vaccination. You can get the Tdap booster dose no matter when you got your last regular tetanus booster shot (Td). Also, you need to get Tdap even if you were vaccinated as a child or have been sick with pertussis in the past.

Why Is the Focus on Protecting Babies from Pertussis?

Babies are at greatest risk for getting pertussis and then having serious complications from it, including death. About half of babies younger than 1 year old who get pertussis need care in the hospital, and 1 out of 100 babies who get treatment in the hospital die.

There are two strategies to protect babies until they're old enough to receive vaccines and build their own immunity against this disease.

First, vaccinate pregnant women with Tdap during each pregnancy, preferably between 27 through 36 weeks of pregnancy. By getting Tdap during pregnancy, mothers build antibodies that are transferred to the newborn, providing protection against pertussis in early life, before the baby can start getting DTaP vaccines at 2 months old. Tdap also helps protect mothers, making them less likely to transmit pertussis to their babies.

Second, make sure everyone around the baby is up-to-date with their pertussis vaccines. This includes parents, siblings, grandparents (including those 65 years and older), other family members, babysitters, etc. They should be up-to-date with the age-appropriate vaccine (DTaP or Tdap) at least two weeks before coming into close contact with the baby. Unless pregnant, only one dose of Tdap is recommended in a lifetime.

These two strategies should reduce infection in babies.

It's also critical that healthcare professionals are up-to-date with a one-time Tdap booster dose, especially those who care for babies.

If I've Had Whooping Cough, Do I Still Need a Pertussis Booster?

Yes. Getting sick with pertussis or getting pertussis vaccines doesn't provide lifelong protection, which means you can still get pertussis and pass it onto others, including babies.

Are Most Coughs Pertussis and Does Everyone with Pertussis "Whoop?"

There are a lot of causes behind a person's cough and not every cough is pertussis. In general, pertussis starts off with cold-like symptoms and maybe a mild cough or fever. But after 1 to 2 weeks, severe coughing can begin. Unlike the common cold, pertussis can become a series of coughing fits that continues for weeks. The best way to know if you have pertussis is to see your doctor, who can make a diagnosis and prescribe antibiotics if needed.

The name "whooping cough" comes from the sound people make gasping for air after a pertussis coughing fit. However, not everyone with pertussis will cough and many who cough will not "whoop."

Teens and adults, especially those who haven't been vaccinated, may have a prolonged cough that keeps them up at night. Those who do get the coughing fits say it's the worst cough of their lives. And the cough may last for weeks or months, causing major disruptions to daily life and complications like broken ribs and ruptured blood vessels.

Babies may not cough at all. Instead, they may have life-threatening pauses (apnea) in breathing or struggle to breathe. Any time someone is struggling to breathe, it is important to get them to a doctor right away.

Are Pertussis Bacteria Changing and Causing an Increase in Pertussis Cases?

CDC is evaluating potential causes of increasing rates of pertussis, including changes in disease-causing bacteria types ("strains"). Unlike a foodborne illness where one strain causes an outbreak, multiple types or strains of pertussis bacteria can be found causing disease at any given time, including during outbreaks. Research is underway to determine if any of the recent genetic changes to pertussis bacteria may be related to the increase in disease in the United States.

Chapter 13

Viral Infections

Chapter Contents

Section 13.1

Adenovirus Infections

This section includes text excerpted from "About Adenoviruses," Centers for Disease Control and Prevention (CDC), April 20, 2015.

What Are Adenovirus Infections?

Adenoviruses are common causes of respiratory illness, but most infections are not severe. They can cause cold-like symptoms, sore throat, bronchitis, pneumonia, diarrhea, and pink eye (conjunctivitis). You can get an adenovirus infection at any age, but infants and people with weakened immune systems are more likely than others to develop severe illness from adenoviruses.

Symptoms

Adenoviruses can cause a wide range of illnesses such as:

- Common cold
- Sore throat (pharyngitis)
- Bronchitis
- Pneumonia
- Diarrhea
- Pink eye (conjunctivitis)
- Fever
- Bladder inflammation or infection (cystitis)
- Inflammation of stomach and intestines (gastroenteritis)
- Neurologic disease

Adenoviruses rarely cause serious illness or death. However, infants and people with weakened immune systems, or existing respiratory or cardiac disease, are at higher risk of developing severe illness from an adenovirus infection.

Transmission

Adenoviruses are usually spread from an infected person to others through:

- close personal contact, such as touching or shaking hands
- the air by coughing and sneezing
- touching an object or surface with adenoviruses on it, then touching your mouth, nose, or eyes before washing your hands

Some adenoviruses can spread through an infected person's stool, for example, during diaper changing. Adenovirus can also spread through the water, such as swimming pools, but this is less common.

Sometimes the virus can be shed for months after a person recovers from an adenovirus infection. This "virus shedding" usually occurs without any symptoms, even though the person can still spread adenovirus to other people.

Prevention

There is currently no adenovirus vaccine available to the general public.

A vaccine against adenovirus types 4 and 7 was approved by the U.S. Food and Drug Administration (FDA) in March 2011, for U.S. military personnel only.

You can protect yourself and others from adenoviruses and other respiratory illnesses by following a few simple steps:

- Wash your hands often with soap and water.
- Cover your mouth and nose when coughing or sneezing.
- Avoid touching your eyes, nose, or mouth with unwashed hands.
- Avoid close contact with people who are sick.
- Stay home when you are sick.

Frequent hand washing is especially important in childcare settings and healthcare facilities.

Adenoviruses are resistant to many common disinfectant products and can remain infectious for long periods on surfaces, objects, and in water of swimming pools and small lakes. It is important to keep adequate levels of chlorine in swimming pools to prevent outbreaks of conjunctivitis caused by adenoviruses.

Treatment

There is no specific treatment for people with adenovirus infection. Most adenovirus infections are mild and may require only care to help relieve symptoms.

Section 13.2

Chickenpox (Varicella)

This section contains text excerpted from the following sources: Text beginning with the heading "What Is Chickenpox?" is excerpted from "Chickenpox," Vaccines.gov, U.S. Department of Health and Human Services (HHS), April 18, 2015; Text beginning with the heading "What Are the Symptoms of Chickenpox?" is excerpted from "Chickenpox and the Vaccine (Shot) to Prevent It," Centers for Disease Control and Prevention (CDC), November 10, 2014.

What Is Chickenpox?

Chickenpox is caused by varicella zoster virus. The main symptom of chickenpox is a rash that turns into itchy, fluid-filled blisters and spreads all over the body. Other typical symptoms that may begin to appear 1 to 2 days before the rash include high fever, tiredness, loss of appetite and headache.

Chickenpox is very contagious and spreads easily from infected people. It can spread from either a cough or a sneeze. It can also spread by contact with virus particles that come from the blisters on the skin, either by touching them or by breathing in virus particles.

A person with chickenpox is contagious 1 to 2 days before the rash appears until all blisters have formed scabs. It takes from 10 to 21 days after exposure for someone to develop chickenpox.

Chickenpox is usually mild, but it can lead to complications, such as severe skin infection, bone and joint infections, dehydration, pneumonia, brain damage, or death. It is not possible to predict who will have a mild case of chickenpox and who will have a serious or even deadly case of disease.

After a person recovers from chickenpox, the virus stays in the body and can reactivate years later to cause a painful condition called shingles.

Who Gets Chickenpox?

Anyone who is not immune from either previous chickenpox virus infection or from vaccination can get chickenpox. Certain groups of people are more likely to have more severe illness with serious complications. These include adults, infants, adolescents, and people whose immune systems have been weakened because of illness or medications.

Chickenpox used to be very common in the United States. About 4 million people would get the disease each year. Also, about 10,600 people were hospitalized and 100 to 150 died each year because of chickenpox.

Thanks to vaccination, serious cases and deaths from chickenpox have declined dramatically. Since the United States started using the vaccine in 1996, the number of hospitalizations decreased by 84% and deaths from chickenpox have gone down more than 90%.

What Are the Symptoms of Chickenpox?

Chickenpox usually causes the following symptoms:

- An itchy rash of blisters
- Fever
- Headache
- Feeling tired

Is It Serious?

Chickenpox is usually mild in children, but the itching can be very uncomfortable. Children with chickenpox can miss up to one week of school or childcare.

Before the vaccine was available, about 4 million people got chickenpox each year in the United States. About 10,600 of those people were hospitalized, and 100 to 150 died each year.

In some cases, chickenpox can cause serious problems, such as:

- Skin infections
- Dehydration (not having enough water in the body)

- Pneumonia (an infection in the lungs)
- Swelling of the brain

How Does Chickenpox Spread?

Chickenpox spreads easily through the air when a person who has chickenpox coughs or sneezes. It can also spread by touching an infected person's blisters. Chickenpox can be spread 1 to 2 days before the infected person gets a rash until all the blisters have formed scabs.

Why Not Let My Child Get Chickenpox Naturally and Build Natural Immunity?

Chickenpox can be a mild disease, but it isn't always. There's no way to know who will have a mild case and who will become very sick. When your child gets his or her chickenpox shots, he or she is getting immunity from chickenpox without the risk of serious complications of the disease.

Why Should My Child Get the Chickenpox Shot?

The chickenpox shot:

- Protects your child from chickenpox, a potentially serious and even deadly disease
- Prevents your child from feeling itchy and uncomfortable from chickenpox
- Keeps your child from missing school or childcare (and keeps you from missing work to care for your sick child)

Is the Chickenpox Shot Safe?

Yes. The chickenpox shot is very safe, and it works very well to prevent chickenpox. Vaccines, like any medicine, can have side effects, but most children who get the chickenpox shot have no side effects.

What Are the Side Effects?

Most children don't have any side effects from the shot. However, some children may develop a reaction and symptoms may include:

- Soreness, redness, or swelling where the shot was given

- Fever
- Mild rash

There are two types of chickenpox shots. Talk to your child's doctor about which one your child will get.

Section 13.3

Chikungunya

This section includes text excerpted from "Chikungunya Virus," Centers for Disease Control and Prevention (CDC), August 3, 2015.

What Is Chikungunya?

Chikungunya virus is transmitted to people by mosquitoes. The most common symptoms of chikungunya virus infection are fever and joint pain. Other symptoms may include headache, muscle pain, joint swelling, or rash. Outbreaks have occurred in countries in Africa, Asia, Europe, and the Indian and Pacific Oceans. In late 2013, chikungunya virus was found for the first time in the Americas on islands in the Caribbean. There is a risk that the virus will be imported to new areas by infected travelers. There is no vaccine to prevent or medicine to treat chikungunya virus infection. Travelers can protect themselves by preventing mosquito bites. When traveling to countries with chikungunya virus, use insect repellent, wear long sleeves and pants, and stay in places with air conditioning or that use window and door screens.

Prevention

- No vaccine exists to prevent chikungunya virus infection or disease.
- Prevent chikungunya virus infection by avoiding mosquito bites (see below). The mosquitoes that spread the chikungunya virus bite mostly during the daytime.

Protect Yourself from Mosquito Bites

- Use air conditioning or window/door screens to keep mosquitoes outside. If you are not able to protect yourself from mosquitoes inside your home or hotel, sleep under a mosquito bed net.
- Help reduce the number of mosquitoes outside your home or hotel room by emptying standing water from containers such as flowerpots or buckets.
- When weather permits, wear long-sleeved shirts and long pants.
- Use insect repellents

Transmission

Through Mosquito Bites

- Chikungunya virus is transmitted to people through mosquito bites. Mosquitoes become infected when they feed on a person already infected with the virus. Infected mosquitoes can then spread the virus to other people through bites.
- Chikungunya virus is most often spread to people by *Aedes aegypti* and *Aedes albopictus* mosquitoes. These are the same mosquitoes that transmit dengue virus. They bite during the day and at night.

Rarely, from Mother to Child

- Chikungunya virus is transmitted rarely from mother to newborn around the time of birth.
- To date, no infants have been found to be infected with chikungunya virus through breastfeeding. Because of the benefits of breastfeeding, mothers are encouraged to breastfeed even in areas where chikungunya virus is circulating.

Rarely, through Infected Blood

- In theory, the virus could be spread through a blood transfusion. To date, there are no known reports of this happening.

Symptoms

- Most people infected with chikungunya virus will develop some symptoms.

- Symptoms usually begin 3–7 days after being bitten by an infected mosquito.
- The most common symptoms are fever and joint pain.
- Other symptoms may include headache, muscle pain, joint swelling, or rash.
- Chikungunya disease does not often result in death, but the symptoms can be severe and disabling.
- Most patients feel better within a week. In some people, the joint pain may persist for months.
- People at risk for more severe disease include newborns infected around the time of birth, older adults (≥65 years), and people with medical conditions such as high blood pressure, diabetes, or heart disease.
- Once a person has been infected, he or she is likely to be protected from future infections.

Diagnosis

- The symptoms of chikungunya are similar to those of dengue and Zika, diseases spread by the same mosquitoes that transmit chikungunya.
- See your healthcare provider if you develop the symptoms described above and have visited an area where chikungunya is found.
- If you have recently traveled, tell your healthcare provider when and where you traveled.
- Your healthcare provider may order blood tests to look for chikungunya or other similar viruses like dengue and Zika.

Treatment

- There is no vaccine to prevent or medicine to treat chikungunya virus.
- Treat the symptoms:
    - Get plenty of rest.
    - Drink fluids to prevent dehydration.

    - Take medicine such as acetaminophen (Tylenol®) or paracetamol to reduce fever and pain.
    - Do not take aspirin and other non-steroidal anti-inflammatory drugs (nonsteroidal anti-inflammatory drugs (NSAIDS) until dengue can be ruled out to reduce the risk of bleeding).
    - If you are taking medicine for another medical condition, talk to your healthcare provider before taking additional medication.
- If you have chikungunya, prevent mosquito bites for the first week of your illness.
- During the first week of infection, chikungunya virus can be found in the blood and passed from an infected person to a mosquito through mosquito bites.
- An infected mosquito can then spread the virus to other people.

Section 13.4

Common Cold

This section contains text excerpted from the following sources: Text beginning with the heading "Protect Yourself and Others from Common Colds" is excerpted from "Common Colds: Protect Yourself and Others," Centers for Disease Control and Prevention (CDC), February 8, 2016; Text beginning with the heading "Diagnosis and Treatment" is excerpted from "Common Cold and Runny Nose," Centers for Disease Control and Prevention (CDC), March 16, 2016.

What Are Common Colds?

Sore throat and runny nose are usually the first signs of a cold, followed by coughing and sneezing. Most people recover in 7–10 days or so. You can help reduce your risk of getting a cold by washing your hands often and avoid touching your face with unwashed hands.

Common colds are the main reason that children miss school and adults miss work. Each year in the United States, there are millions of cases of the common cold. Adults have an average of 2–3 colds per year, and children have even more.

Most people get colds in the winter and spring, but it is possible to get a cold any time of the year. Symptoms usually include sore throat, runny nose, coughing, sneezing, watery eyes, headaches and body aches. Most people recover within about 7–10 days. However, people with weakened immune systems, asthma, or respiratory conditions may develop serious illness, such as pneumonia.

Causes of the Common Cold

Many different viruses can cause the common cold, but rhinoviruses are the most common. Rhinoviruses can also trigger asthma attacks and have been linked to sinus and ear infections. Other viruses that can cause colds include respiratory syncytial virus, human parainfluenza viruses, and human metapneumovirus.

Viruses that cause colds can spread from infected people to others through the air and close personal contact. You can also get infected through contact with stool (poop) or respiratory secretions from an infected person. This can happen when you shake hands with someone who has a cold, or touch a doorknob that has viruses on it, then touch your eyes, mouth, or nose.

How to Protect Yourself and Others

You can help reduce your risk of getting a cold:

- **Wash your hands often with soap and water**

  Wash them for 20 seconds, and help young children do the same. If soap and water are not available, use an alcohol-based hand sanitizer. Viruses that cause colds can live on your hands, and regular hand washing can help protect you from getting sick.

- **Avoid touching your eyes, nose, and mouth with unwashed hands**

  Viruses that cause colds can enter your body this way and make you sick.

- **Stay away from people who are sick**

  Sick people can spread viruses that cause the common cold through close contact with others.

If you have a cold, you should follow these tips to prevent spreading it to other people:

- Stay at home while you are sick
- Avoid close contact with others, such as hugging, kissing, or shaking hands
- Move away from people before coughing or sneezing
- Cough and sneeze into a tissue then throw it away, or cough and sneeze into your upper shirt sleeve, completely covering your mouth and nose
- Wash your hands after coughing, sneezing, or blowing your nose
- Disinfect frequently touched surfaces, and objects such as toys and doorknobs

There is no vaccine to protect you against the common cold.

How to Feel Better

There is no cure for a cold. To feel better, you should get lots of rest and drink plenty of fluids. Over-the-counter medicines may help ease symptoms but will not make your cold go away any faster. Always read the label and use medications as directed. Talk to your doctor before giving your child nonprescription cold medicines, since some medicines contain ingredients that are not recommended for children.

Antibiotics will not help you recover from a cold. They do not work against viruses, and they may make it harder for your body to fight future bacterial infections if you take them unnecessarily.

Rest, over-the-counter medicines and other self-care methods may help you or your child feel better. Remember, always use over-the-counter products as directed. Many over-the-counter products are not recommended for children of certain ages.

When to See a Doctor

You should call your doctor if you or your child has one or more of these conditions:

- a temperature higher than 100.4° F
- symptoms that last more than 10 days
- symptoms that are severe or unusual

If your child is younger than 3 months of age and has a fever, you should always call your doctor right away. Your doctor can determine if you or your child has a cold and can recommend therapy to help with symptoms.

Diagnosis and Treatment

Antibiotics are not needed to treat a cold or runny nose, which almost always gets better on its own. Your healthcare professional will determine what type of illness you or your child has by asking about symptoms and doing a physical examination. Sometimes they will also swab the inside of your nose or mouth.

Since the common cold is caused by viruses, antibiotics will not help it get better and may even cause harm in both children and adults. Your healthcare professional can give you tips to help with symptoms like fever and coughing.

Prevention

There are steps you can take to help prevent getting a cold, including:

- Practice good hand hygiene
- Avoid close contact with people who have colds or other upper respiratory infections

Section 13.5

Croup

Text in this section is excerpted from "Croup," © 1995–2016. The Nemours Foundation/KidsHealth®. Reprinted with permission.

What Is Croup?

Croup is a condition that causes swelling and irritation of the upper airways—the voice box (larynx) and windpipe (trachea). It's caused by the same viruses that cause the common cold. Kids with croup have a "barky" cough or hoarseness, especially when crying.

Croup is most common in kids 6 months to 3 years old, but some older children also get croup. Most cases happen in the fall and early winter.

There are two types of croup: viral croup and spasmodic croup. Both types cause a barking cough.

- **Viral croup** always includes other signs of a cold, such as a runny nose, fever, and fatigue. The virus goes away within 3 to 7 days after it began.
- **Spasmodic croup** may happen in a child with a mild cold. The barking cough usually begins at night and isn't accompanied by fever. Spasmodic croup has a tendency to come back again.

Most cases of croup are mild and can be treated at home. Rarely, croup can be severe and even life-threatening.

Signs and Symptoms

At first, a child may have cold symptoms, like a stuffy or runny nose and a fever. As the upper airways become inflamed and swollen, the child may become hoarse, with a harsh, barking cough. This loud cough often sounds like a seal barking.

If the upper airway continues to swell, it becomes hard for a child to breathe. The child may make a high-pitched or squeaking noise while breathing in—this is called stridor. A child also might breathe very fast or have retractions (when the skin between the ribs pulls in during breathing). In the most serious cases, a child may appear pale or have a bluish color around the mouth due to a lack of oxygen.

Symptoms of croup are often worse at night and when a child is upset or crying.

Diagnosis

Doctors usually diagnose croup by listening for the telltale barking cough and stridor. They will also ask questions, for example whether your child has had any recent illnesses with a fever, runny nose, and congestion, and if your child has a history of croup or upper airway problems.

If the child's croup is severe and slow to get better after treatment, the child may be sent to an emergency room (ER). A neck X-ray may be done to rule out other reasons for the breathing problems, such as:

- an object stuck in the throat
- a peritonsillar abscess (collection of pus at the back of the mouth)
- epiglottitis (swelling of the epiglottis, the flap of tissue that covers the windpipe)

An X-ray of a child with croup usually will show the top of the airway narrowing to a point, which doctors call a "steeple sign."

Treatment

Most cases of viral croup are mild and can be treated at home. Breathing in moist air may help kids feel better, and pain medicine (ibuprofen or acetaminophen) may make them more comfortable. Kids should drink plenty of fluids to prevent dehydration, and rest often.

The best way to expose a child to moist air is to use a cool-mist humidifier or run a hot shower to create a steam-filled bathroom where the child can sit with an adult for 10 minutes. Breathing in the mist will sometimes stop a child from severe coughing. In the cooler weather, taking the child outside for a few minutes to breath in the cool air may ease symptoms. You also can try taking your child for a drive with the car windows slightly lowered.

In certain kids, doctors will prescribe steroids to decrease airway swelling. For severe cases, kids will be put on a breathing treatment that contains a medicine called epinephrine. This medicine quickly reduces swelling in the airways. Sometimes kids with croup will need to stay in a hospital until they're breathing better.

When to Call the Doctor

Most kids recover from croup with no additional problems. But some kids, especially those who were born premature, or have asthma or other lung diseases, may have a higher chance of developing complications from croup.

Call your doctor or get immediate medical attention if your child has:

- trouble breathing, including rapid or labored breathing
- retractions, when the skin between the ribs pulls in with each breath
- stridor, high-pitched or squeaking noise when inhaling
- a pale or bluish color around the mouth

- drooling or difficulty swallowing
- is very tired or sleepy, difficult to wake
- dehydration (signs include a dry or sticky mouth, few or no tears, sunken eyes, thirst, no urine or only a little dark yellow urine for 8 to 12 hours)

Section 13.6

Fifth Disease

This section includes text excerpted from "Parvovirus B19 and Fifth Disease," Centers for Disease Control and Prevention (CDC), November 2, 2015.

What Is Fifth Disease?

Fifth disease is a mild rash illness caused by parvovirus B19. This disease, also called erythema infectiosum, got its name because it was fifth in a list of historical classifications of common skin rash illnesses in children. It is more common in children than adults. A person usually gets sick with fifth disease within 4 to 14 days after getting infected with parvovirus B19.

Signs and Symptoms

The first symptoms of fifth disease are usually mild and may include:

- fever,
- runny nose, and
- headache.

Then you can get a rash on your face and body

After several days, you may get a red rash on your face called "slapped cheek" rash. This rash is the most recognized feature of fifth disease. It is more common in children than adults.

Some people may get a second rash a few days later on their chest, back, buttocks, or arms and legs. The rash may be itchy, especially on the soles of the feet. It can vary in intensity and usually goes away in 7 to 10 days, but it can come and go for several weeks. As it starts to go away, it may look lacy.

You may also have painful or swollen joints

People with fifth disease can also develop pain and swelling in their joints (polyarthropathy syndrome). This is more common in adults, especially women. Some adults with fifth disease may only have painful joints, usually in the hands, feet, or knees, and no other symptoms. The joint pain usually lasts 1 to 3 weeks, but it can last for months or longer. It usually goes away without any long-term problems.

Transmission

Parvovirus B19—which causes fifth disease—spreads through respiratory secretions (such as saliva, sputum, or nasal mucus) when an infected person coughs or sneezes. You are most contagious when it seems like you have "just a cold" and before you get the rash or joint pain and swelling. After you get the rash you are not likely to be contagious, so then it is usually safe for you or your child to go back to work or school.

People with fifth disease who have weakened immune systems may be contagious for a longer amount of time.

Parvovirus B19 can also spread through blood or blood products. A pregnant woman who is infected with parvovirus B19 can pass the virus to her baby.

Once you recover from fifth disease, you develop immunity that generally protects you from parvovirus B19 infection in the future.

Diagnosis

Healthcare providers can often diagnose fifth disease just by seeing "slapped cheek" rash on a patient's face. A blood test can also be done to determine if you are susceptible or immune to parvovirus B19 infection or if you were recently infected. The blood test may be particularly helpful for pregnant women who may have been exposed to parvovirus B19 and are suspected to have fifth disease.

Prevention

There is no vaccine or medicine that can prevent parvovirus B19 infection. You can reduce your chance of being infected or infecting others by:

- washing your hands often with soap and water

- covering your mouth and nose when you cough or sneeze
- not touching your eyes, nose, or mouth
- avoiding close contact with people who are sick
- staying home when you are sick

After you get the rash, you are probably not contagious. So it is usually then safe for you to go back to work or for your child to return to school or a child care center.

Healthcare providers who are pregnant should know about potential risks to their baby and discuss this with their doctor.

All healthcare providers and patients should follow strict infection control practices to prevent parvovirus B19 from spreading.

Treatment

Fifth disease is usually mild and will go away on its own. Children and adults who are otherwise healthy usually recover completely. Treatment usually involves relieving symptoms, such as fever, itching, and joint pain and swelling.

People who have complications from fifth disease should see their healthcare provider for medical treatment.

Section 13.7

Hand, Foot, and Mouth Disease

This section includes text excerpted from "Hand, Foot, and Mouth Disease (HFMD)," Centers for Disease Control and Prevention (CDC), August 18, 2015.

What Is a Hand, Foot, and Mouth Disease?

Hand, foot, and mouth disease is a common viral illness that usually affects infants and children younger than 5 years old. However, it can sometimes occur in adults. Symptoms of hand, foot, and mouth disease include fever, mouth sores, and a skin rash.

Signs and Symptoms

Hand, foot, and mouth disease is a common viral illness that usually affects infants and children younger than 5 years old. However, it can sometimes occur in adults. It usually starts with a fever, reduced appetite, sore throat, and a feeling of being unwell (malaise). One or two days after the fever starts, painful sores can develop in the mouth (herpangina). They begin, often in the back of the mouth, as small red spots that blister and can become ulcers. A skin rash with red spots, and sometimes with blisters, may also develop over one or two days on the palms of the hands and soles of the feet; it may also appear on the knees, elbows, buttocks or genital area.

Some people, especially young children, may get dehydrated if they are not able to swallow enough liquids because of painful mouth sores.

Not everyone will get all of these symptoms. Some people, especially adults, may show no symptoms at all, but they can still pass the virus to others.

Complications

Health complications from hand, foot, and mouth disease are not common.

- Viral or "aseptic" meningitis can occur with hand, foot, and mouth disease, but it is rare. It causes fever, headache, stiff neck, or back pain and may require the infected person to be hospitalized for a few days.
- Encephalitis (inflammation of the brain) or polio-like paralysis can occur, but this is even rarer.
- Fingernail and toenail loss have been reported, occurring mostly in children within a few weeks after having hand, foot, and mouth disease. At this time, it is not known whether nail loss was a result of the disease in reported cases. However, in the reports reviewed, the nail loss was temporary, and the nail grew back without medical treatment.

Causes

Hand, foot, and mouth disease is caused by viruses that belong to the Enterovirus genus (group), including polioviruses, coxsackieviruses, echoviruses, and enteroviruses.

- Coxsackievirus A16 is the most common cause of hand, foot, and mouth disease in the United States, but other coxsackieviruses can also cause the illness.
- Enterovirus 71 has also been associated with cases and outbreaks of hand, foot, and mouth disease. Less often, enterovirus 71 has been associated with severe disease, such as encephalitis.

Transmission

The viruses that cause hand, foot, and mouth disease can be found in an infected person's:

- nose and throat secretions (such as saliva, sputum, or nasal mucus),
- blister fluid, and
- feces (stool).

An infected person may spread the viruses that cause hand, foot, and mouth disease to another person through:

- close personal contact,
- the air (through coughing or sneezing),
- contact with feces,
- contact with contaminated objects and surfaces.

For example, you might get infected by kissing someone who has hand, foot, and mouth disease or by touching a doorknob that has viruses on it then touching your eyes, mouth or nose.

It is possible to get infected with the viruses that cause hand, foot, and mouth disease if you swallow recreational water, such as water in swimming pools. However, this is not very common. This is more likely to happen if the water becomes contaminated with feces from a person who has hand, foot, and mouth disease and is not properly treated with chlorine.

Generally, a person with hand, foot, and mouth disease is most contagious during the first week of illness. People can sometimes be contagious for days or weeks after symptoms go away. Some people, especially adults, may not develop any symptoms, but they can still spread the virus to others. This is why people should always try to maintain good hygiene (e.g., handwashing) so they can minimize their chance of spreading or getting infections.

You should stay home while you are sick with hand, foot, and mouth disease. Talk with your healthcare provider if you are not sure when you should return to work or school. The same applies to children returning to daycare.

Hand, foot, and mouth disease is not transmitted to or from pets or other animals.

Diagnosis

Hand, foot, and mouth disease is one of many infections that cause mouth sores. Healthcare providers can usually identify mouth sores caused by hand, foot, and mouth disease by considering:

- how old the patient is,
- what symptoms the patient has, and
- how the rash and mouth sores look.

Depending on how severe the symptoms are, samples from the throat or feces (stool) may be collected and sent to a laboratory to test for the virus.

Prevention

There is no vaccine to protect against the viruses that cause hand, foot, and mouth disease.

A person can lower their risk of being infected by:

- Washing hands often with soap and water, especially after changing diapers and using the toilet.
- Cleaning and disinfecting frequently touched surfaces and soiled items, including toys.
- Avoiding close contact such as kissing, hugging, or sharing eating utensils or cups with people with hand, foot, and mouth disease.

If a person has mouth sores, it might be painful to swallow. However, it is important for people with hand, foot, and mouth disease to drink enough liquids to prevent dehydration (loss of body fluids). If a person cannot swallow enough liquids, they may need to receive them through an Intravenous (IV) in their vein.

Treatment

There is no specific treatment for hand, foot, and mouth disease. However, some things can be done to relieve symptoms, such as:

- Taking over-the-counter medications to relieve pain and fever (Caution: Aspirin should not be given to children.)
- Using mouthwashes or sprays that numb mouth pain

People who are concerned about their symptoms should contact their healthcare provider.

Section 13.8

Infectious Mononucleosis

This section includes text excerpted from "Epstein-Barr Virus and Infectious Mononucleosis," Centers for Disease Control and Prevention (CDC), September 14, 2016.

What Is Infectious Mononucleosis?

Infectious mononucleosis, also called "mono," is a contagious disease. Epstein-Barr virus (EBV) is the most common cause of infectious mononucleosis, but other viruses can also cause this disease. It is common among teenagers and young adults, especially college students. At least 25% of teenagers and young adults who get infected with EBV will develop infectious mononucleosis.

Symptoms

Typical symptoms of infectious mononucleosis usually appear 4 to 6 weeks after you get infected with EBV. Symptoms may develop slowly and may not all occur at the same time.

These symptoms include:

- extreme fatigue
- fever

- sore throat
- head and body aches
- swollen lymph nodes in the neck and armpits
- swollen liver or spleen or both
- rash

Enlarged spleen and a swollen liver are less common symptoms. For some people, their liver or spleen or both may remain enlarged even after their fatigue ends.

Most people get better in 2 to 4 weeks; however, some people may feel fatigued for several more weeks. Occasionally, the symptoms of infectious mononucleosis can last for 6 months or longer.

Transmission

EBV is the most common cause of infectious mononucleosis, but other viruses can cause this disease. Typically, these viruses spread most commonly through bodily fluids, especially saliva. However, these viruses can also spread through blood and semen during sexual contact, blood transfusions, and organ transplantations.

Prevention and Treatment

There is no vaccine to protect against infectious mononucleosis. You can help protect yourself by not kissing or sharing drinks, food, or personal items, like toothbrushes, with people who have infectious mononucleosis.

You can help relieve symptoms of infectious mononucleosis by:

- drinking fluids to stay hydrated
- getting plenty of rest
- taking over-the-counter medications for pain and fever

If you have infectious mononucleosis, you should not take ampicillin or amoxicillin. Based on the severity of the symptoms, a healthcare provider may recommend treatment of specific organ systems affected by infectious mononucleosis.

Because your spleen may become enlarged as a result of infectious mononucleosis, you should avoid contact sports until you fully recover. Participating in contact sports can be strenuous and may cause the spleen to rupture.

Diagnosing Infectious Mononucleosis

Healthcare providers typically diagnose infectious mononucleosis based on symptoms.

Laboratory tests are not usually needed to diagnose infectious mononucleosis. However, specific antibody tests may be needed to identify the cause of illness in people who do not have a typical case of infectious mononucleosis.

The blood work of patients who have infectious mononucleosis due to EBV infection may show:

- more white blood cells (lymphocytes) than normal
- unusual looking white blood cells (atypical lymphocytes)
- fewer than normal neutrophils or platelets
- abnormal liver function

Section 13.9

Influenza

This section contains text excerpted from the following sources: Text beginning with the heading "Influenza Symptoms" is excerpted from "Flu Symptoms and Complications," Centers for Disease Control and Prevention (CDC), May 23, 2016; Text beginning with the heading "Influenza Is Dangerous for Children" is excerpted from "Children, the Flu, and the Flu Vaccine," Centers for Disease Control and Prevention (CDC), August 5, 2016.

What Is Influenza?

Influenza (also known as the flu) is a contagious respiratory illness caused by flu viruses. It can cause mild to severe illness, and at times can lead to death. The flu is different from a cold. The flu usually comes on suddenly. People who have the flu often feel some or all of these symptoms:

- Fever or feeling feverish/chills
- Cough

- Sore throat
- Runny or stuffy nose
- Muscle or body aches
- Headaches
- Fatigue (tiredness)
- Some people may have vomiting and diarrhea, though this is more common in children than adults.

Flu Complications

Most people who get influenza will recover in several days to less than two weeks, but some people will develop complications as a result of the flu. A wide range of complications can be caused by influenza virus infection of the upper respiratory tract (nasal passages, throat) and lower respiratory tract (lungs). While anyone can get sick with flu and become severely ill, some people are more likely to experience severe flu illness. Young children, adults aged 65 years and older, pregnant women, and people with certain chronic medical conditions are among those groups of people who are at high risk of serious flu complications, possibly requiring hospitalization and sometimes resulting in death. For example, people with chronic lung disease are at higher risk of developing severe pneumonia.

Sinus and ear infections are examples of moderate complications from flu, while pneumonia is a serious flu complication that can result from either influenza virus infection alone or from co-infection of flu virus and bacteria. Other possible serious complications triggered by flu can include inflammation of the heart (myocarditis), brain (encephalitis) or muscle (myositis, rhabdomyolysis) tissues, and multi-organ failure (for example, respiratory and kidney failure). Flu virus infection of the respiratory tract can trigger an extreme inflammatory response in the body and can lead to sepsis, the body's life-threatening response to infection. Flu also can make chronic medical problems worse. For example, people with asthma may experience asthma attacks while they have the flu, and people with chronic heart disease may experience a worsening of this condition triggered by flu.

Influenza Is Dangerous for Children

Influenza ("the flu") is more dangerous than the common cold for children. Each year, many children get sick with seasonal influenza; some of those illnesses result in death.

- Children commonly need medical care because of influenza, especially before they turn 5 years old.
- Severe influenza complications are most common in children younger than 2 years old.
- Children with chronic health problems like asthma, diabetes and disorders of the brain or nervous system are at especially high risk of developing serious flu complications.
- Each year an average of 20,000 children under the age of 5 are hospitalized because of influenza complications.
- Flu seasons vary in severity, however some children die from flu each year. Since 2004–2005, flu-related deaths in children reported to Centers for Disease Control and Prevention (CDC) during regular flu seasons have ranged from 37 deaths to 171 deaths.

The Single Best Way to Protect Your Children from the Flu Is to Get Them Vaccinated Each Year

The seasonal flu vaccine protects against the influenza viruses that research indicates will be most common during the upcoming season. Traditional flu vaccines (called "trivalent" vaccines) are made to protect against three flu viruses; an influenza A (H1N1) virus, an influenza A (H3N2) virus, and an influenza B virus. In addition, there are flu vaccines made to protect against four flu viruses (called "quadrivalent" vaccines). These vaccines protect against the same three viruses as the trivalent vaccine and an additional B virus.

What Kinds of Flu Vaccines Are Available for Children?

Different products are approved for different age groups, including children as young as 6 months of age.

Note that while there is a quadrivalent nasal spray vaccine that is FDA approved for the U.S. market, Advisory Committee on Immunization Practices (ACIP) and CDC recommend that nasal spray vaccine not be used during the 2016–2017 season because of concerns about how well it works.

Your child's healthcare provider will know which vaccines are right for your child.

- CDC recommends that everyone 6 months of age and older get a seasonal flu vaccine.

Keep in mind that vaccination is especially important for certain people who are high risk or who are in close contact with high risk persons. This includes children at high risk for developing complications from influenza illness, and adults who are close contacts of those children.

There Are Special Vaccination Instructions for Children Aged 6 Months through 8 Years of Age

Some children 6 months through 8 years of age require two doses of influenza vaccine. Children 6 months through 8 years getting vaccinated for the first time, and those who have only previously gotten one dose of vaccine, should get two doses of vaccine this season. All children who have previously gotten two doses of vaccine (at any time) only need one dose of vaccine this season. The first dose should be given as soon as vaccine becomes available.

The second dose should be given at least 28 days after the first dose. The first dose "primes" the immune system; the second dose provides immune protection. Children who only get one dose but need two doses can have reduced or no protection from a single dose of flu vaccine.

If your child needs the two doses, begin the process early. This will ensure that your child is protected before influenza starts circulating in your community.

Be sure to get your child a second dose if he or she needs one. It usually takes about two weeks after the second dose for protection to begin.

Some Children Are at Especially High Risk

Children at greatest risk of serious flu-related complications include the following:

1. **Children younger than 6 months old**

   These children are too young to be vaccinated. The best way to protect them is to make sure people around them are vaccinated.

2. **Children aged 6 months up to their 5th birthday**

   It is estimated that each year in the United States, there are more than 20,000 children younger than 5 years old who are hospitalized due to flu. Even children in this age group who are otherwise healthy are at risk simply because of their age.

In addition, children 2 years of age up to their 5th birthday are more likely than healthy older children to be taken to a doctor, an urgent care center, or the emergency room because of flu. To protect their health, all children 6 months and older should be vaccinated against the flu each year. Vaccinating young children, their families, and other caregivers can also help protect them from getting sick.

3. **American Indian and Alaskan Native children**

   These children are more likely to have severe flu illness that results in hospitalization or death.

4. **Children aged 6 months through 18 years with chronic health problems, including:**

   - Asthma
   - Neurological and neurodevelopmental conditions [including disorders of the brain, spinal cord, peripheral nerve, and muscle such as cerebral palsy, epilepsy (seizure disorders), stroke, intellectual disability (mental retardation), moderate to severe developmental delay, muscular dystrophy, or spinal cord injury].
   - Chronic lung disease (such as chronic obstructive pulmonary disease [COPD] and cystic fibrosis)
   - Heart disease (such as congenital heart disease, congestive heart failure and coronary artery disease)
   - Blood disorders (such as sickle cell disease)
   - Endocrine disorders (such as diabetes mellitus)
   - Kidney disorders
   - Liver disorders
   - Metabolic disorders (such as inherited metabolic disorders and mitochondrial disorders)
   - Weakened immune system due to disease or medication (such as people with human immunodeficiency virus (HIV) or acquired immune deficiency syndrome (AIDS), or cancer, or those on chronic steroids); and
   - Children who are receiving long-term aspirin therapy

Section 13.10

Measles

This section contains text excerpted from the following sources: Text under the heading "Top Four Things Parents Need to Know about Measles" is excerpted from "Measles (Rubeola)," Centers for Disease Control and Prevention (CDC), February 20, 2015; Text beginning with the heading "Protect your Child with Measles Vaccine" is excerpted from "Measles: Make Sure Your Child Is Fully Immunized," Centers for Disease Control and Prevention (CDC), April 21, 2016.

Top Four Things to Know about Measles

You may be hearing a lot about measles lately, and all of this news on TV, social media, Internet, newspapers and magazines may leave you wondering what you as a parent really need to know about this disease. Centers for Disease Control and Prevention (CDC) has put together a list of the most important facts about measles for parents like you.

1. Measles Can Be Serious

Some people think of measles as just a little rash and fever that clears up in a few days, but measles can cause serious health complications, especially in children younger than 5 years of age. There is no way to tell in advance the severity of the symptoms your child will experience.

- About 1 in 4 people in the United States who get measles will be hospitalized
- 1 out of every 1,000 people with measles will develop brain swelling, which could lead to brain damage
- 1 or 2 out of 1,000 people with measles will die, even with the best care

Some of the more common measles symptoms include:

- Fever
- Rash

- Runny nose
- Red eyes

2. Measles Is Very Contagious

Measles spreads through the air when an infected person coughs or sneezes. It is so contagious that if one person has it, 9 out of 10 people around him or her will also become infected if they are not protected. Your child can get measles just by being in a room where a person with measles has been, even up to two hours after that person has left. An infected person can spread measles to others even before knowing he/she has the disease—from four days before developing the measles rash through four days afterward.

3.Your Child Can Still Get Measles in United States

Measles was declared eliminated from the United States in 2000 thanks to a highly effective vaccination program. Eliminated means that the disease is no longer constantly present in this country. However, measles is still common in many parts of the world, including some countries in Europe, Asia, the Pacific, and Africa. Worldwide, an estimated 20 million people get measles and 146,000 people, mostly children, die from the disease each year.

Even if your family does not travel internationally, you could come into contact with measles anywhere in your community. Every year, measles is brought into the United States by unvaccinated travelers (Americans or foreign visitors) who get measles while they are in other countries. Anyone who is not protected against measles is at risk.

4. You Have the Power to Protect Your Child against Measles with a Safe and Effective Vaccine

The best protection against measles is measles-mumps-rubella (MMR) vaccine. MMR vaccine provides long-lasting protection against all strains of measles. Your child needs two doses of MMR vaccine for best protection:

- The first dose at 12 through 15 months of age
- The second dose 4 through 6 years of age

If your family is traveling overseas, the vaccine recommendations are a little different:

- If your baby is 6 through 11 months old, he or she should receive 1 dose of MMR vaccine before leaving.
- If your child is 12 months of age or older, he or she will need 2 doses of MMR vaccine (separated by at least 28 days) before departure.

Protect your Child with Measles Vaccine

You can protect your child against measles with a combination vaccine that provides protection against three diseases: measles, mumps, and rubella (MMR). The MMR vaccine is proven to be very safe and effective. CDC recommends that children get two doses:

- the first dose at 12 through 15 months of age, and
- the second dose before entering school at 4 through 6 years of age.

Your child's doctor may offer the measles, mumps, rubella and varicella (MMRV) vaccine, which protects against measles, mumps, rubella, and varicella (chickenpox). MMRV vaccine is licensed for children 12 months through 12 years of age. It may be used in place of MMR vaccine if a child needs to have varicella vaccine in addition to measles, mumps, and rubella vaccines. Your child's doctor can help you decide which vaccine to use.

Section 13.11

Mumps

This section contains text excerpted from the following sources: Text beginning with the heading "What Is Mumps?" is excerpted from "Mumps," Vaccines.gov, U.S. Department of Health and Human Services (HHS), April 20, 2015; Text beginning with the heading "What Are the Symptoms of Mumps?" is excerpted from "Mumps and the Vaccine (Shot) to Prevent It," Centers for Disease Control and Prevention (CDC), November 10, 2014.

What Is Mumps?

Mumps is a contagious disease that is caused by the mumps virus. Most people with mumps will have swelling of their salivary glands, which causes the puffy cheeks and a tender, swollen jaw. Other symptoms may include fever, headache, muscle aches, tiredness, and loss of appetite. Symptoms usually appear about 16 to 18 days after being exposed to someone who was contagious.

Mumps virus spreads in the air from an infected person's cough or sneeze. A child also can get infected with mumps by coming in contact with an object, like a toy, that has mumps virus on it. An infected person is most likely to spread mumps one to two days before symptoms of swollen glands appear. Infected people can spread mumps for up to five days after symptoms appear.

Complications can occur and might be more severe in teenagers and adults. Mumps can cause inflammation of the brain (encephalitis), inflammation of the tissue covering the brain and spinal cord (meningitis), deafness, inflammation of the testicles (called orchitis), inflammation of the ovaries (oophoritis), and, in rare cases, death.

About one out of three people with mumps may have no symptoms, or symptoms may be very mild.

Who Gets Mumps?

Anyone who is not immune from either previous mumps infection or from vaccination can get mumps.

Before the routine vaccination program was introduced in the United States, mumps was a common illness in infants, children, and young adults. Because most people have now been vaccinated, mumps has become a rare disease in the United States.

Mumps outbreaks can still occur in highly vaccinated U.S. communities, particularly in close-contact settings such as schools, colleges, and camps. However, high vaccination coverage helps to limit the size, duration, and spread of mumps outbreaks.

What Are the Symptoms of Mumps?

Mumps usually causes the following symptoms for about 7 to 10 days:

- Fever
- Headache
- Muscle aches
- Tiredness
- Loss of appetite (not wanting to eat)
- Swollen glands under the ears or jaw

Some people who get mumps do not have symptoms. Others may feel sick but will not have swollen glands.

Is It Serious?

In most children, mumps is pretty mild. But it can cause serious, lasting problems, including:

- Meningitis (infection of the covering of the brain and spinal cord)
- Deafness (temporary or permanent)
- Encephalitis (swelling of the brain)
- Orchitis (swelling of the testicles) in males who have reached puberty
- Oophoritis (swelling of the ovaries) and/or mastitis (swelling of the breasts) in females who have reached puberty

In rare cases, mumps is deadly.

How Does Mumps Spread?

Mumps spreads when an infected person coughs or sneezes. Mumps can spread before swollen glands appear and for 5 days afterward.

Why Should My Child Get the MMR Shot?

The measles-mumps-rubella (MMR) vaccine shot:

- Protects your child from mumps, a potentially serious disease (and also protects against measles and rubella)
- Prevents your child from getting a fever and swollen glands under the ears or jaw from mumps
- Keeps your child from missing school or childcare (and keeps you from missing work to care for your sick child)

Is the MMR Shot Safe?

Yes. The MMR shot is very safe, and it is effective at preventing mumps (as well as measles and rubella). Vaccines, like any medicine, can have side effects. But most children who get the MMR shot have no side effects.

What Are the Side Effects?

Most children don't have any side effects from the shot. The side effects that do occur are usually very mild, such as a fever or rash. More serious side effects are rare. These may include high fever that could cause a seizure (in about 1 person out of every 3,000 that get the shot) and temporary pain and stiffness in joints (mostly in teens and adults).

Section 13.12

Rabies

This section contains text excerpted from the following sources: Text beginning with the heading "Kids and Rabies" is excerpted from "Kids and Rabies," Centers for Disease Control and Prevention (CDC), September 26, 2014; Text beginning with the heading "Be Cautious While Hiking, Camping, and Playing Outdoors" is excerpted from "Protect Your Family from Rabies," Centers for Disease Control and Prevention (CDC), July 28, 2014.

Kids and Rabies

Rabies is a dangerous virus that is found in the saliva of animals. It can infect and kill animals and humans. Every 10 minutes, someone dies from rabies. Even though anyone can get rabies, more than half of the people who get rabies are kids under the age of 15.

People usually get rabies when they are bitten by an animal that has the virus. When it's likely that you or a child is at serious risk for rabies, get help right away. Symptoms of rabies might not show up for months, but it is important to receive proper care very soon. When symptoms of rabies appear, people often die within a few days.

Early symptoms of rabies in people can include:

- fever
- headache
- weakness

As it gets worse, symptoms may include:

- difficulty sleeping
- anxiety
- confusion
- tingling sensation (usually at the site of the bite)
- excitation (being too excited)
- hallucinations (seeing things that aren't there)

- agitation
- salivating (drooling) more than usual
- difficulty swallowing
- fear of water

Below, you will learn about things you can do that will help make sure you never get rabies. Once you've read to the end, encourage a child to read through the information with you. Then visit the Kids and Rabies Website to learn more about rabies and to take a fun test of your rabies knowledge.

Help Your Pets Stay Rabies Free

Most people who have pets, such as dogs and cats, are very close to their animal companions. You might even have children and pets that are very close to each other. But there are times when pets are also in close contact with wild animals. If your pet is bitten by a wild animal that has rabies, your pet can get sick and die. It could also cause you or a child to get rabies from your sick pet.

When a human gets rabies, it's often because a pet got rabies first. The good news is that there are things children and adults alike can do to help make sure your pets never get rabies. That way, they will stay healthy and won't cause humans to get rabies.

Things you should do include:

- Take your pets to a veterinarian on a regular basis. They will keep your pets up-to-date on their rabies shots, which helps protect them from rabies.
- Talk to your veterinarian about spaying or neutering your pet. This helps cut down on the number of stray animals.
- Call animal control to remove all stray animals from your neighborhood. These animals may not have gotten their rabies shot and can give other animals and people rabies.
- Remind kids not to go near stray animals and remind them to tell an adult if they see a pet wandering around without any person watching them closely.
- Keep your pets indoors. When a dog goes outside, make sure an adult is there to watch it and keep it safe. Make sure children know not to take their pet outside without an adult around.

- Do not feed or put water for your pets outside. Keep your garbage covered. These items may cause wild animals to come near your yard or house.

Stay Away from Wild Animals

Most of the time, rabies is found in wild animals. The main animals that get rabies include raccoons, skunks, foxes and bats.

If you see a wild animal acting strangely, stay away from it. Help kids to understand that they should avoid wild animals at all times. Some things to look for are:

- General sickness
- Problems swallowing
- Lots of drool or saliva
- An animal that appears more tame than you would expect
- An animal that bites at everything
- An animal that's having trouble moving or may even be paralyzed

Animals that act this way may need to be helped by people who know how to take care of wild animals. Call animal control and make sure the animal gets the help it needs.

Sometimes, people may come across a dead animal. Never pick up or touch dead animals and make sure children know to stay away from dead animals. Animals who have died can still give people rabies, especially if they have only been dead for a short time. If a dead animal is spotted, call animal control to properly take care of the animal's body.

Get Help If An Animal Bites You

Animals can sometimes bite people even when you try to avoid them. If an animal bites you, seek help immediately. Let kids know that they should tell an adult immediately if they are bitten by an animal. Show them how to wash with soap and water so that they will know what to do if they are bitten. They should then be taken to a doctor who will know what to do next.

Most of the time, people know when an animal bites them. But that's not always the case with bats, which are one of the main animals that can give you rabies. Bats have small teeth that might not always be felt when they bite and they don't always leave bite marks that are easily seen.

Bats can be found indoors or out. Make sure children know to tell an adult when:

- a bat comes near or touches them
- a bat flies into their room or place where they sleep
- they find a dead bat
- they hear others talk about touching a living or dead bat

Be Cautious While Hiking, Camping, and Playing Outdoors

During the summer, many Americans love to spend time in the outdoors. Few people will ever be exposed to a rabies-suspect animal or need to see a doctor due to a potential exposure. Teach children and others never to handle live or dead wild animals, as well as unfamiliar domestic animals. Tell them to report any unusual animal behavior to an adult right away, because it could mean that the animal is very sick.

Some might have concerns about the presence of bats in locations such as camps. While bats have been known to expose people to rabies, most bats in a natural setting are not rabid and, in many camp situations, the presence or sighting of bats is common and normal.

However, precautions can be taken at campsites and along trails to help minimize the risk of exposure to bats for your child or family members:

- When possible, prevent bats from entering campground living quarters and other occupied spaces. Animal care and wildlife conservation agencies can provide further information on "bat-proofing."
- Screens or mosquito netting can provide a useful barrier against direct bat contact.
- Teach children and other camp attendees never to handle live or dead bats, as well as unfamiliar wild or domestic animals (even if they appear friendly). Tell children to report any contact or unusual animal behavior to an adult or camp official right away.

Talk with Your Family about the Seriousness of Rabies

While very few people die from rabies, life-threatening situations can arise when potential exposures occur and preventive measures are not undertaken. Each year 30,000 to 40,000 persons in the United States require post-exposure prophylaxis (PEP) due to potential exposures to rabies.

To help ensure your loved ones do not face similar risks, use the above information to talk with your children and other family members about the dangers of rabies, the threat of exposure from wild animals and the things they need to do to stay healthy and rabies free.

Section 13.13

Rotavirus Disease

This section includes text excerpted from "Rotavirus," Centers for Disease Control and Prevention (CDC), August 12, 2016.

What Is Rotavirus?

Rotavirus is a contagious virus that can cause gastroenteritis (inflammation of the stomach and intestines). Symptoms include severe watery diarrhea, often with vomiting, fever, and abdominal pain. Infants and young children are most likely to get rotavirus disease. They can become severely dehydrated and need to be hospitalized and can even die.

Symptoms

Rotavirus disease is most common in infants and young children. However, older children and adults also can get sick from rotavirus. Once a person has been exposed to rotavirus, it takes about 2 days for the symptoms to appear.

Children who get infected may have severe watery diarrhea, often with vomiting, fever, and abdominal pain. Vomiting and watery diarrhea can last from 3 to 8 days. Additional symptoms may include loss of appetite and dehydration (loss of body fluids), which can be especially dangerous for infants and young children.

Symptoms of dehydration include:

- decrease in urination,
- dry mouth and throat and
- feeling dizzy when standing up.

Adults who get rotavirus disease tend to have milder symptoms.

Children, even those that are vaccinated, may get sick from rotavirus more than once. That is because neither natural infection with rotavirus nor rotavirus vaccination provides full protection from future infections. Usually a person's first time getting rotavirus causes the most severe symptoms. However, vaccinated children are much less likely to get sick from rotavirus, and if they do get sick, their symptoms are usually less severe than unvaccinated children.

Transmission

Rotavirus spreads easily among infants and young children. Children can spread the virus both before and after they become sick with diarrhea. They can also pass rotavirus to family members and other people with whom they have close contact.

People who are infected with rotavirus shed rotavirus in their feces (poop)—this is often how the virus spreads from a person's body to other people and into the environment. They shed the virus most when they are sick and during the first 3 days after they recover.

The virus spreads by the fecal-oral route; this means the virus is shed by an infected person and then enters a susceptible person's mouth to cause infection. Rotavirus can be spread by contaminated:

- Hands
- Objects (toys, surfaces)
- Food
- Water

Children are most likely to get rotavirus in the winter and spring (December through June).

Prevention

Rotavirus spreads easily. Good hygiene like hand washing and cleanliness are important, but are not enough to control the spread of the disease.

Rotavirus vaccine is the best way to protect your child against rotavirus illness. Most children (about 9 out of 10) who get the vaccine will be protected from severe rotavirus illness. While about 7 out of 10 children will be protected from rotavirus illness. CDC recommends routine vaccination of infants with either of the two available vaccines:

- RotaTeq® (RV5), which is given in 3 doses at ages 2 months, 4 months, and 6 months; or
- Rotarix® (RV1), which is given in 2 doses at ages 2 months and 4 months.

Both rotavirus vaccines are given orally.

Rotavirus vaccines do not prevent diarrhea or vomiting caused by other viruses or pathogens.

Treatment

There is no specific medicine to treat rotavirus infection, but your doctor may recommend medicines to treat symptoms. There is no antiviral drug to treat it, and antibiotic drugs will not help because antibiotics fight bacteria not viruses.

Rotavirus infection can cause severe vomiting and diarrhea. This can lead to dehydration (loss of body fluids). Infants and young children, older adults, and people with other illnesses are most at risk of dehydration.

Symptoms of dehydration include decrease in urination, dry mouth and throat and feeling dizzy when standing up. A dehydrated child may also:

- cry with few or no tears and
- be unusually sleepy or fussy.

The best way to protect against dehydration is to drink plenty of liquids. Oral rehydration solutions that you can get over the counter in U.S. food and drug stores are most helpful for mild dehydration. Severe dehydration may require hospitalization for treatment with intravenous (IV) fluids, which are given to patients directly through their veins. If you or someone you are caring for is severely dehydrated, contact your doctor.

Section 13.14

Rubella (German Measles)

This section contains text excerpted from the following sources: Text beginning with the heading "What Is Rubella?" is excerpted from "Rubella and the Vaccine (Shot) to Prevent It," Centers for Disease Control and Prevention (CDC), November 10, 2014; Text beginning with the heading "Rubella Is Dangerous for Pregnant Women and Unborn Babies" is excerpted from "Rubella: Make Sure Your Child Gets Vaccinated," Centers for Disease Control and Prevention (CDC), January 19, 2016.

What Is Rubella?

Rubella, sometimes called "German measles," is a disease caused by a virus. The infection is usually mild with fever and a rash. But, if a pregnant woman gets infected, the virus can cause serious birth defects.

What Are the Symptoms of Rubella?

In children, rubella usually causes the following symptoms that last 2 or 3 days:

- Rash that starts on the face and spreads to the rest of the body
- Low fever (less than 101 degrees)

Before the rash appears, older children and adults may also have:

- Swollen glands
- Cold-like symptoms
- Aching joints (especially in young women)

About half of the people who get rubella do not have symptoms.

Is It Serious?

Rubella is usually mild in children. Complications are not common, but they occur more often in adults. In rare cases, rubella can cause serious problems, including brain infections and bleeding problems.

Rubella is most dangerous for a pregnant woman's unborn baby. Infection during pregnancy can cause miscarriage, or birth defects like deafness, blindness, intellectual disability, and heart defects. As many as 85 out of 100 babies born to mothers who had rubella in the first 3 months of pregnancy will have a birth defect.

How Does Rubella Spread?

Rubella spreads when an infected person coughs or sneezes.

The disease is most contagious when the infected person has a rash. But it can spread up to 7 days before the rash appears. People without symptoms can still spread rubella.

Rubella Is Dangerous for Pregnant Women and Unborn Babies

The most serious complication from rubella infection is the harm it can cause a pregnant woman's unborn baby. If an unvaccinated pregnant woman gets infected with rubella virus she can have a miscarriage, or her baby can die just after birth. Also, she can pass the virus to her unborn baby who can develop serious birth defects such as:

- heart problems,
- loss of hearing and eyesight,
- intellectual disability, and
- liver or spleen damage.

Serious birth defects are more common if a woman is infected early in her pregnancy, especially in the first trimester.

Children should be vaccinated on schedule to protect them from rubella infection and to prevent them from spreading rubella to a pregnant woman and her unborn baby.

Protect Your Child, and Others, with Rubella Vaccine

The best way to protect your child from rubella is to get him or her vaccinated on schedule. Children should be vaccinated against rubella to protect them from infection and to prevent them from spreading rubella to a pregnant woman and her unborn baby, as well those who cannot get vaccinated because they have a health condition or are too young.

Rubella vaccine is usually given as part of a combination vaccine called MMR, which protects against three diseases: measles, mumps, and rubella. MMR vaccine is safe and effective and has been widely used in the United States for more than 30 years.

Children should get 2 doses of MMR vaccine:

- the first dose at 12 through 15 months of age and
- the second dose at 4 through 6 years of age, before entering school.

Your child's doctor may also offer the MMRV vaccine, which protects against four diseases: measles, mumps, rubella, and varicella (chickenpox).

Talk to your child's healthcare professional for help deciding which vaccine to use.

Section 13.15

Zika Virus

This section contains text excerpted from the following sources: Text beginning with the heading "What We Know about Zika" is excerpted from "What Parents Should Know about Zika," Centers for Disease Control and Prevention (CDC), May 4, 2016; Text under the heading "Tips to Protect Yourself and Others from Zika Virus" is excerpted from "Protect Yourself and Others," Centers for Disease Control and Prevention (CDC), July 25, 2016.

What We Know about Zika

- **Infants and children can be infected with Zika.**
    - The primary way that infants and children get Zika is through bites of two types of mosquitoes.
    - To date, no cases of Zika have been reported from breastfeeding. Because of the benefits of breastfeeding, mothers are encouraged to breastfeed, even in areas where Zika virus is found.
    - Common symptoms of Zika are fever, rash, joint pain, and red eyes. Symptoms usually go away within a few days to one week. Many people infected with Zika don't have symptoms.

- There is no vaccine or medicine for Zika.

- **Birth defects, including microcephaly, and other problems have been reported in babies born to women infected with Zika during pregnancy.**
  - Zika virus can be passed from a woman to her fetus during pregnancy or around the time of birth. We are studying how Zika virus affects pregnancies.
  - Since May 2015, Brazil has had a large outbreak of Zika. During this outbreak, Brazilian officials reported an increase in the number of babies born with microcephaly in areas with Zika. Recently, CDC concluded that Zika virus infection during pregnancy is a cause of microcephaly and other severe fetal brain defects.
  - Pregnancy loss and other pregnancy problems have been reported in women infected with Zika during pregnancy. Zika has been linked with other birth defects, including eye defects, hearing loss, and impaired growth.
  - Not all babies whose mothers had Zika during pregnancy are born with health problems. Researchers are working to better understand how often having Zika during pregnancy causes problems.
  - Infection with Zika virus at later times, including around the time of birth or in early childhood, has not been linked to microcephaly.

- **Microcephaly happens for many reasons, and many times the cause is unknown.**
  - Genetic conditions, certain infections, and toxins can cause microcephaly. If your child has microcephaly, his or her doctor or other healthcare provider will look for the underlying reason. However, for about half of children with microcephaly, the underlying cause is never discovered.
  - If you have a child with microcephaly, it is unlikely that it had to do with Zika if you did not travel to an area with Zika during pregnancy.
  - Although head size reflects brain size, head size does not always predict short- or long-term health effects. While some children with microcephaly can have seizures, vision or

hearing problems, and developmental disabilities, others do not have health problems.

What We Don't Know about Zika

- We do not know how often Zika is passed from a woman to her fetus during pregnancy or around the time of birth.
- We do not know whether the timing of the woman's Zika virus infection during pregnancy, or the severity of a woman's symptoms, affect her pregnancy.
- We do not know the long-term health outcomes for infants and children with Zika virus infection.

What Parents Can Do

- **Prevent mosquito bites.**

To protect your child from mosquito bites:

- Dress your child in clothing that covers arms and legs.
- Cover crib, stroller, and baby carrier with mosquito netting.
- Do not use insect repellent on babies under 2 months of age.
- Do not use products containing oil of lemon eucalyptus or para-menthane-diol on children younger than 3 years old.
- In children older than 2 months, do not apply insect repellent onto a child's hands, eyes, mouth, or to irritated or broken skin.
- Never spray insect repellent directly on a child's face. Instead, spray it on your hands and then apply sparingly, taking care to avoid the eyes and mouth.
- Control mosquitoes inside and outside your home.

- **If your child has symptoms, take him or her to see a doctor or other healthcare provider.**

For children with Zika symptoms of fever, rash, joint pain, or red eyes who have traveled to or resided in an affected area, contact your child's healthcare provider and describe where you have traveled.

- Fever (≥100.4° F) in a baby less than 2 months old always requires evaluation by a medical professional. If your baby is less than 2 months old and has a fever, call your healthcare provider or get medical care.

Tips to Protect Yourself and Others from Zika Virus

Use the tips below to protect yourself and others from Zika

- Following these tips will help to protect you, your partner, your family, your friends, and your community from Zika. The more steps you take, the more protected you are.

Prevent mosquito bites

- Zika virus is spread to people mainly through the bite of an infected mosquito.
- Mosquitoes that spread Zika virus bite mostly during the day, but they can also bite at night.
- The best way to prevent Zika is to protect yourself from mosquito bites.

Plan for travel

- Currently, outbreaks are occurring in many countries and territories.
- Zika virus will continue to spread and it will be difficult to determine how and where the virus will spread over time.

What you can do

- Check travel notices.
- Plan for travel (both before and after your trip)

Chapter 14

Parasitic and Fungal Infections

Chapter Contents

Section 14.1

Ascariasis and Hookworm Infection

This section contains text excerpted from the following sources: Text beginning with the heading "What Is Ascariasis?" is excerpted from "Ascariasis FAQs," Centers for Disease Control and Prevention (CDC), January 10, 2013; Text beginning with the heading "What Is Hookworm?" is excerpted from "Hookworm FAQs," Centers for Disease Control and Prevention (CDC), December 16, 2014.

What Is Ascariasis?

Ascaris is an intestinal parasite of humans. It is the most common human worm infection. The larvae and adult worms live in the small intestine and can cause intestinal disease.

How Is Ascariasis Spread?

Ascaris lives in the intestine and *Ascaris* eggs are passed in the feces of infected persons. If the infected person defecates outside (near bushes, in a garden, or field), or if the feces of an infected person are used as fertilizer, then eggs are deposited on the soil. They can then mature into a form that is infective. Ascariasis is caused by ingesting infective eggs. This can happen when hands or fingers that have contaminated dirt on them are put in the mouth or by consuming vegetables or fruits that have not been carefully cooked, washed or peeled.

Who Is at Risk for Infection?

Infection occurs worldwide in warm and humid climates, where sanitation and hygiene are poor, including in temperate zones during warmer months. Persons in these areas are at risk if soil contaminated with human feces enters their mouths or if they eat vegetables or fruit that have not been carefully washed, peeled or cooked. Ascariasis is now uncommon in the United States.

What Are the Symptoms of Ascariasis?

People infected with *Ascaris* often show no symptoms. If symptoms do occur they can be light and include abdominal discomfort. Heavy infections can cause intestinal blockage and impair growth in children. Other symptoms such as cough are due to migration of the worms through the body.

How Is Ascariasis Diagnosed?

Healthcare providers can diagnose ascariasis by taking a stool sample and using a microscope to look for the presence of eggs. Some people notice infection when a worm is passed in their stool or is coughed up. If this happens, bring in the worm specimen to your healthcare provider for diagnosis.

How Can I Prevent Infection?

- Avoid contact with soil that may be contaminated with human feces, including with human fecal matter ("night soil") used to fertilize crops.
- Wash your hands with soap and warm water before handling food.
- Teach children the importance of washing hands to prevent infection.
- Wash, peel, or cook all raw vegetables and fruits before eating, particularly those that have been grown in soil that has been fertilized with manure.

What Is the Treatment for Ascariasis?

Anthelmintic medications (drugs that rid the body of parasitic worms), such as albendazole and mebendazole, are the drugs of choice for treatment. Infections are generally treated for 1–3 days. The recommended medications are effective.

What Is Preventive Treatment?

In developing countries, groups at higher risk for soil-transmitted helminth infections (hookworm, *Ascaris*, and whipworm) are often treated without a prior stool examination. Treating in this way is called preventive treatment (or "preventive chemotherapy"). The high-risk groups identified by the World Health Organization are preschool and school-age children, women of childbearing age (including pregnant women in the 2nd and 3rd trimesters and lactating women) and adults in occupations where there is a high risk of heavy infections. School-age children are often treated through school-health programs and preschool children and pregnant women at visits to health clinics.

What Is Mass Drug Administration (MDA)?

The soil-transmitted helminths (hookworm, *Ascaris*, and whipworm) and four other "neglected tropical diseases" (river blindness, lymphatic filariasis, schistosomiasis and trachoma) are sometimes treated through mass drug administrations. Since the drugs used are safe and inexpensive or donated, entire risk groups are offered preventive treatment. Mass drug administrations are conducted periodically (often annually), commonly with drug distributors who go door-to-door. Multiple neglected tropical diseases are often treated simultaneously using MDAs.

What Is Hookworm?

Hookworm is an intestinal parasite of humans. The larvae and adult worms live in the small intestine can cause intestinal disease. The two main species of hookworm infecting humans are *Ancylostoma duodenale* and *Necator americanus*.

How Is Hookworm Spread?

Hookworm eggs are passed in the feces of an infected person. If an infected person defecates outside (near bushes, in a garden, or field) or if the feces from an infected person are used as fertilizer, eggs are deposited on soil. They can then mature and hatch, releasing larvae (immature worms). The larvae mature into a form that can penetrate the skin of humans. Hookworm infection is transmitted primarily by walking barefoot on contaminated soil. One kind of hookworm (*Ancylostoma duodenale*) can also be transmitted through the ingestion of larvae.

Who Is at Risk for Infection?

People living in areas with warm and moist climates and where sanitation and hygiene are poor are at risk for hookworm infection if they walk barefoot or in other ways allow their skin to have direct contact with contaminated soil. Soil is contaminated by an infected person defecating outside or when human feces ("night soil") are used as fertilizer. Children who play in contaminated soil may also be at risk.

What Are the Signs and Symptoms of Hookworm?

Itching and a localized rash are often the first signs of infection. These symptoms occur when the larvae penetrate the skin. A person with a light infection may have no symptoms. A person with a heavy infection may experience abdominal pain, diarrhea, loss of appetite, weight loss, fatigue and anemia. The physical and cognitive growth of children can be affected.

How Is Hookworm Diagnosed?

Healthcare providers can diagnose hookworm by taking a stool sample and using a microscope to look for the presence of hookworm eggs.

How Can I Prevent Infection?

Do not walk barefoot in areas where hookworm is common and where there may be fecal contamination of the soil. Avoid other skin-to-soil contact and avoid ingesting such soil. Fecal contamination occurs when people defecate outdoors or use human feces as fertilizer.

The infection of others can be prevented by not defecating outdoors or using human feces as fertilizer, and by effective sewage disposal systems.

What Is the Treatment for Hookworm?

Hookworm infections are generally treated for 1–3 days with medication prescribed by your healthcare provider. The drugs are effective and appear to have few side effects. Iron supplements may be prescribed if you have anemia.

What Is Preventive Treatment?

In developing countries, groups at higher risk for soil-transmitted helminth infections (hookworm, *Ascaris*, and whipworm) are often treated without a prior stool examination. Treating in this way is called preventive treatment (or "preventive chemotherapy"). The high-risk groups identified by the World Health Organization are preschool and school-age children, women of childbearing age (including pregnant women in the 2nd and 3rd trimesters and lactating women) and adults in occupations where there is a high risk of heavy infections. School-age children are often treated through school-health programs and preschool children and pregnant women at visits to health clinics.

Section 14.2

Baylisascaris Infection

This section includes text excerpted from "Baylisascaris FAQs," Centers for Disease Control and Prevention (CDC), October 11, 2012. Reviewed October 2016.

What Is Baylisascaris?

Baylisascaris worms are intestinal parasites found in a wide variety of animals. Different species of Baylisascaris are associated with different animal hosts. For example, *Baylisascaris procyonis* is found in raccoons and *Baylisascaris columnaris* is an intestinal parasite found in skunks. Cases of *Baylisascaris* infection in people are not frequently reported, but can be severe. *Baylisascaris procyonis* is thought to pose the greatest risk to humans because of the often close association of raccoons to human dwellings.

In What Parts of the World Is Baylisascaris Found?

Baylisascaris procyonis has been identified in the United States, Europe, and Japan. Some evidence of infection in animals has been reported in South America.

In the United States, infected raccoons have been found in a number of states, especially in the mid-Atlantic, northeastern and Midwestern states and parts of California.

How Do People Get Infected?

People become infected by ingesting infectious eggs. Most infections are in children and others who are more likely to put dirt or animal waste in their mouth by mistake.

How Can I Prevent Baylisascaris Infection?

Eggs passed in raccoon feces are not immediately infectious. In the environment, eggs take 2 to 4 weeks to become infectious. If raccoons have set up a den or a latrine in your yard, raccoon feces and material contaminated with raccoon feces should be removed carefully and burned, buried, or sent to a landfill. Care should be taken to avoid contaminating hands and clothes. Treat decks, patios, and other surfaces with boiling water or a propane flame-gun (exercise proper precautions). Prompt removal and destruction of raccoon feces before the eggs become infectious will reduce risk for exposure and possible infection.

Do not keep, feed, or adopt wild animals, including raccoons, as pets.

Washing your hands after working or playing outdoors is good practice for preventing a number of diseases.

What Are the Signs and Symptoms of Baylisascaris Infection?

The incubation period (time from exposure to symptoms) is usually 1 to 4 weeks. If present, signs and symptoms can include:

- Nausea
- Tiredness
- Liver enlargement
- Loss of coordination
- Lack of attention to people and surroundings
- Loss of muscle control
- Blindness
- Coma

What Should I Do If I Think I Am Infected with Baylisascaris?

You should discuss your concerns with your healthcare provider, who will examine you and ask you questions (for example, about your interactions with raccoons or other wild animals). *Baylisascaris* infection is difficult to diagnosis in humans. There are no widely available tests, so the diagnosis is often made by ruling out other diseases.

How Is Baylisascaris Infection Treated?

A healthcare provider can discuss treatment options with you. No drug has been found to be completely effective against *Baylisascaris* infection in people. Albendazole has been recommended for some cases.

If I Have Baylisascaris Infection, Should My Family Members Be Tested for the Infection?

Baylisascaris infection is not contagious, so one person cannot give the infection to another. However, if your family may have been exposed the same way you were (such as contact with or exposure to an environment contaminated with raccoon or exotic pet feces), they should consult with a healthcare provider.

Section 14.3

Cryptosporidiosis

This section contains text excerpted from the following sources: Text beginning with the heading "What Is Cryptosporidiosis?" is excerpted from "General Information for the Public," Centers for Disease Control and Prevention (CDC), April 20, 2015; Text under the heading "Prevention and Control" is excerpted from "Prevention and Control-General Public," Centers for Disease Control and Prevention (CDC), October 7, 2015.

What Is Cryptosporidiosis?

Cryptosporidiosis is a disease that causes watery diarrhea. It is caused by microscopic germs—parasites called *Cryptosporidium*. *Cryptosporidium*, or "Crypto" for short, can be found in water, food, soil or on surfaces or dirty hands that have been contaminated with the feces of humans or animals infected with the parasite. During 2001–2010,

Crypto was the leading cause of waterborne disease outbreaks, linked to recreational water in the United States. The parasite is found in every region of the United States and throughout the world.

How Is Cryptosporidiosis Spread?

Crypto lives in the gut of infected humans or animals. An infected person or animal sheds Crypto parasites in their poop. An infected person can shed 10,000,000 to 100,000,000 Crypto germs in a single bowel movement. Shedding of Crypto in poop begins when symptoms like diarrhea begin and can last for weeks after symptoms stop. Swallowing as few as 10 Crypto germs can cause infection.

Crypto can be spread by:

- Swallowing recreational water (for example, the water in swimming pools, fountains, lakes, rivers) contaminated with Crypto
- Crypto's high tolerance to chlorine enables the parasite to survive for long periods of time in chlorinated drinking and swimming pool water
- Drinking untreated water from a lake or river that is contaminated with Crypto
- Swallowing water, ice, or beverages contaminated with poop from infected humans or animals
- Eating undercooked food or drinking unpasteurized/raw apple cider or milk that gets contaminated with Crypto
- Touching your mouth with contaminated hands
- Hands can become contaminated through a variety of activities, such as touching surfaces or objects (e.g., toys, bathroom fixtures, changing tables, diaper pails) that have been contaminated by poop from an infected person, changing diapers, caring for an infected person, and touching an infected animal

Crypto is not spread through contact with blood.

What Are the Symptoms of Cryptosporidiosis, When Do They Begin, And How Long Do They Last?

Symptoms of Crypto generally begin 2 to 10 days (average 7 days) after becoming infected with the parasite. Symptoms include:

- Watery diarrhea

- Stomach cramps or pain
- Dehydration
- Nausea
- Vomiting
- Fever
- Weight loss

Symptoms usually last about 1 to 2 weeks (with a range of a few days to 4 or more weeks) in people with healthy immune systems.

The most common symptom of cryptosporidiosis is watery diarrhea. Some people with Crypto will have no symptoms at all.

Who Is Most at Risk for Cryptosporidiosis?

People who are most likely to become infected with *Cryptosporidium* include:

- Children who attend childcare centers, including diaper-aged children
- Childcare workers
- Parents of infected children
- People who take care of other people with Crypto
- International travelers
- Backpackers, hikers, and campers who drink unfiltered, untreated water
- People who drink from untreated shallow, unprotected wells
- People, including swimmers, who swallow water from contaminated sources
- People who handle infected calves or other ruminants like sheep

Contaminated water might include water that has not been boiled or filtered, as well as contaminated recreational water sources (e.g., swimming pools, lakes, rivers, ponds, and streams). Several community-wide outbreaks have been linked to drinking tap water or recreational water contaminated with *Cryptosporidium*. Crypto's high tolerance to chlorine enables the parasite to survive for long periods of time in chlorinated drinking and swimming pool water. This means anyone swallowing contaminated water could get ill.

- Young children and pregnant women may be more likely to get dehydrated because of their diarrhea so they should drink plenty of fluids while ill.
- People with severely weakened immune systems are at risk for more serious disease. Symptoms may be more severe and could lead to serious or life-threatening illness. Examples of people with weakened immune systems include those with acquired immune deficiency syndrome (AIDS); those with inherited diseases that affect the immune system; and cancer and transplant patients who are taking certain immunosuppressive drugs.

What Should I Do If I Think I Might Have Cryptosporidiosis?

For diarrhea whose cause has not been determined, the following actions may help relieve symptoms: Individuals who have health concerns should talk to their healthcare provider.

- Drink plenty of fluids to remain well hydrated and avoid dehydration. Serious health problems can occur if the body does not maintain proper fluid levels. For some people, diarrhea can be severe resulting in hospitalization due to dehydration.
- Maintain a well-balanced diet. Doing so may help speed recovery.
- Avoid beverages that contain caffeine, such as tea, coffee, and many soft drinks.
- Avoid alcohol, as it can lead to dehydration.

Contact your healthcare provider if you suspect that you have cryptosporidiosis.

How Is Cryptosporidiosis Diagnosed?

Cryptosporidiosis is a diarrheal disease that is spread through contact with the stool of an infected person or animal. The disease is diagnosed by examining stool samples. People infected with Crypto can shed the parasite irregularly in their poop (for example, one day they shed parasite, the next day they don't, the third day they do) so patients may need to give three samples collected on three different days to help make sure that a negative test result is accurate and really means they do not have Crypto. Healthcare providers should specifically request testing for Crypto. Routine ova and parasite testing does not normally include Crypto testing.

What Is the Treatment for Cryptosporidiosis?

Most people with healthy immune systems will recover from cryptosporidiosis without treatment. The following actions may help relieve symptoms. Individuals who have health concerns should talk to their healthcare provider.

- Drink plenty of fluids to remain well hydrated and avoid dehydration. Serious health problems can occur if the body does not maintain proper fluid levels. For some people, diarrhea can be severe resulting in hospitalization due to dehydration.
- Maintain a well-balanced diet. Doing so may help speed recovery.
- Avoid beverages that contain caffeine, such as tea, coffee, and many soft drinks.
- Avoid alcohol, as it can lead to dehydration.

Over-the-counter anti-diarrheal medicine might help slow down diarrhea, but a healthcare provider should be consulted before such medicine is taken.

A drug called nitazoxanide has been U.S. Food and Drug Administration (FDA)-approved for treatment of diarrhea caused by *Cryptosporidium* in people with healthy immune systems and is available by prescription. Consult with your healthcare provider for more information about potential advantages and disadvantages of taking nitazoxanide.

Infants, young children, and pregnant women may be more likely than others to suffer from dehydration. Losing a lot of fluids from diarrhea can be dangerous—and especially life-threatening in infants. These people should drink extra fluids when they are sick. Severe dehydration may require hospitalization for treatment with fluids given through your vein (intravenous or IV fluids). If you are pregnant or a parent and you suspect you or your child are severely dehydrated, contact a healthcare provider about fluid replacement options.

Prevention and Control

The following recommendations are intended to help prevent and control cryptosporidiosis in members of the general public.

Practice Good Hygiene

Everywhere

- Wet hands with clean, running water and apply soap. Lather all surfaces of hands and scrub for at least 20 seconds. Rinse with clean, running water and dry with a clean towel or air:
  - before preparing or eating food,
  - after using the toilet,
  - after changing diapers or cleaning up a child who has used the toilet,
  - before and after caring for someone who is ill with diarrhea,
  - after handling an animal, particularly young livestock, or its stool,
  - after gardening, even if wearing gloves.

Alcohol-based hand sanitizers do not effectively kill Cryptosporidium. At child care facilities:

- Exclude children who are ill with diarrhea from child care settings until the diarrhea has stopped.

At the pool:

- Protect others by not swimming if ill with diarrhea.
- If cryptosporidiosis is diagnosed, do not swim for at least 2 weeks after diarrhea stops.
- Do not swallow the water.
- Take young children on bathroom breaks every 60 minutes or check their diapers every 30–60 minutes.

Avoid Water That Might Be Contaminated

- Do not drink untreated water from lakes, rivers, springs, ponds, streams, or shallow wells.
- Follow advice given during local drinking water advisories.
- If the safety of drinking water is in doubt (e.g., during an outbreak, or if water treatment is unknown) use at least one of the following:
- Commercially bottled water,

- Water that has been previously boiled for 1 minute and left to cool. At elevations above 6,500 feet (1,981 meters), boil for 3 minutes.
- Use a filter designed to remove *Cryptosporidium.*
- The label might read 'NSF 53' or 'NSF 58'.
- Filter labels that read "absolute pore size of 1 micron or smaller" are also effective.
- If the safety of drinking water is in doubt, (e.g., during an outbreak or if water treatment is unknown), use bottled, boiled, or filtered water to wash fruits and vegetables that will be eaten raw.

Practice Extra Caution While Traveling

- Do not use or drink inadequately treated water or use ice when traveling in countries where the water might be unsafe.
- Avoid eating uncooked foods when traveling in countries where the food supply might be unsafe.

Section 14.4

Giardiasis

This section includes text excerpted from "Giardia," Centers for Disease Control and Prevention (CDC), July 21, 2015.

What Is Giardiasis?

Giardiasis is a diarrheal disease caused by the microscopic parasite *Giardia.* A parasite is an organism that feeds off of another to survive. Once a person or animal (for example, cats, dogs, cattle, deer, and beavers) has been infected with *Giardia*, the parasite lives in the intestines and is passed in feces (poop). Once outside the body, *Giardia* can sometimes survive for weeks or months. *Giardia* can be found within every region of the United States and around the world.

How Do You Get Giardiasis and How Is It Spread?

Giardiasis can be spread by:

- Swallowing *Giardia* picked up from surfaces (such as bathroom handles, changing tables, diaper pails, or toys) that contain feces (poop) from an infected person or animal
- Drinking water or using ice made from water sources where *Giardia* may live (for example, untreated or improperly treated water from lakes, streams, or wells)
- Swallowing water while swimming or playing in water where *Giardia* may live, especially in lakes, rivers, springs, ponds, and streams
- Eating uncooked food that contains *Giardia* organisms
- Having contact with someone who is ill with giardiasis
- Traveling to countries where giardiasis is common

Anything that comes into contact with feces (poop) from infected humans or animals can become contaminated with the *Giardia* parasite. People become infected when they swallow the parasite. It is not possible to become infected through contact with blood.

What Are the Symptoms of Giardiasis?

Giardia infection can cause a variety of intestinal symptoms, which include:

- Diarrhea
- Gas or flatulence
- Greasy stool that can float
- Stomach or abdominal cramps
- Upset stomach or nausea
- Dehydration

These symptoms may also lead to weight loss. Some people with *Giardia* infection have no symptoms at all.

How long After Infection Do Symptoms Appear?

Symptoms of giardiasis normally begin 1 to 3 weeks after becoming infected.

How Long Will Symptoms Last?

In otherwise healthy people, symptoms of giardiasis may last 2 to 6 weeks. Occasionally, symptoms last longer. Medications can help decrease the amount of time symptoms last.

Who Is Most at Risk of Getting Giardiasis?

Though giardiasis is commonly thought of as a camping or backpacking-related disease and is sometimes called "Beaver Fever," anyone can get giardiasis. People more likely to become infected include:

- Children in childcare settings, especially diaper-aged children
- Close contacts of people with giardiasis (for example, people living in the same household) or people who care for those sick with giardiasis
- People who drink water or use ice made from places where *Giardia* may live (for example, untreated or improperly treated water from lakes, streams, or wells)
- Backpackers, hikers, and campers who drink unsafe water or who do not practice good hygiene (for example, proper handwashing)
- People who swallow water while swimming and playing in recreational water where *Giardia* may live, especially in lakes, rivers, springs, ponds, and streams
- International travelers

What Should I Do If I Think I May Have Giardiasis?

Contact your healthcare provider.

How Is Giardiasis Diagnosed?

Your healthcare provider will ask you to submit stool (poop) samples to see if you are infected. Because testing for giardiasis can be difficult, you may be asked to submit several stool specimens collected over several days.

What Is the Treatment for Giardiasis?

Many prescription drugs are available to treat giardiasis. Although the *Giardia* parasite can infect all people, infants and pregnant women may be more likely to experience dehydration from the diarrhea caused by giardiasis. To prevent dehydration, infants and pregnant women should drink a lot of fluids while ill. Dehydration can be life threatening for infants, so it is especially important that parents talk to their healthcare providers about treatment options for their infants.

What Can I Do to Prevent and Control Giardiasis?

To prevent and control infection with the *Giardia* parasite, it is important to:

- Practice good hygiene
- Avoid water (drinking or recreational) that may be contaminated
- Avoid eating food that may be contaminated

Section 14.5

Hymenolepis (Dwarf Tapeworm) Infection

This section includes text excerpted from "Hymenolepiasis FAQs," Centers for Disease Control and Prevention (CDC), January 10, 2012. Reviewed October 2016.

What Is Hymenolepis nana Infection?

The dwarf tapeworm or *Hymenolepis nana* is found worldwide. Infection is most common in children, in persons living in institutional settings, and in people who live in areas where sanitation and personal hygiene is inadequate.

How Did I Get Infected?

One becomes infected by accidentally ingesting dwarf tapeworm eggs. This can happen by ingesting fecally contaminated foods or water, by touching your mouth with contaminated fingers, or by ingesting contaminated soil. People can also become infected if they accidentally ingest an infected arthropod (intermediate host, such as a small beetle or mealworm) that has gotten into food.

Adult dwarf tapeworms are very small in comparison with other tapeworms and may reach 15–40 mm (up to 2 inches) in length. The adult dwarf tapeworm is made up of many small segments, called proglottids As the dwarf tapeworm matures inside the intestine, these segments break off and pass into the stool. An adult dwarf tapeworm can live for 4–6 weeks. However, once you are infected, the dwarf tapeworm may reproduce inside the body (autoinfection) and continue the infection.

What Are the Symptoms of a Dwarf Tapeworm Infection?

Most people who are infected do not have any symptoms. Those who have symptoms may experience nausea, weakness, loss of appetite, diarrhea, and abdominal pain. Young children, especially those with a heavy infection, may develop a headache, itchy bottom, or have difficulty sleeping. Sometimes infection is misdiagnosed as a pinworm infection.

Contrary to popular belief, a dwarf tapeworm infection does not generally cause weight loss. You cannot feel the dwarf tapeworm inside your body.

How Is Dwarf Tapeworm Infection Diagnosed?

Diagnosis is made by identifying dwarf tapeworm eggs in stool. Your healthcare provider will ask you to submit stool specimens collected over several days to see if you are infected.

Is a Dwarf Tapeworm Infection Serious?

No. Infection with the dwarf tapeworm is generally not serious. However, prolonged infection can lead to more severe symptoms; therefore, medical attention is needed to eliminate the dwarf tapeworm.

How Is a Dwarf Tapeworm Infection Treated?

Treatment is available. A prescription drug called praziquantel is given. The medication causes the dwarf tapeworm to dissolve within the intestine. Praziquantel is generally well tolerated. Sometimes more than one treatment is necessary.

Can Infection Be Spread to Other Family Members?

Yes. Eggs are infectious (meaning they can re-infect you or infect others) immediately after being shed in feces.

How Can Dwarf Tapeworm Infection Be Prevented?

To reduce the likelihood of infection you should:

- Wash your hands with soap and warm water after using the toilet, changing diapers, and before preparing foods.
- Teach children the importance of washing hands to prevent infection.
- When traveling in countries where food is likely to be contaminated, wash, peel or cook all raw vegetables and fruits with safe water before eating.

Section 14.6

Pediculosis capitis *(Head Lice)*

This section contains text excerpted from the following sources: Text beginning with the heading "What Are Head Lice?" is excerpted from "Parasites – Lice – Head Lice," Centers for Disease Control and Prevention (CDC), August 28, 2015; Text beginning with the heading "Is Mayonnaise Effective for Treating Head Lice?" is excerpted from "Parasites – Lice – Head Lice," Centers for Disease Control and Prevention (CDC), September 24, 2013.

What Are Head Lice?

The head louse, or *Pediculus humanus capitis*, is a parasitic insect that can be found on the head, eyebrows, and eyelashes of people. Head lice feed on human blood several times a day and live close to the human scalp. Head lice are not known to spread disease.

Who Is at Risk for Getting Head Lice?

Head lice are found worldwide. In the United States, infestation with head lice is most common among pre-school children attending child care, elementary schoolchildren, and the household members of infested children. Although reliable data on how many people in the United States get head lice each year are not available, an estimated 6 million to 12 million infestations occur each year in the United States among children 3 to 11 years of age. In the United States, infestation with head lice is much less common among African-Americans than among persons of other races, possibly because the claws of the of the head louse found most frequently in the United States are better adapted for grasping the shape and width of the hair shaft of other races.

Head lice move by crawling; they cannot hop or fly. Head lice are spread by direct contact with the hair of an infested person. Anyone who comes in head-to-head contact with someone who already has head lice is at greatest risk. Spread by contact with clothing (such as hats, scarves, coats) or other personal items (such as combs, brushes, or towels) used by an infested person is uncommon. Personal hygiene or cleanliness in the home or school has nothing to do with getting head lice.

Where Are Head Lice Commonly Found?

Head lice and head lice nits are found almost exclusively on the scalp, particularly around and behind the ears and near the neckline at the back of the head. Head lice or head lice nits sometimes are found on the eyelashes or eyebrows but this is uncommon. Head lice hold tightly to hair with hook-like claws at the end of each of their six legs. Head lice nits are cemented firmly to the hair shaft and can be difficult to remove even after the nymphs hatch and empty casings remain.

What Are the Signs and Symptoms of Head Lice Infestation?

- Tickling feeling of something moving in the hair.
- Itching, caused by an allergic reaction to the bites of the head louse.
- Irritability and difficulty sleeping; head lice are most active in the dark.

- Sores on the head caused by scratching. These sores can sometimes become infected with bacteria found on the person's skin.

How Did My Child Get Head Lice?

Head-to-head contact with an already infested person is the most common way to get head lice. Head-to-head contact is common during play at school, at home, and elsewhere (sports activities, playground, slumber parties, camp).

Although uncommon, head lice can be spread by sharing clothing or belongings. This happens when lice crawl, or nits attached to shed hair hatch, and get on the shared clothing or belongings. Examples include:

- sharing clothing (hats, scarves, coats, sports uniforms) or articles (hair ribbons, barrettes, combs, brushes, towels, stuffed animals) recently worn or used by an infested person;
- or lying on a bed, couch, pillow, or carpet that has recently been in contact with an infested person.

Dogs, cats, and other pets do not play a role in the spread of head lice.

How Is a Head Lice Infestation Diagnosed?

The diagnosis of a head lice infestation is best made by finding a live nymph or adult louse on the scalp or hair of a person. Because nymphs and adult lice are very small, move quickly, and avoid light, they can be difficult to find. Use of a magnifying lens and a fine-toothed comb may be helpful to find live lice. If crawling lice are not seen, finding nits firmly attached within a ¼-inch of base of the hair shafts strongly suggests, but does not confirm, that a person is infested and should be treated. Nits that are attached more than ¼-inch from the base of the hair shaft are almost always dead or already hatched. Nits are often confused with other things found in the hair such as dandruff, hair spray droplets, and dirt particles. If no live nymphs or adult lice are seen, and the only nits found are more than ¼-inch from the scalp, the infestation is probably old and no longer active and does not need to be treated.

If you are not sure if a person has head lice, the diagnosis should be made by their healthcare provider, local health department, or other person trained to identify live head lice.

How Is A Head Lice Infestation Treated?

Treatment for head lice is recommended for persons diagnosed with an active infestation. All household members and other close contacts should be checked; those persons with evidence of an active infestation should be treated. Some experts believe prophylactic treatment is prudent for persons who share the same bed with actively-infested individuals. All infested persons (household members and close contacts) and their bedmates should be treated at the same time.

Do Head Lice Spread Disease?

Head lice should not be considered as a medical or public health hazard. Head lice are not known to spread disease. Head lice can be an annoyance because their presence may cause itching and loss of sleep. Sometimes the itching can lead to excessive scratching that can sometimes increase the chance of a secondary skin infection.

Can Head Lice Be Spread by Sharing Sports Helmets and Headphones?

Head lice are spread most commonly by direct contact with thc hair of an infested person. Spread by contact with inanimate objects and personal belongings may occur but is very uncommon. Head lice feet are specially adapted for holding onto human hair. Head lice would have difficulty attaching firmly to smooth or slippery surfaces like plastic, metal, polished synthetic leathers, and other similar materials.

Can Wigs or Hair Pieces Spread Lice?

Head lice and their eggs (nits) soon perish if separated from their human host. Adult head lice can live only a day or so off the human head without blood for feeding. Nymphs (young head lice) can live only for several hours without feeding on a human. Nits (head lice eggs) generally die within a week away from their human host and cannot hatch at a temperature lower than that close to the human scalp. For these reasons, the risk of transmission of head lice from a wig or other hairpiece is extremely small, particularly if the wig or hairpiece has not been worn within the preceding 48 hours by someone who is actively infested with live head lice.

Can Swimming Spread Lice?

Data show that head lice can survive underwater for several hours but are unlikely to be spread by the water in a swimming pool. Head lice have been seen to hold tightly to human hair and not let go when submerged under water. Chlorine levels found in pool water do not kill head lice.

Head lice may be spread by sharing towels or other items that have been in contact with an infested person's hair, although such spread is uncommon. Children should be taught not to share towels, hair brushes, and similar items either at poolside or in the changing room.

Swimming or washing the hair within 1–2 days after treatment with some head lice medicines might make some treatments less effective. Seek the advice of your healthcare provider or health department if you have questions.

Is There a Treatment Recommendation for Certain Age Groups?

Before treating young children, please consult the child's doctor, or the health department for the recommended treatment based on the child's age and weight.

Is It Necessary to Remove All the Nits?

No. The two treatments 9 days apart are designed to eliminate all live lice, and any lice that may hatch from eggs that were laid after the first treatment.

Many nits are more than ¼-inch from the scalp. Such nits are usually not viable and very unlikely to hatch to become crawling lice, or may in fact be empty shells, also known as casings. Nits are cemented to hair shafts and are very unlikely to be transferred successfully to other people.

However, parents may choose to remove all nits found on hair for aesthetic reasons or to reduce the chance of unnecessary retreatment.

Where Can I Go to Have the Nits Removed from Hair?

Centers for Disease Control and Prevention (CDC) does not make recommendations about businesses that may offer such services. Your healthcare provider or local health department may be able to provide additional guidance. Removal of all nits after successful treatment with a pediculicide is not necessary to prevent further spread of head lice. Removal of nits after treatment with a pediculicide may be done for aesthetic reasons, or to reduce diagnostic confusion and the chance of unnecessary retreatment. Because pediculicides are not 100% ovicidal (i.e., do not kill all the egg stages), some experts recommend the manual removal of nits that are attached less than 1 cm of the base of the hair shaft.

Why Do Some Experts Recommend Bagging Items for Two Weeks?

Head lice survive less than one or two days if they fall off the scalp and cannot feed. Head lice eggs (nits) cannot hatch and usually die within a week if they do not remain under ideal conditions of heat and humidity similar to those found close to the human scalp. Therefore, because a nit must incubate under conditions equivalent to those found near the human scalp, it is very unlikely to hatch away from the head. In addition, if the egg were to hatch, the newly emerged nymph would die within several hours if it did not feed on human blood.

However, although rarely necessary, some experts recommend that items that may be contaminated by an infested person and that cannot be laundered or dry-cleaned should be sealed in plastic bag and stored for 2 weeks to kill any lice that already are present or that might hatch from any nits that may be present on the items.

Should Household Sprays Be Used to Kill Adult Lice?

No. Using fumigant sprays or fogs is NOT recommended. Fumigant sprays and fogs can be toxic if inhaled or absorbed through the skin and they are not necessary to control head lice.

Do I Need to Have My Home Fumigated?

No. Use of insecticide sprays or fogs is NOT recommended. Fumigant spray and fogs can be toxic if inhaled or absorbed through the skin and they are not necessary to control head lice.

Routine house cleaning, including vacuuming of carpeting, rugs, furniture, car seats, and other fabric covered items, as well as laundering of linens and clothing worn or used by the infested person is sufficient. Only items that have been in contact with the head of the infested person in the 48 hours before treatment need be considered for cleaning.

Should I Have a Pest Control Company Spray My House?

No. Use of insecticide sprays or fogs is NOT recommended. Fumigant spray and fogs can be toxic if inhaled or absorbed through the skin and they are not necessary to control head lice.

Routine vacuuming of floors and furniture is sufficient to remove lice or nits that may have fallen off the head of an infested person.

Section 14.7

Enterobiasis (Pinworm Infection)

This section includes text excerpted from "Pinworm Infection FAQs," Centers for Disease Control and Prevention (CDC), January 10, 2013.

What Is a Pinworm?

A pinworm ("threadworm") is a small, thin, white roundworm (nematode) called *Enterobius vermicularis* that sometimes lives in the colon and rectum of humans. Pinworms are about the length of a staple. While an infected person sleeps, female pinworms leave the intestine through the anus and deposit their eggs on the surrounding skin.

What Are the Symptoms of a Pinworm Infection?

Pinworm infection (called enterobiasis or oxyuriasis) causes itching around the anus which can lead to difficulty sleeping and restlessness. Symptoms are caused by the female pinworm laying her eggs. Symptoms of pinworm infection usually are mild and some infected people have no symptoms.

Who Is at Risk for Pinworm Infection?

Pinworm infection occurs worldwide and affects persons of all ages and socioeconomic levels. It is the most common worm infection in the United States. Pinworm infection occurs most commonly among:

- school-aged and preschool-aged children,
- institutionalized persons, and
- household members and caretakers of persons with pinworm infection.

Pinworm infection often occurs in more than one person in household and institutional settings. Child care centers often are the site of cases of pinworm infection.

How Is Pinworm Infection Spread?

Pinworm infection is spread by the fecal-oral route, that is by the transfer of infective pinworm eggs from the anus to someone's mouth, either directly by hand or indirectly through contaminated clothing, bedding, food, or other articles.

Pinworm eggs become infective within a few hours after being deposited on the skin around the anus and can survive for 2 to 3 weeks on clothing, bedding, or other objects. People become infected, usually unknowingly, by swallowing (ingesting) infective pinworm eggs that are on fingers, under fingernails, or on clothing, bedding, and other contaminated objects and surfaces. Because of their small size, pinworm eggs sometimes can become airborne and ingested while breathing.

Can My Family Become Infected with Pinworms from Swimming Pools?

Pinworm infections are rarely spread through the use of swimming pools. Pinworm infections occur when a person swallows pinworm eggs picked up from contaminated surfaces or fingers. Although chlorine levels found in pools are not high enough to kill pinworm eggs, the presence of a small number of pinworm eggs in thousands of gallons of water (the amount typically found in pools) makes the chance of infection unlikely.

My Little Kids Like to Co-Bathe–Could This Be How They Are Becoming Infected?

During this treatment time and two weeks after final treatment, it is a good idea to avoid co-bathing and the reuse or sharing of washcloths.

Showering may be preferred to avoid possible contamination of bath water. Careful handling and frequent changing of underclothing, night clothes, towels, and bedding can help reduce infection, reinfection, and environmental contamination with pinworm eggs. These items should be laundered in hot water, especially after each treatment of the infected person and after each usage of washcloths until infection is cleared.

How Is Pinworm Infection Diagnosed?

Itching during the night in a child's perianal area strongly suggests pinworm infection. Diagnosis is made by identifying the worm or its eggs. Worms can sometimes be seen on the skin near the anus or on underclothing, pajamas, or sheets about 2 to 3 hours after falling asleep.

Pinworm eggs can be collected and examined using the "tape test" as soon as the person wakes up. This "test" is done by firmly pressing the adhesive side of clear, transparent cellophane tape to the skin around the anus. The eggs stick to the tape and the tape can be placed on a slide and looked at under a microscope. Because washing/bathing or having a bowel movement can remove eggs from the skin, this test should be done as soon as the person wakes up in the morning before they wash, bathe, go to the toilet, or get dressed. The "tape test" should be done on three consecutive mornings to increase the chance of finding pinworm eggs.

Because itching and scratching of the anal area is common in pinworm infection, samples taken from under the fingernails may also contain eggs. Pinworm eggs rarely are found in routine stool or urine samples.

How Is Pinworm Infection Treated?

Pinworm can be treated with either prescription or over-the-counter medications. A healthcare provider should be consulted before treating a suspected case of pinworm infection.

Treatment involves two doses of medication with the second dose being given 2 weeks after the first dose. All household contacts and caretakers of the infected person should be treated at the same time. Reinfection can occur easily so strict observance of good hand hygiene is essential (e.g., proper handwashing, maintaining clean short fingernails, avoiding nail biting, avoiding scratching the perianal area).

Daily morning bathing and daily changing of underwear helps removes a large proportion of eggs. Showering may be preferred to avoid possible contamination of bath water. Careful handling and frequent changing of underclothing, night clothes, towels, and bedding can help reduce infection, reinfection, and environmental contamination with pinworm eggs. These items should be laundered in hot water, especially after each treatment of the infected person and after each usage of washcloths until infection is cleared.

Should Family and Other Close Contacts of Someone with Pinworm Also Be Treated for Pinworm?

Yes. The infected person and all household contacts and caretakers of the infected person should be treated at the same time.

Section 14.8

Scabies

This section includes text excerpted from "Scabies Frequently Asked Questions (FAQs)," Centers for Disease Control and Prevention (CDC), November 2, 2010. Reviewed October 2016.

What Is Scabies?

Scabies is an infestation of the skin by the human itch mite (*Sarcoptes scabiei var. hominis*). The microscopic scabies mite burrows into the upper layer of the skin where it lives and lays its eggs. The most common symptoms of scabies are intense itching and a pimple-like skin rash. The scabies mite usually is spread by direct, prolonged, skin-to-skin contact with a person who has scabies.

Scabies is found worldwide and affects people of all races and social classes. Scabies can spread rapidly under crowded conditions where close body and skin contact is frequent. Institutions such as nursing homes, extended-care facilities, and prisons are often sites of scabies outbreaks. Child care facilities also are a common site of scabies infestations.

What Is Crusted (Norwegian) Scabies?

Crusted scabies is a severe form of scabies that can occur in some persons who are immunocompromised (have a weak immune system), elderly, disabled, or debilitated. It is also called Norwegian scabies. Persons with crusted scabies have thick crusts of skin that contain large numbers of scabies mites and eggs. Persons with crusted scabies are very contagious to other persons and can spread the infestation easily both by direct skin-to-skin contact and by contamination of items such as their clothing, bedding, and furniture. Persons with crusted scabies may not show the usually signs and symptoms of scabies such as the characteristic rash or itching (pruritus). Persons with crusted scabies should receive quick and aggressive medical treatment for their infestation to prevent outbreaks of scabies.

How Soon after Infestation Do Symptoms of Scabies Begin?

If a person has never had scabies before, symptoms may take as long as 4–6 weeks to begin. It is important to remember that an infested person can spread scabies during this time, even if he/she does not have symptoms yet.

In a person who has had scabies before, symptoms usually appear much sooner (1–4 days) after exposure.

What Are the Signs and Symptoms of Scabies Infestation?

The most common signs and symptoms of scabies are intense itching (pruritus), especially at night, and a pimple-like (papular) itchy rash. The itching and rash each may affect much of the body or be limited to common sites such as the wrist, elbow, armpit, webbing between the fingers, nipple, penis, waist, belt-line, and buttocks. The rash also can include tiny blisters (vesicles) and scales. Scratching the rash can cause skin sores; sometimes these sores become infected by bacteria.

Tiny burrows sometimes are seen on the skin; these are caused by the female scabies mite tunneling just beneath the surface of the skin. These burrows appear as tiny raised and crooked (serpiginous) grayish-white or skin-colored lines on the skin surface. Because mites are often few in number (only 10–15 mites per person), these burrows may be difficult to find. They are found most often in the webbing between the fingers, in the skin folds on the wrist, elbow, or knee, and on the penis, breast, or shoulder blades.

The head, face, neck, palms, and soles often are involved in infants and very young children, but usually not adults and older children.

Persons with crusted scabies may not show the usual signs and symptoms of scabies such as the characteristic rash or itching (pruritus).

How Did I Get Scabies?

Scabies usually is spread by direct, prolonged, skin-to-skin contact with a person who has scabies. Contact generally must be prolonged; a quick handshake or hug usually will not spread scabies. Scabies sometimes is spread indirectly by sharing articles such as clothing, towels, or bedding used by an infested person; however, such indirect spread can occur much more easily when the infested person has crusted scabies.

How Is Scabies Infestation Diagnosed?

Diagnosis of a scabies infestation usually is made based on the customary appearance and distribution of the rash and the presence of burrows. Whenever possible, the diagnosis of scabies should be confirmed by identifying the mite, mite eggs, or mite fecal matter (scybala). This can be done by carefully removing a mite from the end of its burrow using the tip of a needle or by obtaining skin scraping to examine under a microscope for mites, eggs, or mite fecal matter. It is important to remember that a person can still be infested even if mites, eggs, or fecal matter cannot be found; typically fewer than 10–15 mites can be present on the entire body of an infested person who is otherwise healthy. However, persons with crusted scabies can be infested with thousands of mites and should be considered highly contagious.

Can Scabies Be Treated?

Yes. Products used to treat scabies are called *scabicides* because they kill scabies mites; some also kill eggs. Scabicides to treat human scabies are available only with a doctor's prescription; no "over-the-counter" (non-prescription) products have been tested and approved for humans.

Always follow carefully the instructions provided by the doctor and pharmacist, as well as those contained in the box or printed on the label. When treating adults and older children, scabicide cream or lotion is applied to all areas of the body from the neck down to the feet and toes; when treating infants and young children, the cream or lotion also is applied to the head and neck. The medication should be left on the body for the recommended time before it is washed off. Clean clothes should be worn after treatment.

All persons should be treated at the same time in order to prevent reinfestation. Retreatment may be necessary if itching continues more than 2–4 weeks after treatment or if new burrows or rash continue to appear.

Never use a scabicide intended for veterinary or agricultural use to treat humans!

Who Should Be Treated for Scabies?

Anyone who is diagnosed with scabies, as well as his or her sexual partners and other contacts who have had prolonged skin-to-skin contact with the infested person, should be treated. Treatment is recommended for members of the same household as the person with scabies, particularly those persons who have had prolonged skin-to-skin contact with the infested person. All persons should be treated at the same time to prevent reinfestation.

Retreatment may be necessary if itching continues more than 2–4 weeks after treatment or if new burrows or rash continue to appear.

How Soon After Treatment Will I Feel Better?

If itching continues more than 2–4 weeks after initial treatment or if new burrows or rash continue to appear (if initial treatment includes more than one application or dose, then the 2–4 time period begins after the last application or dose), retreatment with scabicide may be necessary; seek the advice of a physician.

Did I Get Scabies from My Pet?

No. Animals do not spread human scabies. Pets can become infested with a different kind of scabies mite that does not survive or reproduce on humans but causes "mange" in animals. If an animal with "mange" has close contact with a person, the animal mite can get under the person's skin and cause temporary itching and skin irritation. However, the animal mite cannot reproduce on a person and will die on its own in a couple of days. Although the person does not need to be treated, the animal should be treated because its mites can continue to burrow into the person's skin and cause symptoms until the animal has been treated successfully.

Can Scabies Be Spread by Swimming in a Public Pool?

Scabies is spread by prolonged skin-to-skin contact with a person who has scabies. Scabies sometimes also can be spread by contact with items such as clothing, bedding, or towels that have been used by a person with scabies, but such spread is very uncommon unless the infested person has crusted scabies.

Scabies is very unlikely to be spread by water in a swimming pool. Except for a person with crusted scabies, only about 10–15 scabies mites are present on an infested person; it is extremely unlikely that any would emerge from under wet skin.

Although uncommon, scabies can be spread by sharing a towel or item of clothing that has been used by a person with scabies.

How Can I Remove Scabies Mites from My House or Carpet?

Scabies mites do not survive more than 2–3 days away from human skin. Items such as bedding, clothing, and towels used by a person with scabies can be decontaminated by machine-washing in hot water and drying using the hot cycle or by dry-cleaning. Items that cannot be washed or dry-cleaned can be decontaminated by removing from any body contact for at least 72 hours.

Because persons with crusted scabies are considered very infectious, careful vacuuming of furniture and carpets in rooms used by these persons is recommended.

Fumigation of living areas is unnecessary.

How Can I Remove Scabies Mites from My Clothes?

Scabies mites do not survive more than 2–3 days away from human skin. Items such as bedding, clothing, and towels used by a person with scabies can be decontaminated by machine-washing in hot water and drying using the hot cycle or by dry-cleaning. Items that cannot be washed or dry-cleaned can be decontaminated by removing from any body contact for at least 72 hours.

Because persons with crusted scabies are considered very infectious, careful vacuuming of furniture and carpets in rooms used by these persons is recommended.

Fumigation of living areas is unnecessary.

If I Come in Contact with A Person Who Has Scabies, Should I Treat Myself?

No. If a person thinks he or she might have scabies, he/she should contact a doctor. The doctor can examine the person, confirm the diagnosis of scabies, and prescribe an appropriate treatment. Products used to treat scabies in humans are available only with a doctor's prescription.

Sleeping with any scabies infested person presents a high risk for transmission. The longer a person has skin-to-skin exposure, the greater is the likelihood for transmission to occur. Although briefly shaking hands with a person who has non-crusted scabies could be considered as presenting a relatively low risk, holding the hand of a person with scabies for 5–10 minutes could be considered to present a relatively high risk of transmission. However, transmission can occur even after brief skin-to-skin contact, such as a handshake, with a person who has crusted scabies. In general, a person who has skin-to-skin contact with a person who has crusted scabies would be considered a good candidate for treatment.

To determine when prophylactic treatment should be given to reduce the risk of transmission, early consultation should be sought with a healthcare provider who understands:

1. the type of scabies (i.e., non-crusted vs crusted) to which a person has been exposed;
2. the degree and duration of skin exposure that a person has had to the infested patient;
3. whether the exposure occurred before or after the patient was treated for scabies; and,
4. whether the exposed person works in an environment where he/she would be likely to expose other people during the asymptomatic incubation period. For example, a nurse or caretaker who works in a nursing home or hospital often would be treated prophylactically to reduce the risk of further scabies transmission in the facility.

Section 14.9

Cercarial Dermatitis (Swimmer's Itch)

This section includes text excerpted from "Swimmer's Itch FAQs," Centers for Disease Control and Prevention (CDC), January 10, 2012. Reviewed October 2016.

What Is Swimmer's Itch?

Swimmer's itch, also called cercarial dermatitis, appears as a skin rash caused by an allergic reaction to certain microscopic parasites that infect some birds and mammals. These parasites are released from infected snails into fresh and salt water (such as lakes, ponds, and oceans). While the parasite's preferred host is the specific bird or mammal, if the parasite comes into contact with a swimmer, it burrows into the skin causing an allergic reaction and rash. Swimmer's itch is found throughout the world and is more frequent during summer months.

What Are the Signs and Symptoms of Swimmer's Itch?

Symptoms of swimmer's itch may include:

- tingling, burning, or itching of the skin
- small reddish pimples
- small blisters

Within minutes to days after swimming in contaminated water, you may experience tingling, burning, or itching of the skin. Small reddish pimples appear within twelve hours. Pimples may develop into small blisters. Scratching the areas may result in secondary bacterial infections. Itching may last up to a week or more, but will gradually go away.

Because swimmer's itch is caused by an allergic reaction to infection, the more often you swim or wade in contaminated water, the more likely you are to develop more serious symptoms. The greater the number of exposures to contaminated water, the more intense and immediate symptoms of swimmer's itch will be.

Be aware that swimmer's itch is not the only rash that may occur after swimming in fresh or salt water.

Do I Need to See My Healthcare Provider for Treatment?

Most cases of swimmer's itch do not require medical attention. If you have a rash, you may try the following for relief:

- Use corticosteroid cream
- Apply cool compresses to the affected areas
- Bathe in Epsom salts or baking soda
- Soak in colloidal oatmeal baths
- Apply baking soda paste to the rash (made by stirring water into baking soda until it reaches a paste-like consistency)
- Use an anti-itch lotion

Though difficult, try not to scratch. Scratching may cause the rash to become infected. If itching is severe, your healthcare provider may suggest prescription-strength lotions or creams to lessen your symptoms.

Can Swimmer's Itch Be Spread from Person-to-Person?

Swimmer's itch is not contagious and cannot be spread from one person to another.

Who Is at Risk for Swimmer's Itch?

Anyone who swims or wades in infested water may be at risk. Larvae are more likely to be present in shallow water by the shoreline. Children are most often affected because they tend to swim, wade, and play in the shallow water more than adults. Also, they are less likely to towel dry themselves when leaving the water.

Once an Outbreak of Swimmer's Itch Has Occurred in Water, Will the Water Always Be Unsafe?

No. Many factors must be present for swimmer's itch to become a problem in water. Since these factors change (sometimes within a swim season), swimmer's itch will not always be a problem. However, there is no way to know how long water may be unsafe. Larvae generally survive for 24 hours once they are released from the snail. However, an infected snail will continue to produce cercariae throughout the remainder of its life. For future snails to become infected, migratory birds or mammals in the area must also be infected so the lifecycle can continue.

Is It Safe to Swim in My Swimming Pool?

Yes. As long as your swimming pool is well maintained and chlorinated, there is no risk of swimmer's itch. The appropriate snails must be present in order for swimmer's itch to occur.

What Can Be Done to Reduce the Risk of Swimmer's Itch?

To reduce the likelihood of developing swimmer's itch:

- Do not swim in areas where swimmer's itch is a known problem or where signs have been posted warning of unsafe water.
- Do not swim near or wade in marshy areas where snails are commonly found.
- Towel dry or shower immediately after leaving the water.
- Do not attract birds (e.g., by feeding them) to areas where people are swimming.
- Encourage health officials to post signs on shorelines where swimmer's itch is a current problem.

Section 14.10

Dermatophytes (Tinea and Ringworm)

This section includes text excerpted from "Ringworm," Centers for Disease Control and Prevention (CDC), December 4, 2015.

What Is Ringworm?

Ringworm is a common infection of the skin and nails that is caused by fungus. The infection is called "ringworm" because it can cause an itchy, red, circular rash. Ringworm is also called "tinea" or "dermatophytosis." The different types of ringworm are usually named for the location of the infection on the body.

Areas of the body that can be affected by ringworm include:

- Feet (tinea pedis, commonly called "athlete's foot")
- Groin, inner thighs, or buttocks (tinea cruris, commonly called "jock itch")
- Scalp (tinea capitis)
- Beard (tinea barbae)
- Hands (tinea manuum)
- Toenails or fingernails (tinea unguium, also called "onychomycosis") Click here for more information about fungal nail infections. Note: please link this last sentence to the new nail infections page.
- Other parts of the body such as arms or legs (tinea corporis)

Approximately 40 different species of fungi can cause ringworm; the scientific names for the types of fungi that cause ringworm are *Trichophyton, Microsporum,* and *Epidermophyton.*

Who Gets Ringworm?

Ringworm is very common. Anyone can get ringworm, but people who have weakened immune systems may be especially at risk for infection and may have problems fighting off a ringworm infection. People who use public showers or locker rooms, athletes (particularly those who are involved in contact sports such as wrestling), people who wear tight shoes and have excessive sweating, and people who have close contact with animals may also be more likely to come in contact with the fungi that cause ringworm.

What Are Symptoms of Ringworm Infections?

Ringworm can affect skin on almost any part of the body as well as fingernails and toenails. The symptoms of ringworm often depend on which part of the body is infected, but they generally include:

- Itchy skin
- Ring-shaped rash

- Red, scaly, cracked skin
- Hair loss

Symptoms typically appear between 4 and 14 days after the skin comes in contact with the fungi that cause ringworm.

Symptoms of ringworm by location on the body:

- Feet (tinea pedis or "athlete's foot"): The symptoms of ringworm on the feet include red, swollen, peeling, itchy skin between the toes (especially between the pinky toe and the one next to it). The sole and heel of the foot may also be affected. In severe cases, the skin on the feet can blister.
- Scalp (tinea capitis): Ringworm on the scalp usually looks like a scaly, itchy, red, circular bald spot. The bald spot can grow in size and multiple spots might develop if the infection spreads. Ringworm on the scalp is more common in children than it is in adults.
- Groin (tinea cruris or "jock itch"): Ringworm on the groin looks like scaly, itchy, red spots, usually on the inner sides of the skin folds of the thigh.
- Beard (tinea barbae): Symptoms of ringworm on the beard include scaly, itchy, red spots on the cheeks, chin, and upper neck. The spots might become crusted over or filled with pus, and the affected hair might fall out.

How Can I Prevent Ringworm?

- Keep your skin clean and dry.
- Wear shoes that allow air to circulate freely around your feet.
- Don't walk barefoot in areas like locker rooms or public showers.
- Clip your fingernails and toenails short and keep them clean.
- Change your socks and underwear at least once a day.
- Don't share clothing, towels, sheets, or other personal items with someone who has ringworm.
- Wash your hands with soap and running water after playing with pets. If you suspect that your pet has ringworm, take it to see a veterinarian. If your pet has ringworm, follow the steps below to prevent spreading the infection.

- If you're an athlete involved in close contact sports, shower immediately after your practice session or match, and keep all of your sports gear and uniform clean. Don't share sports gear (helmet, etc.) with other players.

My Pet Has Ringworm and I'm Worried about Ringworm in My House. What Should I Do?

Ringworm can easily transfer from animals to humans.5 You can take the following steps to protect yourself and your pet:

For people

Do

- Wash your hands with soap and running water after playing with or petting your pet.
- Wear gloves and long sleeves if you must handle animals with ringworm, and always wash your hands after handling the animal.
- Vacuum the areas of the home that the infected pet commonly visits. This will help to remove infected fur or flakes of skin.
- Disinfect areas the pet has spent time in, including surfaces and bedding.
- The spores of this fungus can be killed with common disinfectants like diluted chlorine bleach (1/4 c per gallon water), benzalkonium chloride, or strong detergents.
- Never mix cleaning products. This may cause harmful gases.

Do not handle animals with ringworm if your immune system is weak in any way (if you have HIV/AIDS, are undergoing cancer treatment, or are taking medications that suppress the immune system, for example).

For pets

Protect your pet's health

- If you suspect that your pet has ringworm, make sure it is seen by a veterinarian so treatment can be started.
- If one of your pets has ringworm, make sure you have every pet in the household checked for ringworm infection.

What Is Diagnosis of Ringworm?

Your healthcare provider can usually diagnose ringworm by looking at the affected skin and asking questions about your symptoms. He or she may also take a small skin scraping to be examined under a microscope or sent to a laboratory for a fungal culture.

What Is Treatment for Ringworm?

The treatment for ringworm depends on its location on the body and how serious the infection is. Some forms of ringworm can be treated with non-prescription ("over-the-counter") medications, but other forms of ringworm need treatment with prescription antifungal medication.

- **Ringworm on the skin** like athlete's foot (tinea pedis) and jock itch (tinea cruris) can usually be treated with non-prescription antifungal creams, lotions, or powders applied to the skin for 2 to 4 weeks. There are many non-prescription products available to treat ringworm, including:
    - Clotrimazole (Lotrimin, Mycelex)
    - Miconazole (Aloe Vesta Antifungal, Azolen, Baza Antifungal, Carrington Antifungal, Critic Aid Clear, Cruex Prescription Strength, DermaFungal, Desenex, Fungoid Tincture, Micaderm, Micatin, Micro-Guard, Miranel, Mitrazol, Podactin, Remedy Antifungal, Secura Antifungal)
    - Terbinafine (Lamisil)
    - Ketoconazole (Xolegel)

For non-prescription creams, lotions, or powders, follow the directions on the package label. Contact your healthcare provider if your infection doesn't go away or gets worse.

- **Ringworm on the scalp** (tinea capitis) usually needs to be treated with prescription antifungal medication taken by mouth for 1 to 3 months. Creams, lotions, or powders don't work for ringworm on the scalp. Prescription antifungal medications used to treat ringworm on the scalp include:
    - Griseofulvin (Grifulvin V, Gris-PEG)
    - Terbinafine
    - Itraconazole (Onmel, Sporanox)
    - Fluconazole (Diflucan)

You should contact your healthcare provider if:

- Your infection gets worse or doesn't go away after using non-prescription medications.
- You or your child has ringworm on the scalp. Ringworm on the scalp needs to be treated with prescription antifungal medication.

Section 14.11

Toxocariasis

This section includes text excerpted from "Toxocariasis FAQs," Centers for Disease Control and Prevention (CDC), January 10, 2013.

What Is Toxocariasis?

Toxocariasis is an infection transmitted from animals to humans (zoonosis) caused by the parasitic roundworms commonly found in the intestine of dogs (*Toxocara canis*) and cats (*T. cati*).

Who Is at Risk for Toxocariasis?

Anyone can become infected with *Toxocara.* Young children and owners of dogs or cats have a higher chance of becoming infected.

Approximately 13.9% of the United States population has antibodies to *Toxocara*. This suggests that tens of millions of Americans may have been exposed to the *Toxocara* parasite.

How Can I Get Toxocariasis?

Dogs and cats that are infected with *Toxocara* can shed *Toxocara* eggs in their feces. You or your children can become infected by accidentally swallowing dirt that has been contaminated with dog or cat feces that contain infectious *Toxocara* eggs. Although it is rare, people can also become infected from eating undercooked meat containing *Toxocara* larvae.

What Are the Clinical Manifestations of Toxocariasis?

Many people who are infected with *Toxocara* do not have symptoms and do not ever get sick. Some people may get sick from the infection, and may develop:

- **Ocular toxocariasis:** Ocular toxocariasis occurs when *Toxocara* larvae migrate to the eye. Symptoms and signs of ocular toxocariasis include vision loss, eye inflammation or damage to the retina. Typically, only one eye is affected.
- **Visceral toxocariasis:** Visceral toxocariasis occurs when *Toxocara* larvae migrate to various body organs, such as the liver or central nervous system. Symptoms of visceral toxocariasis include fever, fatigue, coughing, wheezing, or abdominal pain.

How Serious Is Infection with Toxocara?

In most cases, *Toxocara* infections are not serious, and many people, especially adults infected by a small number of larvae (immature worms), may not notice any symptoms. The most severe cases are rare, but are more likely to occur in young children, who often play in dirt, or eat dirt (pica) contaminated by dog or cat feces.

How Is Toxocariasis Spread?

The most common *Toxocara* parasite of concern to humans is *T. canis*, which puppies usually contract from the mother before birth or from her milk. The larvae mature rapidly in the puppy's intestine; when the pup is 3 or 4 weeks old, they begin to produce large numbers of eggs that contaminate the environment through the animal's feces. Over a 2 to 4 week time period, infective larvae develop in the eggs. Toxocariasis is not spread by person-to-person contact like a cold or the flu.

What Should I Do If I Think I Have Toxocariasis?

See your healthcare provider to discuss the possibility of infection and, if necessary, to be examined. Your provider may take a sample of your blood for testing.

What Is the Treatment for Toxocariasis?

Visceral toxocariasis is treated with antiparasitic drugs. Treatment of ocular toxocariasis is more difficult and usually consists of measures to prevent progressive damage to the eye.

How Do I Prevent Toxocariasis?

- Take your pets to the veterinarian to prevent infection with *Toxocara*. Your veterinarian can recommend a testing and treatment plan for deworming.
- Wash your hands with soap and water after playing with your pets or other animals, after outdoor activities, and before handling food.
- Teach children the importance of washing hands to prevent infection.
- Do not allow children to play in areas that are soiled with pet or other animal feces.
- Clean your pet's living area at least once a week. Feces should be either buried or bagged and disposed of in the trash. Wash your hands after handling pet waste.
- Teach children that it is dangerous to eat dirt or soil.

Chapter 15

Other Diseases Associated with Infections

Chapter Contents

Section 15.1

Encephalitis and Meningitis

This section includes text excerpted from "Meningitis and Encephalitis Fact Sheet," National Institute of Neurological Disorders and Stroke (NINDS), February 23, 2016.

What Are Meningitis and Encephalitis?

Infections, and less commonly other causes, in the brain and spinal cord can cause dangerous inflammation. This inflammation can produce a wide range of symptoms, including fever, headache, seizures, change in behavior or confusion and, in extreme cases, can cause brain damage, stroke, or even death.

Infection of the meninges, the membranes that surround the brain and spinal cord, is called meningitis. Inflammation of the brain itself is called *encephalitis*. *Myelitis* refers to inflammation of the spinal cord. When both the brain and the spinal cord are involved, the condition is called *encephalomyelitis*.

What Causes Meningitis and Encephalitis?

Infectious causes of meningitis and encephalitis include bacteria, viruses, fungi, and parasites. Many of these affect healthy people. For others, environmental and exposure history, recent travel or immunocompromised state (such as human immunodeficiency virus (HIV), diabetes, steroids, chemotherapy) are important elements. There are also non-infectious causes such as autoimmune causes and medications.

Who Is at Risk for Encephalitis and Meningitis?

Anyone can get encephalitis or meningitis. People with weakened immune systems, including those persons with HIV or those taking immunosuppressant drugs, are at increased risk.

How Are These Disorders Transmitted?

Some forms of bacterial meningitis and encephalitis are contagious and can be spread through contact with saliva, nasal discharge, feces, or respiratory and throat secretions (often spread through kissing, coughing, or sharing drinking glasses, eating utensils, or such personal items as toothbrushes, lipstick, or cigarettes). For example, people sharing a household, at a daycare center, or in a classroom with an infected person can become infected. College students living in dormitories—in particular, college freshmen—have a higher risk of contracting meningococcal meningitis than college students overall. Children who have not been given routine vaccines are at increased risk of developing certain types of bacterial meningitis.

Because these diseases can occur suddenly and progress rapidly, anyone who is suspected of having either meningitis or encephalitis should immediately contact a doctor or go to the hospital.

What Are the Signs and Symptoms?

The hallmark signs of meningitis are sudden fever, severe headache, nausea/vomiting, double vision, drowsiness, sensitivity to bright light, and a stiff neck; encephalitis can be characterized by fever, seizures, change in behavior, confusion and disorientation, and related neurological signs depending on which part of the brain is affected by the encephalitic process, as some of these are quite focal (locally centered) while others are more global.

Meningitis often appears with flu-like symptoms that develop over 1–2 days. Distinctive rashes are typically seen in some forms of the disease. Meningococcal meningitis may be associated with kidney and adrenal gland failure and shock.

Individuals with encephalitis often show mild flu-like symptoms. In more severe cases, patients may experience problems with speech or hearing, double vision, hallucinations, personality changes, loss of consciousness, loss of sensation in some parts of the body, muscle weakness, partial paralysis in the arms and legs, sudden severe dementia, seizures, and memory loss.

Important signs of meningitis or encephalitis to watch for in an infant include fever, lethargy, not waking for feeding, vomiting, body stiffness, unexplained or unusual irritability, and a full or bulging fontanel (the soft spot on the top of the head).

How Are Meningitis and Encephalitis Diagnosed?

Following a physical exam and medical history to review activities of the past several days/weeks (such as recent exposure to insects or animals, any contact with ill persons, recent travel, or preexisting medical conditions and medications list), the doctor may order various diagnostic tests to confirm the presence of infection and inflammation. Early diagnosis is vital, as symptoms can appear suddenly and escalate to brain damage, hearing and/or speech loss, blindness, or even death.

A neurological examination involves a series of tests designed to assess motor and sensory function, nerve function, hearing and speech, vision, coordination and balance, mental status, and changes in mood or behavior.

Laboratory screening of blood, urine, and body secretions can help detect and identify brain and/or spinal cord infection and determine the presence of antibodies and foreign proteins. Such tests can also rule out metabolic conditions that have similar symptoms.

Analysis of the cerebrospinal fluid that surrounds and protects the brain and spinal cord can detect infections in the brain and/or spinal cord, acute and chronic inflammation, and other diseases.

Brain imaging can reveal signs of brain inflammation, internal bleeding or hemorrhage, or other brain abnormalities.

Electroencephalography, or EEG, can identify abnormal brain waves by monitoring electrical activity in the brain through the skull. Among its many functions, EEG is used to help diagnose seizures or patterns that may suggest specific viral infections such as herpes virus, and to detect subclinical seizures which may contribute to abnormalities in level of consciousness in critically ill individuals.

How Are These Infections Treated?

Persons who are suspected of having meningitis or encephalitis should receive immediate, aggressive medical treatment. Both diseases can progress quickly and have the potential to cause severe, irreversible neurological damage.

Meningitis

Early treatment of bacterial meningitis is important to its outcome, with antibiotics that can cross the protective blood-brain lining. Appropriate antibiotic treatment for most types of meningitis can reduce the risk of dying from the disease to below 15 percent.

Infected sinuses may need to be drained. Corticosteroids such as prednisone may be ordered to relieve brain pressure and swelling and to prevent hearing loss that is common in patients with *Haemophilus influenza meningitis*. Lyme disease is treated with intravenous antibiotics.

Unlike bacteria, viruses cannot be killed by antibiotics; generally there is no specific treatment for viruses except for the herpes virus, which can be treated with the antiviral drug acyclovir. The physician may prescribe anticonvulsants such as dilantin or phenytoin to prevent seizures and corticosteroids to reduce brain inflammation. If inflammation is severe, pain medicine and sedatives may be prescribed to make the person more comfortable.

Acute disseminated encephalomyelitis is treated with steroids. Fungal meningitis is treated with intravenous antifungal medications.

Encephalitis

Antiviral drugs used to treat viral encephalitis include acyclovir and ganciclovir.

Anticonvulsants may be prescribed to stop or prevent seizures. Corticosteroids can reduce brain swelling. Individuals with breathing difficulties may require artificial respiration.

Autoimmune causes of encephalitis are treated with additional immunosuppressant drugs and screening for tumors when appropriate.

Individuals should receive evaluation for comprehensive rehabilitation that might include cognitive rehabilitation, physical, speech, and occupational therapy once the acute illness is under control.

Can Meningitis and Encephalitis Be Prevented?

Avoid sharing food, utensils, glasses, and other objects with a person who may be exposed to or have the infection. Wash hands often with soap and rinse under running water.

Effective vaccines are available to prevent pneumonia, *H. influenza*, pneumococcal meningitis, and infection with other bacteria that can cause meningococcal meningitis.

People who live, work, or go to school with someone who has been diagnosed with bacterial meningitis may be asked to take antibiotics for a few days as a preventive measure.

To lessen the risk of being bitten by an infected mosquito or other insect, people should limit outdoor activities at night, wear long-sleeved clothing when outdoors, use insect repellents that are most effective for that particular region of the country, and rid lawn and outdoor areas of free-standing pools of water, in which mosquitoes breed. Do not over-apply repellants, particularly on young children and especially infants, as chemicals such as DEET may be absorbed through the skin.

What Is the Prognosis for These Infections?

Outcome generally depends on the particular infectious agent involved, the severity of the illness, and how quickly treatment is given. In most cases, people with very mild encephalitis or meningitis can make a full recovery, although the process may be slow.

Individuals who experience only headache, fever, and stiff neck may recover in 2–4 weeks. Those with bacterial meningitis typically show some relief 48–72 hours following initial treatment but are more likely to experience complications caused by the disease. In more serious cases, these diseases can cause hearing and/or speech loss, blindness, permanent brain and nerve damage, behavioral changes, cognitive disabilities, lack of muscle control, seizures, and memory loss. These patients may need long-term therapy, medication, and supportive care. The recovery from encephalitis is variable depending on the cause and extent of brain inflammation.

Section 15.2

Pneumonia

This section includes text excerpted from "Pneumonia Can Be Prevented—Vaccines Can Help," Centers for Disease Control and Prevention (CDC), November 9, 2015.

What Is Pneumonia?

Pneumonia is an infection of the lungs that can cause mild to severe illness in people of all ages. Common signs of pneumonia can include cough, fever, and trouble breathing.

Who Is At Risk for Pneumonia?

Certain people are more likely to become ill with pneumonia:

- Children younger than 5 years old
- People who have underlying medical conditions (like asthma, diabetes or heart disease)

- People who smoke cigarettes
- Adults 65 years or older

Encourage friends and loved ones with certain health conditions, like diabetes and asthma, to get vaccinated.

Causes and Types of Pneumonia

Pneumonia can be caused by viruses, bacteria, and fungi. In the United States, common causes of viral pneumonia are influenza and respiratory syncytial virus (RSV), and a common cause of bacterial pneumonia is *Streptococcus pneumoniae* (pneumococcus). However, clinicians are not always able to find out which germ caused someone to get sick with pneumonia.

When someone develops pneumonia in the community (not in a hospital), it's called community-acquired pneumonia. Pneumonia developed during or following a stay in a healthcare facility (like hospitals, long-term care facilities, and dialysis centers) is called healthcare-associated pneumonia, which includes hospital-acquired pneumonia and ventilator-associated pneumonia. The bacteria and viruses that most commonly cause pneumonia in the community are different from those in healthcare settings.

Pneumonia Can Be Prevented—Vaccines Can Help

Pneumonia, an infection of the lungs, needlessly affects millions of people worldwide each year. Pneumonia infections can often be prevented and can usually be treated.

Globally, pneumonia kills nearly 1 million children younger than 5 years of age each year. This is greater than the number of deaths from any infectious disease, such as HIV infection, malaria or tuberculosis.

Pneumonia isn't just a public health issue in developing countries though. Each year in the United States, about 1 million people have to seek care in a hospital due to pneumonia, and about 50,000 people die from the disease. Most of the people affected by pneumonia in the United States are adults.

Many of these deaths—both globally and in the United States—could be prevented with vaccines and appropriate treatment (like antibiotics and antivirals).

Lower Your Risk with Vaccines

In the United States, there are vaccines that help prevent infection by some of the bacteria and viruses that can cause pneumonia:

- *Haemophilus influenzae* type b (Hib)
- Influenza (flu)
- Measles
- Pertussis (whooping cough)
- Pneumococcus
- Varicella (chickenpox)

These vaccines are safe, but side effects can occur. Most side effects are mild or moderate, meaning they do not affect daily activities.

Protect Your Health with These Healthy Living Practices

Try to stay away from sick people. If you are sick, stay away from others as much as possible to keep from getting them sick. You can also help prevent respiratory infections by:

- Washing your hands regularly
- Cleaning surfaces that are touched a lot
- Coughing or sneezing into a tissue or into your elbow or sleeve
- Limiting contact with cigarette smoke
- Treating and preventing conditions like diabetes

Section 15.3

Reye Syndrome

This section includes text excerpted from "Reye's Syndrome," National Institute of Neurological Disorders and Stroke (NINDS), September 25, 2009. Reviewed October 2016.

What Is Reye Syndrome?

Reye syndrome (RS) is primarily a children's disease, although it can occur at any age. It affects all organs of the body but is most harmful to the brain and the liver—causing an acute increase of pressure within the brain and, often, massive accumulations of fat in the liver and other organs. RS is defined as a two-phase illness because it generally occurs in conjunction with a previous viral infection, such as the flu or chickenpox. The disorder commonly occurs during recovery from a viral infection, although it can also develop 3 to 5 days after the onset of the viral illness. RS is often misdiagnosed as encephalitis, meningitis, diabetes, drug overdose, poisoning, sudden infant death syndrome, or psychiatric illness. Symptoms of RS include persistent or recurrent vomiting, listlessness, personality changes such as irritability or combativeness, disorientation or confusion, delirium, convulsions, and loss of consciousness. If these symptoms are present during or soon after a viral illness, medical attention should be sought immediately. The symptoms of RS in infants do not follow a typical pattern; for example, vomiting does not always occur. Epidemiologic evidence indicates that aspirin (salicylate) is the major preventable risk factor for Reye syndrome. The mechanism by which aspirin and other salicylates trigger Reye syndrome is not completely understood. A "Reye-like" illness may occur in children with genetic metabolic disorders and other toxic disorders. A physician should be consulted before giving a child any aspirin or anti-nausea medicines during a viral illness, which can mask the symptoms of RS.

Is There Any Treatment?

There is no cure for RS. Successful management, which depends on early diagnosis, is primarily aimed at protecting the brain against irreversible damage by reducing brain swelling, reversing the metabolic injury, preventing complications in the lungs, and anticipating cardiac arrest. It has been learned that several inborn errors of metabolism mimic RS in that the first manifestation of these errors may be an encephalopathy with liver dysfunction. These disorders must be considered in all suspected cases of RS. Some evidence suggests that treatment in the end stages of RS with hypertonic intravenous (IV) glucose solutions may prevent progression of the syndrome.

What Is the Prognosis?

Recovery from RS is directly related to the severity of the swelling of the brain. Some people recover completely, while others may sustain varying degrees of brain damage. Those cases in which the disorder progresses rapidly and the patient lapses into a coma have a poorer prognosis than those with a less severe course. Statistics indicate that when RS is diagnosed and treated in its early stages, chances of recovery are excellent. When diagnosis and treatment are delayed, the chances for successful recovery and survival are severely reduced. Unless RS is diagnosed and treated successfully, death is common, often within a few days.

Part Three

Medical Conditions Appearing in Childhood

Chapter 16

Allergies in Children

Chapter Contents

Section 16.1

Allergic Reactions in Kids

This section contains text excerpted from the following sources: Text under the heading "About Allergies" is excerpted from "Fighting Allergy Season with Medications," U.S. Food and Drug Administration (FDA), May 7, 2014; Text beginning with the heading "Allergy and Your Child" is excerpted from "Allergy Relief for Your Child," U.S. Food and Drug Administration (FDA), May 26, 2016.

About Allergies

An allergy is a heightened immune system reaction to a substance that your body has identified as an invader. If you have allergies and encounter a trigger—called an "allergen"—your immune system fights it by making antibodies, which causes your body to release chemicals called histamines. Histamines are responsible for symptoms such as repetitive sneezing and itchy, watery eyes.

Allergic rhinitis affects more than 30 million children and adults in the United States and more than 500 million people worldwide. It may be seasonal or year-round.

The seasonal allergy, often called "hay fever," typically occurs in the spring, summer or fall. If you have this, you may suffer from repetitive sneezing, and stuffy or runny nose and itching in the nose, eyes or on the roof of the mouth. Eye inflammation can occur when your eyes react to allergens with symptoms of reddening, itching and swelling.

Plant pollens usually cause seasonal allergies. Pollen allergies are common, and allergy-causing pollen can come from trees, weeds and grasses, according to the National Institute of Allergy and Infectious Diseases. Trees and grasses are typical spring culprits in the United States, while ragweed and other weeds ramp up in late summer and early fall.

Indoor substances, such as dust mites, often cause the year-round type of allergies. Molds can cause seasonal and year-round allergies.

Allergy and Your Child

Children are magnets for colds. But when the sniffles and sneezing won't go away for weeks, the culprit may be something else: allergies.

Long-lasting sneezing, with a stuffy or runny nose, may signal the presence of allergic rhinitis—the collection of symptoms that affect the nose when you have an allergic reaction to something you breathe in and that lands on the lining inside the nose.

Allergies may be seasonal or they can strike year-round (perennial). In most parts of the United States, plant pollens are often the cause of seasonal allergic rhinitis—more commonly called hay fever. Indoor substances, such as mold, dust mites, and pet dander, may cause the perennial kind.

Up to 40 percent of children suffer from allergic rhinitis, according to the National Institute of Allergy and Infectious Diseases (NIAID). And children are more likely to develop allergies if one or both parents have allergies.

The U.S. Food and Drug Administration (FDA) regulates both over-the-counter (OTC) and prescription medicines that offer allergy relief as well as allergen extracts used to diagnose and treat allergies. And parents should take particular care when giving these products to children.

Immune System Reaction

An allergy is the body's reaction to a specific substance, or allergen. Our immune system responds to the invading allergen by releasing histamine and other chemicals that typically trigger symptoms in the nose, lungs, throat, sinuses, ears, eyes, skin, or stomach lining.

In some children, allergies can also trigger symptoms of asthma—a disease that causes wheezing or difficulty breathing.

If a child has allergies and asthma, "not controlling the allergies can make asthma worse," says Anthony Durmowicz, M.D., a pediatric pulmonary doctor in FDA's Division of Pulmonary, Allergy, and Rheumatology Products.

Avoiding the Culprit

If your child has seasonal allergies, you may want to pay attention to pollen counts and try to keep your child inside when the levels are high.

- In the late summer and early fall, during ragweed pollen season, pollen levels are highest in the morning.
- In the spring and summer, during the grass pollen season, pollen levels are highest in the evening.

- Some molds, another allergy trigger, may also be seasonal. For example, leaf mold is more common in the fall.
- Sunny, windy days can be especially troublesome for pollen allergy sufferers.

It may also help to keep windows closed in your house and car and run the air conditioner.

Allergy Medicines

For most children, symptoms may be controlled by avoiding the allergen, if known, and using OTC medicines. But if a child's symptoms are persistent and not relieved by OTC medicines, it is wise to see a healthcare professional to assess your child's symptoms and see if other treatments, including prescription medicines, may be appropriate. There are seven options available (see table below) to help bring your child relief. Although some allergy medicines are approved for use in children as young as 6 months, Dianne Murphy, M.D., director of FDA's Office of Pediatric Therapeutics, has some cautions. "Always read the label to make sure the product is appropriate for your child's age," Murphy says. "Just because a product's box says that it is intended for children does not mean it is intended for children of all ages."

Another reason to carefully read the label is that even though the big print may say the product is for a certain symptom (sneezing, allergy, cough, etc.), different products may have the same medicine (active ingredient). So it might seem that you are buying different products to treat different symptoms, but in fact the same medicine could be in all the products. The result: You might accidentally be giving too much of one type of medicine to your child.

More Child-Friendly Medicines

Recent pediatric legislation, including a combination of incentives and requirements for drug companies, has significantly increased research and development of drugs for children and has led to more products with new pediatric information in their labeling. Since 1997, a combination of legislative activities has helped generate studies in children for 600 products.

Many of the older drugs were only tested in adults, says Durmowicz. "But we now have more information available for the newer allergy medications," he adds. "With the passing of this legislation, there should be more confidence in pediatric dosing and safety with the newer drugs."

The legislation also requires drugs for children to be in a child-friendly formulation, adds Durmowicz. So if the drug was initially developed as a capsule, it has to also be made in a form that a child can take, such as a liquid with cherry flavoring, rapidly dissolving tablets, or strips for placing under the tongue.

In February 2016, FDA approved a generic version of Flonase Allergy Relief, an over-the-counter-allergy symptom reliever nasal spray for the temporary relief of the symptoms of hay fever or other upper respiratory allergies. In March 2016, FDA approved the first generic version of Nasonex spray for the treatment of nasal symptoms of seasonal and perennial allergic rhinitis in adults and children 2 and older.

Section 16.2

Food Allergies

This section includes text excerpted from "Food Allergies in Schools," Centers for Disease Control and Prevention (CDC), June 17, 2015.

What Is a Food Allergy?

A *food allergy* occurs when the body has a specific and reproducible immune response to certain foods. The body's immune response can be severe and life threatening, such as anaphylaxis. Although the immune system normally protects people from germs, in people with food allergies, the immune system mistakenly responds to food as if it were harmful.

Eight foods or food groups account for 90% of serious allergic reactions in the United States: milk, eggs, fish, crustacean shellfish, wheat, soy, peanuts, and tree nuts.

Symptoms of Food Allergy in Children

Symptoms Communicated by Children with Food Allergies

- It feels like something is poking my tongue.

- My tongue (or mouth) is tingling (or burning).
- My tongue (or mouth) itches.
- My tongue feels like there is hair on it.
- My mouth feels funny.
- There's a frog in my throat; there's something stuck in my throat.
- My tongue feels full (or heavy).
- My lips feel tight.
- It feels like there are bugs in there (to describe itchy ears).
- It (my throat) feels thick.
- It feels like a bump is on the back of my tongue (throat).

The symptoms and severity of allergic reactions to food can be different between individuals, and can also be different for one person over time. Anaphylaxis is a sudden and severe allergic reaction that may cause death. Not all allergic reactions will develop into anaphylaxis.

Food Allergies In Schools

- Children with food allergies are two to four times more likely to have asthma or other allergic conditions than those without food allergies.
- The prevalence of food allergies among children increased 18% during 1997–2007, and allergic reactions to foods have become the most common cause of anaphylaxis in community health settings.
- In 2006, about 88% of schools had one or more students with a food allergy.

Treatment and Prevention of Food Allergies in Children

There is no cure for food allergies. Strict avoidance of the food allergen is the only way to prevent a reaction. However, since it is not always easy or possible to avoid certain foods, staff in schools and ECE programs should develop plans to deal with allergic reactions, including anaphylaxis. Early and quick recognition and treatment of allergic reactions that may lead to anaphylaxis can prevent serious health problems or death.

Chapter 17

Blood and Circulatory Disorders in Children

Chapter Contents

Section 17.1

Anemia

This section includes text excerpted from "Anemia," National Heart, Lung, and Blood Institute (NHLBI), May 18, 2012. Reviewed October 2016.

What Is Anemia?

Anemia is a condition in which your blood has a lower than normal number of red blood cells.

Anemia also can occur if your red blood cells don't contain enough hemoglobin. Hemoglobin is an iron-rich protein that gives blood its red color. This protein helps red blood cells carry oxygen from the lungs to the rest of the body.

If you have anemia, your body doesn't get enough oxygen-rich blood. As a result, you may feel tired or weak. You also may have other symptoms, such as shortness of breath, dizziness, or headaches.

Severe or long-lasting anemia can damage your heart, brain, and other organs in your body. Very severe anemia may even cause death.

What Causes Anemia?

The three main causes of anemia are:

- Blood loss
- Lack of red blood cell production
- High rates of red blood cell destruction

Who Is at Risk for Anemia?

Anemia is a common condition. It occurs in all age, racial, and ethnic groups. Both men and women can have anemia. However, women of childbearing age are at higher risk for the condition because of blood loss from menstruation.

Anemia can develop during pregnancy due to low levels of iron and folic acid (folate) and changes in the blood. During the first 6 months of pregnancy, the fluid portion of a woman's blood (the plasma) increases faster than the number of red blood cells. This dilutes the blood and can lead to anemia.

During the first year of life, some babies are at risk for anemia because of iron deficiency. At-risk infants include those who are born too early and infants who are fed breast milk only or formula that isn't fortified with iron. These infants can develop iron deficiency by 6 months of age.

Infants between 1 and 2 years of age also are at risk for anemia. They may not get enough iron in their diets, especially if they drink a lot of cow's milk. Cow's milk is low in the iron needed for growth.

Drinking too much cow's milk may keep an infant or toddler from eating enough iron-rich foods or absorbing enough iron from foods.

Older adults also are at increased risk for anemia. Researchers continue to study how the condition affects older adults. Many of these people have other medical conditions as well.

Major Risk Factors

Factors that raise your risk for anemia include:

- A diet that is low in iron, vitamins, or minerals
- Blood loss from surgery or an injury
- Long-term or serious illnesses, such as kidney disease, cancer, diabetes, rheumatoid arthritis, HIV/AIDS, inflammatory bowel disease (including Crohn's disease), liver disease, heart failure, and thyroid disease
- Long-term infections
- A family history of inherited anemia, such as sickle cell anemia or thalassemia

How Is Anemia Diagnosed?

Your doctor will diagnose anemia based on your medical and family histories, a physical exam, and results from tests and procedures.

Because anemia doesn't always cause symptoms, your doctor may find out you have it while checking for another condition.

How Is Anemia Treated?

Treatment for anemia depends on the type, cause, and severity of the condition. Treatments may include dietary changes or supplements, medicines, procedures, or surgery to treat blood loss.

Section 17.2

Sickle Cell Anemia

This section includes text excerpted from "Tips for Supporting Students with Sickle Cell Disease," Centers for Disease Control and Prevention (CDC), January 30, 2014.

What Is Sickle Cell Disease?

Sickle cell disease (SCD) is an inherited blood disorder (a blood disorder that runs in families). People with SCD produce an abnormal type of hemoglobin (called hemoglobin S (HbS) or sickle hemoglobin). Hemoglobin is a protein in red blood cells that carries oxygen from the lungs to the organs and tissues in the body. The abnormal hemoglobin in SCD can cause the red blood cells to have a sickle or banana shape under certain conditions. People with SCD often have a decreased number of red blood cells, a condition called anemia, which can cause lack of energy, breathlessness, and pale color of the skin and lips. There are many forms of SCD and the most common type is Hb SS, known as sickle cell anemia, which is inherited when a child receives two "S" genes (one from each parent). Hb SC is a form of disease that is inherited when a child receives one sickle cell gene, "S" from one parent and from the other parent, a gene for an abnormal hemoglobin called "C." Another type of SCD, sickle beta-thalassemia, occurs when a child inherits one sickle cell gene and one gene for beta thalassemia (another type of abnormal inherited hemoglobin that causes anemia).

How Does Sickle Cell Disease Affect People?

While normal red blood cells are round like donuts and move freely through blood vessels, sickled blood cells clog the flow of blood and can break apart as they move through blood vessels. Additionally, sickled red blood cells do not deliver oxygen throughout the body as well as normal red blood cells do. As a result people living with sickle cell disease may suffer with:

- Severe pain

- Low number of red blood cells (or anemia)
- Stroke

What Conditions Can Cause Severe Pain (Sickle Cell Disease Crisis)?

One of the biggest challenges posed by SCD is the unpredictable nature of pain and the wide-ranging severity of health problems due to the condition. Some people with SCD may have infrequent problems with pain, whereas others experiencing pain may require hospitalization.

Certain factors are more likely to trigger a painful sickle cell crisis:

- Infections
- Cold and/or damp conditions
- Air pollution
- Dehydration
- Extreme physical activity
- Stress
- Sudden changes in temperature
- Use of alcohol or caffeine
- Smoking

Is Sickle Cell Disease Contagious?

No, you cannot catch sickle cell disease like a cold. Sickle cell disease is a genetically inherited disorder, passed down from a person's parents.

Why Is Your Child out of School So Often?

A person with sickle cell disease needs to be seen by a doctor more frequently than other students, so they may be at a doctor's appointment. At other times, sickle cell disease may cause a person to be in so much pain that he or she cannot attend school.

Why Do People with Sickle Cell Disease Have Yellow Eyes?

Sickle cell causes a person's red blood cells to die more quickly than the red blood cells of a person who does not have sickle cell. Their eyes become yellow due to a substance that is released when the red blood cells break down.

Why Should a Student with Sickle Cell Disease Be Able to Keep a Water Bottle at His or Her Desk or Leave Class More Frequently for Water Fountain and Restroom Breaks?

Water helps to increase a person's vein size and allows sickle-shaped cells to flow through blood vessels more easily. Allowing a student with sickle cell disease to access water freely may help to reduce the pain that can occur with sickle cell disease. As a result of needing to drink so much water, and because sickle cell disease causes kidney problems, the student may need to use the restroom more often.

Why Are Children with Sickle Cell Disease Smaller or Less Physically Developed than Other Children?

Children with sickle cell disease have red blood cells that do not carry oxygen as well as children with normal red blood cells. In order for any child's body to grow and develop, oxygen is needed throughout the body for energy. A child with sickle cell disease will grow and develop at a slower pace because less oxygen is being delivered throughout his or her body by the red blood cells.

When to Seek Medical Care for Students with Sickle Cell Disease

Sudden or worsening symptoms, like chest or abdominal pain, fever (>101 degrees), or any sign of stroke (e.g., weakness or numbness on either side of the body, not able to talk, sudden dizziness or headache, difficulty with memory, blurred vision) require immediate medical help. Remember, always notify parents if their child's health status changes during the school day.

Section 17.3

Thalassemia

This section includes text excerpted from "Facts About Thalassemia," Centers for Disease Control and Prevention (CDC), May 24, 2016.

What Is Thalassemia?

Thalassemia is an inherited (i.e., passed from parents to children through genes) blood disorder caused when the body doesn't make enough of a protein called hemoglobin, an important part of red blood cells. When there isn't enough hemoglobin, the body's red blood cells don't function properly and they last shorter periods of time, so there are fewer healthy red blood cells traveling in the bloodstream.

Red blood cells carry oxygen to all the cells of the body. Oxygen is a sort of food that cells use to function. When there are not enough healthy red blood cells, there is also not enough oxygen delivered to all the other cells of the body, which may cause a person to feel tired, weak or short of breath. This is a condition called anemia. People with thalassemia may have mild or severe anemia. Severe anemia can damage organs and lead to death.

What Are the Different Types of Thalassemia?

When we talk about different "types" of thalassemia, we might be talking about one of two things: the specific part of hemoglobin that is affected (usually either "alpha" or "beta"), or the severity of thalassemia, which is noted by words like trait, carrier, intermedia, or major.

Hemoglobin, which carries oxygen to all cells in the body, is made of two different parts, called alpha and beta. When thalassemia is called "alpha" or "beta," this refers to the part of hemoglobin that isn't being made. If either the alpha or beta part is not made, there aren't enough building blocks to make normal amounts of hemoglobin. Low alpha is called alpha thalassemia. Low beta is called beta thalassemia.

When the words "trait," "minor," "intermedia," or "major" are used, these words describe how severe the thalassemia is. A person who has thalassemia trait may not have any symptoms at all or may have only mild anemia, while a person with thalassemia major may have severe symptoms and may need regular blood transfusions.

In the same way that traits for hair color and body structure are passed down from parents to children, thalassemia traits are passed from parents to children. The type of thalassemia that a person has depends on how many and what type of traits for thalassemia a person has inherited, or received from their parents. For instance, if a person receives a beta thalassemia trait from his father and another from his mother, he will have beta thalassemia major. If a person received an alpha thalassemia trait from her mother and the normal alpha parts from her father, she would have alpha thalassemia trait (also called alpha thalassemia minor). Having a thalassemia trait means that you may not have any symptoms, but you might pass that trait on to your children and increase their risk for having thalassemia.

Sometimes, thalassemias have other names, like Constant Spring, Cooley Anemia, or hemoglobin Bart hydrops fetalis. These names are specific to certain thalassemias—for instance, Cooley Anemia is the same thing as beta thalassemia major.

How Do I Know If I Have Thalassemia?

People with moderate and severe forms of thalassemia usually find out about their condition in childhood, since they have symptoms of severe anemia early in life. People with less severe forms of thalassemia may only find out because they are having symptoms of anemia, or maybe because a doctor finds anemia on a routine blood test or a test done for another reason.

Because thalassemias are inherited, the condition sometimes runs in families. Some people find out about their thalassemia because they have relatives with a similar condition.

People who have family members from certain parts of the world have a higher risk for having thalassemia. Traits for thalassemia are more common in people from Mediterranean countries, like Greece and Turkey, and in people from Asia, Africa, and the Middle East. If you have anemia and you also have family members from these areas, your doctor might test your blood further to find out if you have thalassemia.

How Can I Prevent Thalassemia?

Because thalassemia is passed from parents to children, it is very hard to prevent. However, if you or your partner knows of family members with thalassemia, or if you both have family members from places in the world where thalassemia is common, you can speak to a genetic counselor to determine what your risk would be of passing thalassemia to your children.

Section 17.4

Hemophilia

This section includes text excerpted from "What Is Hemophilia?" National Heart, Lung, and Blood Institute (NHLBI), July 13, 2013.

What Is Hemophilia?

Hemophilia is a rare bleeding disorder in which the blood doesn't clot normally.

If you have hemophilia, you may bleed for a longer time than others after an injury. You also may bleed inside your body (internally), especially in your knees, ankles, and elbows. This bleeding can damage your organs and tissues and may be life threatening.

What Causes Hemophilia?

A defect in one of the genes that determines how the body makes blood clotting factor VIII or IX causes hemophilia. These genes are located on the X chromosomes.

Chromosomes come in pairs. Females have two X chromosomes, while males have one X and one Y chromosome. Only the X chromosome carries the genes related to clotting factors.

A male who has a hemophilia gene on his X chromosome will have hemophilia. When a female has a hemophilia gene on only one of her X chromosomes, she is a "hemophilia carrier" and can pass the gene to her children. Sometimes carriers have low levels of clotting factor and have symptoms of hemophilia, including bleeding. Clotting factors are proteins in the blood that work together with platelets to stop or control bleeding.

Very rarely, a girl may be born with a very low clotting factor level and have a greater risk for bleeding, similar to boys who have hemophilia and very low levels of clotting factor. There are several hereditary and genetic causes of this much rarer form of hemophilia in females.

Some males who have the disorder are born to mothers who aren't carriers. In these cases, a mutation (random change) occurs in the gene as it is passed to the child.

Below are two examples of how the hemophilia gene is inherited.

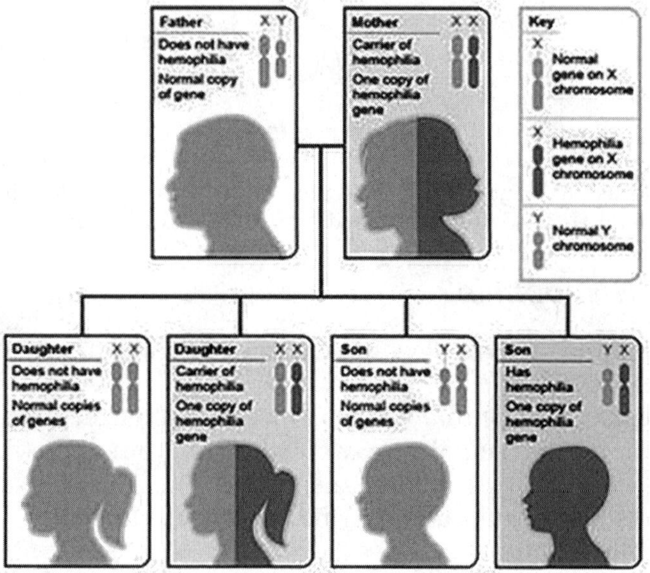

Figure 17.1. *Inheritance Pattern for Hemophilia—Example 1*

(Source: "Hemophilia," National Heart, Lung, and Blood Institute (NHLBI), July 13, 2013.)

Each daughter has a 50 percent chance of inheriting the hemophilia gene from her mother and being a carrier. Each son has a 50 percent chance of inheriting the hemophilia gene from his mother and having hemophilia.

Each daughter will inherit the hemophilia gene from her father and be a carrier. None of the sons will inherit the hemophilia gene from their father; thus, none will have hemophilia.

What Are the Signs and Symptoms of Hemophilia?

The major signs and symptoms of hemophilia are excessive bleeding and easy bruising.

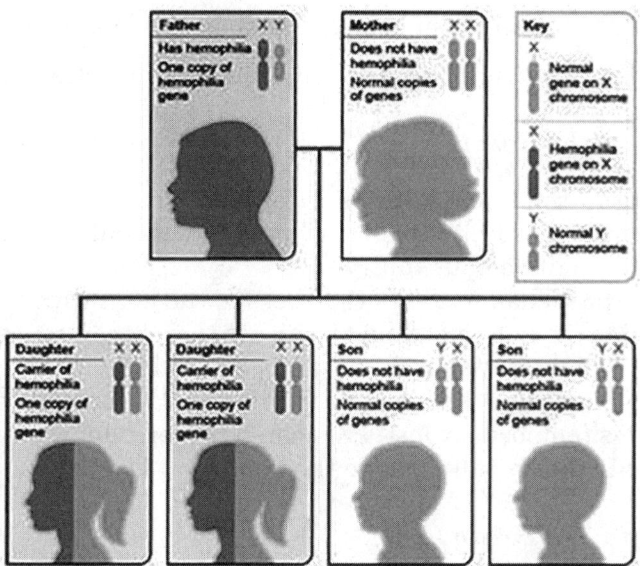

Figure 17.2. *Inheritance Pattern for Hemophilia—Example 2*

(Source: "Hemophilia," National Heart, Lung, and Blood Institute (NHLBI), July 13, 2013.)

Excessive Bleeding

The extent of bleeding depends on how severe the hemophilia is.

Children who have mild hemophilia may not have signs unless they have excessive bleeding from a dental procedure, an accident, or surgery. Males who have severe hemophilia may bleed heavily after circumcision.

Bleeding can occur on the body's surface (external bleeding) or inside the body (internal bleeding).

Signs of external bleeding may include:

- Bleeding in the mouth from a cut or bite or from cutting or losing a tooth
- Nosebleeds for no obvious reason
- Heavy bleeding from a minor cut
- Bleeding from a cut that resumes after stopping for a short time

Signs of internal bleeding may include:

- Blood in the urine (from bleeding in the kidneys or bladder)

- Blood in the stool (from bleeding in the intestines or stomach)
- Large bruises (from bleeding into the large muscles of the body)

Bleeding in the Joints

Bleeding in the knees, elbows, or other joints is another common form of internal bleeding in people who have hemophilia. This bleeding can occur without obvious injury.

At first, the bleeding causes tightness in the joint with no real pain or any visible signs of bleeding. The joint then becomes swollen, hot to touch, and painful to bend.

Swelling continues as bleeding continues. Eventually, movement in the joint is temporarily lost. Pain can be severe. Joint bleeding that isn't treated quickly can damage the joint.

Bleeding in the Brain

Internal bleeding in the brain is a very serious complication of hemophilia. It can happen after a simple bump on the head or a more serious injury. The signs and symptoms of bleeding in the brain include:

- Long-lasting, painful headaches or neck pain or stiffness
- Repeated vomiting
- Sleepiness or changes in behavior
- Sudden weakness or clumsiness of the arms or legs or problems walking
- Double vision
- Convulsions or seizures

How Is Hemophilia Diagnosed?

If you or your child appears to have a bleeding problem, your doctor will ask about your personal and family medical histories. This will reveal whether you or your family members, including women and girls, have bleeding problems. However, some people who have hemophilia have no recent family history of the disease.

You or your child also will likely have a physical exam and blood tests to diagnose hemophilia. Blood tests are used to find out:

- How long it takes for your blood to clot
- Whether your blood has low levels of any clotting factors

- Whether any clotting factors are completely missing from your blood

The test results will show whether you have hemophilia, what type of hemophilia you have, and how severe it is.

Hemophilia A and B are classified as mild, moderate, or severe, depending on the amount of clotting factor VIII or IX in the blood.

Table 17.1. Mild, moderate, or severe hemophilia

Mild hemophilia	5–40 percent of normal clotting factor
Moderate hemophilia	1–5 percent of normal clotting factor
Severe hemophilia	Less than 1 percent of normal clotting factor

The severity of symptoms can overlap between the categories. For example, some people who have mild hemophilia may have bleeding problems almost as often or as severe as some people who have moderate hemophilia.

Severe hemophilia can cause serious bleeding problems in babies. Thus, children who have severe hemophilia usually are diagnosed during the first year of life. People who have milder forms of hemophilia may not be diagnosed until they're adults.

The bleeding problems of hemophilia A and hemophilia B are the same. Only special blood tests can tell which type of the disorder you or your child has. Knowing which type is important because the treatments are different.

Pregnant women who are known hemophilia carriers can have the disorder diagnosed in their unborn babies as early as 12 weeks into their pregnancies.

Women who are hemophilia carriers also can have "preimplantation diagnosis" to have children who don't have hemophilia.

For this process, women have their eggs removed and fertilized by sperm in a laboratory. The embryos are then tested for hemophilia. Only embryos without the disorder are implanted in the womb.

How Is Hemophilia Treated?

Treatment with Replacement Therapy

The main treatment for hemophilia is called replacement therapy. Concentrates of clotting factor VIII (for hemophilia A) or clotting factor

IX (for hemophilia B) are slowly dripped or injected into a vein. These infusions help replace the clotting factor that's missing or low.

Clotting factor concentrates can be made from human blood. The blood is treated to prevent the spread of diseases, such as hepatitis. With the current methods of screening and treating donated blood, the risk of getting an infectious disease from human clotting factors is very small.

To further reduce the risk, you or your child can take clotting factor concentrates that aren't made from human blood. These are called recombinant clotting factors. Clotting factors are easy to store, mix, and use at home—it only takes about 15 minutes to receive the factor.

You may have replacement therapy on a regular basis to prevent bleeding. This is called preventive or prophylactic therapy. Or, you may only need replacement therapy to stop bleeding when it occurs. This use of the treatment, on an as-needed basis, is called demand therapy.

Demand therapy is less intensive and expensive than preventive therapy. However, there's a risk that bleeding will cause damage before you receive the demand therapy.

Section 17.5

Thrombocytopenia

This section includes text excerpted from "What Is Thrombocytopenia?" National Heart, Lung, and Blood Institute (NHLBI), September 25, 2012. Reviewed October 2016.

What Is Thrombocytopenia?

Thrombocytopenia is a condition in which your blood has a lower than normal number of blood cell fragments called platelets.

Platelets are made in your bone marrow along with other kinds of blood cells. They travel through your blood vessels and stick together (clot) to stop any bleeding that may happen if a blood vessel is damaged. Platelets also are called thrombocytes because a clot also is called a thrombus.

What Causes Thrombocytopenia?

Many factors can cause thrombocytopenia (a low platelet count). The condition can be inherited or acquired. "Inherited" means your parents pass the gene for the condition to you. "Acquired" means you aren't born with the condition, but you develop it. Sometimes the cause of thrombocytopenia isn't known.

Who Is at Risk for Thrombocytopenia?

People who are at highest risk for thrombocytopenia includes people who:

- Have certain types of cancer, aplastic anemia, or autoimmune diseases
- Are exposed to certain toxic chemicals
- Have a reaction to certain medicines
- Have certain viruses
- Have certain genetic conditions

What Are the Signs and Symptoms of Thrombocytopenia?

Mild to serious bleeding causes the main signs and symptoms of thrombocytopenia. Bleeding can occur inside your body (internal bleeding) or underneath your skin or from the surface of your skin (external bleeding).

Signs and symptoms can appear suddenly or over time. Mild thrombocytopenia often has no signs or symptoms. Many times, it's found during a routine blood test.

Check with your doctor if you have any signs of bleeding. Severe thrombocytopenia can cause bleeding in almost any part of the body. Bleeding can lead to a medical emergency and should be treated right away.

External bleeding usually is the first sign of a low platelet count. External bleeding may cause purpura or petechiae. Purpura are purple, brown, and red bruises. This bruising may happen easily and often. Petechiae are small red or purple dots on your skin.

Other signs of external bleeding include:

- Prolonged bleeding, even from minor cuts

- Bleeding or oozing from the mouth or nose, especially nosebleeds or bleeding from brushing your teeth
- Abnormal vaginal bleeding (especially heavy menstrual flow)

A lot of bleeding after surgery or dental work also might suggest a bleeding problem.

Heavy bleeding into the intestines or the brain (internal bleeding) is serious and can be fatal. Signs and symptoms include:

- Blood in the urine or stool or bleeding from the rectum. Blood in the stool can appear as red blood or as a dark, tarry color. (Taking iron supplements also can cause dark, tarry stools.)
- Headaches and other neurological symptoms. These problems are very rare, but you should discuss them with your doctor.

How Is Thrombocytopenia Diagnosed?

Your doctor will diagnose thrombocytopenia based on your medical history, a physical exam, and test results. A hematologist also may be involved in your care. This is a doctor who specializes in diagnosing and treating blood diseases and conditions.

Once thrombocytopenia is diagnosed, your doctor will begin looking for its cause.

How Is Thrombocytopenia Treated?

Treatment for thrombocytopenia depends on its cause and severity. The main goal of treatment is to prevent death and disability caused by bleeding.

If your condition is mild, you may not need treatment. A fully normal platelet count isn't necessary to prevent bleeding, even with severe cuts or accidents.

If your thrombocytopenia is severe, your doctor may prescribe treatments such as medicines, blood or platelet transfusions, or splenectomy.

Section 17.6

Thrombophilia (Excessive Blood Clotting)

What Is Thrombophilia?

Thrombophilia, also known as hypercoagulation, is a medical disorder in which excessive blood clotting occurs. In healthy people, a wound that causes bleeding triggers an immediate response in the body. Blood platelets begin to stick together in masses called blood clots. This process is known as coagulation and is the body's primary means of stopping blood loss. Thrombophilia means that the body has an abnormal blood clotting response. Thrombophilia can manifest as an overactive blood clot response, in which blood clots form too easily or too often. It can also refer to persistent blood clots that are not dissolved by the body, or blood clots that form inside blood vessels or arteries.

Causes

Excessive blood clotting disorders can be inherited or acquired. Acquired clotting disorders can result from traumatic injury, surgery, long-term bed rest, obesity, severe dehydration, certain chronic health conditions, and the use of certain medications. Excessive blood clotting can also be caused by sitting for long periods of time during car or airplane trips. Certain medical history factors can also indicate a person's likelihood of having an excessive blood clotting disorder, primarily family members who have been diagnosed with an excessive blood clotting disorder. The majority of pediatric thrombophilia cases occur in children who have a combination of multiple risk factors.

Symptoms and Risks

Symptoms of excessive blood clotting disorders vary depending on where excessive blood clots form in the body.

Chest pain, shortness of breath, and pain in the upper arms, back, neck, or jaw can be symptoms of a blood clot in the heart or lungs. This type of blood clot can result in a heart attack, which restricts or blocks blood flow to part of the heart. An undiagnosed or untreated heart attack can result in serious long-term complications, including death.

Persistent headaches, changes in ability to speak, difficulty understanding others talking, dizziness, or paralysis can indicate a blood clot in the brain. This type of blood clot can result in a stroke. A stroke causes restricted blood flow to the brain, which can result in serious complications including death if left undiagnosed or untreated.

Swelling, pain, redness, or warm skin on the arms or legs can indicate a type of blood clot known as a deep vein thrombosis. These types of blood clots can travel through the blood stream and cause serious complications if they reach the brain, heart, or lungs.

Diagnosis

Excessive blood clotting disorders are diagnosed through physical exam, medical history interview, and diagnostic blood tests. Blood tests for excessive clotting measure the levels of various blood components such as red and white blood cells, platelets, and blood clotting protein factors. Blood tests also analyze the clotting behavior of the blood samples to identify normal or abnormal clotting function. Medical history factors are evaluated to assess a person's risk for excessive blood clotting disorder. Some factors that indicate a possible blood clotting disorder diagnosis include frequent unexplained bruising and/or family members who have been diagnosed with a blood clotting disorder.

Treatment and Prevention

There is no course of prevention for inherited thrombophilia. To reduce the risk of acquired thrombophilia, it is important to follow prescribed treatments for diseases that can result in excessive blood clotting, such as diabetes and certain heart and vascular disorders. Most cases of thrombophilia are treatable with medication that thins the blood to prevent excessive clotting.

References

1. "Excessive Blood Clotting," National Heart, Lung, and Blood Institute. June 11, 2014.
2. "Hypercoagulation," FamilyDoctor.org. March 2014.

3. Raffin, Leslie. "Thrombophilia in Children: Who to Test, How, When, and Why?" n.d.

4. "What Is Excessive Blood Clotting (Hypercoagulation)?" American Heart Association. November 30, 2015.

Section 17.7

von Willebrand Disease

This section includes text excerpted from "Facts about von Willebrand Disease," Centers for Disease Control and Prevention (CDC), March 2, 2016.

What Is von Willebrand Disease?

von Willebrand disease (VWD) is a blood disorder in which the blood does not clot properly. Blood contains many proteins that help the body stop bleeding. One of these proteins is called von Willebrand factor (VWF). People with VWD either have a low level of VWF in their blood or the VWF protein doesn't work the way it should.

Normally, when a person is injured and starts to bleed, the VWF in the blood attaches to small blood cells called platelets. This helps the platelets stick together, like glue, to form a clot at the site of injury and stop the bleeding. When a person has VWD, because the VWF doesn't work the way it should, the clot might take longer to form or not form the way it should, and bleeding might take longer to stop. This can lead to heavy, hard-to-stop bleeding. Although rare, the bleeding can be severe enough to damage joints or internal organs, or even be life-threatening.

Who Is Affected?

VWD is the most common bleeding disorder, found in up to 1% of the U.S. population. This means that 3.2 million (or about 1 in every 100) people in the United States have the disease. Although VWD occurs among men and women equally, women are more likely to notice the symptoms because of heavy or abnormal bleeding during their menstrual periods and after childbirth.

Types of VWD

Type 1

This is the most common and mildest form of VWD, in which a person has lower than normal levels of VWF. A person with Type 1 VWD also might have low levels of factor VIII, another type of blood-clotting protein. This should not be confused with hemophilia, in which there are low levels or a complete lack of factor VIII but normal levels of VWF.

Type 2

With this type of VWD, although the body makes normal amounts of the VWF, the factor does not work the way it should. Type 2 is further broken down into four subtypes?2A, 2B, 2M, and 2N?depending on the specific problem with the person's VWF. Because the treatment is different for each type, it is important that a person know which subtype he or she has.

Type 3

This is the most severe form of VWD, in which a person has very little or no VWF and low levels of factor VIII.

Causes

Most people who have VWD are born with it. It almost always is inherited, or passed down, from a parent to a child. VWD can be passed down from either the mother or the father, or both, to the child.

While rare, it is possible for a person to get VWD without a family history of the disease. This happens when a "spontaneous mutation" occurs. That means there has been a change in the person's gene. Whether the child received the affected gene from a parent or as a result of a mutation, once the child has it, the child can later pass it along to his or her children. Rarely, a person who is not born with VWD can acquire it or have it first occur later in life. This can happen when a person's own immune system destroys his or her VWF, often as a result of use of a medication or as a result of another disease. If VWD is acquired, meaning it was not inherited from a parent, it cannot be passed along to any children.

Signs and Symptoms

The major signs of VWD are:

Frequent or Hard-to-Stop Nosebleeds

People with VWD might have nosebleeds that:

- Start without injury (spontaneous)
- Occur often, usually five times or more in a year
- Last more than 10 minutes
- Need packing or cautery to stop the bleeding

Easy Bruising
People with VWD might experience easy bruising that:

- Occurs with very little or no trauma or injury
- Occurs often (one to four times per month)
- Is larger than the size of a quarter
- Is not flat and has a raised lump

Longer than Normal Bleeding After Injury, Surgery, Childbirth, or Dental Work
People with VWD might have longer than normal bleeding after injury, surgery, or childbirth, for example:

- After a cut to the skin, the bleeding lasts more than 5 minutes
- Heavy or longer bleeding occurs after surgery. Bleeding sometimes stops, but starts up again hours or days later.
- Heavy bleeding occurs during or after childbirth

People with VWD might have longer than normal bleeding during or after dental work, for example:

- Heavy bleeding occurs during or after dental surgery
- The surgery site oozes blood longer than 3 hours after the surgery
- The surgery site needs packing or cautery to stop the bleeding

The amount of bleeding depends on the type and severity of VWD. Other common bleeding events include:

- Blood in the stool (feces) from bleeding into the stomach or intestines
- Blood in the urine from bleeding into the kidneys or bladder
- Bleeding into joints or internal organs in severe cases (Type 3)

Diagnosis

To find out if a person has VWD, the doctor will ask questions about personal and family histories of bleeding. The doctor also will check for unusual bruising or other signs of recent bleeding and order some blood tests that will measure how the blood clots. The tests will provide information about the amount of clotting proteins present in the blood and if the clotting proteins are working properly. Because certain medications can cause bleeding, even among people without a bleeding disorder, the doctor will ask about recent or routine medications taken that could cause bleeding or make bleeding symptoms worse.

Treatments

The type of treatment prescribed for VWD depends on the type and severity of the disease. For minor bleeds, treatment might not be needed.

The most commonly used types of treatment are:

Desmopressin Acetate Injection

This medicine (DDAVP®) is injected into a vein to treat people with milder forms of VWD (mainly type 1). It works by making the body release more VWF into the blood. It helps increase the level of factor VIII in the blood as well.

- Desmopressin Acetate Nasal Spray
- Factor Replacement Therapy
- Antifibrinolytic Drugs

Chapter 18

Cancer in Children

Chapter Contents

Section 18.1

Leukemia

This section contains text excerpted from the following sources: Text under the heading "Overview" is excerpted from "Leukemia—Patient Version," National Cancer Institute (NCI), May 15, 2015; Text beginning with the heading "About Childhood Acute Lymphoblastic Leukemia" is excerpted from "Childhood Acute Lymphoblastic Leukemia Treatment (PDQ®)—Patient Version," National Cancer Institute (NCI), July 28, 2016; Text beginning with the heading "Childhood Acute Myeloid Leukemia and Other Myeloid Malignancies" is excerpted from "Childhood Acute Myeloid Leukemia/Other Myeloid Malignancies Treatment (PDQ®)–Patient Version," National Cancer Institute (NCI), July 28, 2016.

Overview

Leukemia is cancer of the blood cells. Most blood cells form in the bone marrow. In leukemia, immature blood cells become cancer. These cells do not work the way they should and they crowd out the healthy blood cells in the bone marrow.

Different types of leukemia depend on the type of blood cell that becomes cancer. For example, lymphoblastic leukemia is a cancer of the lymphoblasts (white blood cells, which fight infection). White blood cells are the most common type of blood cell to become cancer. But red blood cells (cells that carry oxygen from the lungs to the rest of the body) and platelets (cells that clot the blood) may also become cancer.

Leukemia occurs most often in adults older than 55 years, but it is also the most common cancer in children younger than 15 years.

Leukemia can be either acute or chronic. Acute leukemia is a fast-growing cancer that usually gets worse quickly. Chronic leukemia is a slower-growing cancer that gets worse slowly over time. The treatment and prognosis for leukemia depend on the type of blood cell affected and whether the leukemia is acute or chronic.

About Childhood Acute Lymphoblastic Leukemia

Childhood acute lymphoblastic leukemia (ALL) is a type of cancer in which the bone marrow makes too many immature lymphocytes (a type of white blood cell).

Childhood acute lymphoblastic leukemia (also called ALL or acute lymphocytic leukemia) is a cancer of the blood and bone marrow. This type of cancer usually gets worse quickly if it is not treated.

ALL is the most common type of cancer in children.

Leukemia May Affect Red Blood Cells, White Blood Cells, and Platelets

In a healthy child, the bone marrow makes blood stem cells (immature cells) that become mature blood cells over time. A blood stem cell may become a myeloid stem cell or a lymphoid stem cell.

A myeloid stem cell becomes one of three types of mature blood cells:

- Red blood cells that carry oxygen and other substances to all tissues of the body.
- Platelets that form blood clots to stop bleeding.
- White blood cells that fight infection and disease.

A lymphoid stem cell becomes a lymphoblast cell and then one of three types of lymphocytes (white blood cells):

- B lymphocytes that make antibodies to help fight infection.
- T lymphocytes that help B lymphocytes make the antibodies that help fight infection.
- Natural killer cells that attack cancer cells and viruses.

In a child with ALL, too many stem cells become lymphoblasts, B lymphocytes, or T lymphocytes. These cells are cancer (leukemia) cells. The leukemia cells do not work like normal lymphocytes and are not able to fight infection very well. Also, as the number of leukemia cells increases in the blood and bone marrow, there is less room for healthy white blood cells, red blood cells, and platelets. This may lead to infection, anemia, and easy bleeding.

Past Treatment for Cancer and Certain Genetic Conditions Affect the Risk of Having Childhood ALL

Anything that increases your risk of getting a disease is called a risk factor. Having a risk factor does not mean that you will get cancer; not having risk factors doesn't mean that you will not get cancer. Talk with your child's doctor if you think your child may be at risk.

Possible risk factors for ALL include the following:

- Being exposed to X-rays before birth.
- Being exposed to radiation.
- Past treatment with chemotherapy.
- Having certain changes in the chromosomes or genes.
- Having certain genetic conditions, such as:
- Down syndrome.
- Neurofibromatosis type 1 (NF1).
- Shwachman syndrome.
- Bloom syndrome.
- Ataxia-telangiectasia.

Tests That Examine the Blood and Bone Marrow Are Used to Detect (Find) and Diagnose Childhood ALL

The following tests and procedures may be used to diagnose childhood ALL and find out if leukemia cells have spread to other parts of the body such as the brain or testicles:

- Physical exam and history
- Complete blood count (CBC) with differential
- Blood chemistry studies
- Bone marrow aspiration and biopsy

The following tests may be done on the tissue that is removed:

- Cytogenetic analysis
- Immunophenotyping
- Lumbar puncture
- Chest X-ray
- Testicular biopsy

Childhood Acute Myeloid Leukemia and Other Myeloid Malignancies

Childhood acute myeloid leukemia (AML) is a type of cancer in which the bone marrow makes a large number of abnormal blood cells.

Childhood acute myeloid leukemia (AML) is a cancer of the blood and bone marrow. AML is also called acute myelogenous leukemia, acute myeloblastic leukemia, acute granulocytic leukemia, and acute nonlymphocytic leukemia. Cancers that are acute usually get worse quickly if they are not treated. Cancers that are chronic usually get worse slowly.

Leukemia and other diseases of the blood and bone marrow may affect red blood cells, white blood cells, and platelets.

Normally, the bone marrow makes blood stem cells (immature cells) that become mature blood cells over time. A blood stem cell may become a myeloid stem cell or a lymphoid stem cell. A lymphoid stem cell becomes a white blood cell.

A myeloid stem cell becomes one of three types of mature blood cells:

- Red blood cells that carry oxygen and other substances to all tissues of the body.
- White blood cells that fight infection and disease.
- Platelets that form blood clots to stop bleeding.

In AML, the myeloid stem cells usually become a type of immature white blood cell called myeloblasts (or myeloid blasts). The myeloblasts, or leukemia cells, in AML are abnormal and do not become healthy white blood cells. The leukemia cells can build up in the blood and bone marrow so there is less room for healthy white blood cells, red blood cells, and platelets. When this happens, infection, anemia, or easy bleeding may occur. The leukemia cells can spread outside the blood to other parts of the body, including the central nervous system (brain and spinal cord), skin, and gums. Sometimes leukemia cells form a solid tumor called a granulocytic sarcoma or chloroma.

There are subtypes of AML based on the type of blood cell that is affected. The treatment of AML is different when it is a subtype called acute promyelocytic leukemia (APL) or when the child has Down syndrome.

Other myeloid diseases can affect the blood and bone marrow.

Chronic myelogenous leukemia

In chronic myelogenous leukemia (CML), too many bone marrow stem cells become a type of white blood cell called granulocytes. Some of these bone marrow stem cells never become mature white blood cells. These are called blasts. Over time, the granulocytes and blasts crowd out the red blood cells and platelets in the bone marrow. CML is rare in children.

Juvenile myelomonocytic leukemia

Juvenile myelomonocytic leukemia (JMML) is a rare childhood cancer that occurs more often in children around the age of 2 years and is more common in boys. In JMML, too many bone marrow stem cells become 2 types of white blood cells called myelocytes and monocytes. Some of these bone marrow stem cells never become mature white blood cells. These immature cells, called blasts, are unable to do their usual work. Over time, the myelocytes, monocytes, and blasts crowd out the red blood cells and platelets in the bone marrow. When this happens, infection, anemia, or easy bleeding may occur.

Myelodysplastic syndromes

Myelodysplastic syndromes (MDS) occur less often in children than in adults. In MDS, the bone marrow makes too few red blood cells, white blood cells, and platelets. These blood cells may not mature and enter the blood. The treatment for MDS depends on how low the numbers of red blood cells, white blood cells, or platelets are. Over time, MDS may become AML.

Transient myeloproliferative disorder (TMD) is a type of MDS. This disorder of the bone marrow can develop in newborns who have Down syndrome. It usually goes away on its own within the first 3 weeks of life. Infants who have Down syndrome and TMD have an increased chance of developing AML before the age of 3 years.

Myelodysplastic Syndromes Treatment

Myelodysplastic/Myeloproliferative Neoplasms Treatment

AML or MDS may occur after treatment with certain anticancer drugs and/or radiation therapy.

Cancer treatment with certain anticancer drugs and/or radiation therapy may cause therapy related AML (t-AML) or therapy-related MDS (t-MDS). The risk of these therapy-related myeloid diseases depends on the total dose of the anticancer drugs used and the radiation dose and treatment field. Some patients also have an inherited risk for t-AML and t-MDS. These therapy-related diseases usually occur within 7 years after treatment, but are rare in children.

The risk factors for childhood AML, childhood CML, JMML, and MDS are similar.

Anything that increases your risk of getting a disease is called a risk factor. Having a risk factor does not mean that you will get cancer; not having risk factors doesn't mean that you will not get cancer. Talk with your child's doctor if you think your child may be at risk. These and other factors may increase the risk of childhood AML, childhood CML, JMML, and MDS:

- Having a brother or sister, especially a twin, with leukemia.
- Being Hispanic.
- Being exposed to cigarette smoke or alcohol before birth.
- Having a personal history of aplastic anemia.
- Having a personal or family history of MDS.
- Having a family history of AML.
- Past treatment with chemotherapy or radiation therapy.
- Being exposed to ionizing radiation or chemicals such as benzene.
- Having certain genetic disorders, such as:
  - Down syndrome.
  - Fanconi anemia.
  - Neurofibromatosis type 1.
  - Noonan syndrome.
  - Shwachman-Diamond syndrome.

Signs and symptoms of childhood AML, childhood CML, JMML, or MDS include fever, feeling tired, and easy bleeding or bruising.

These and other signs and symptoms may be caused by childhood AML, childhood CML, JMML, or MDS or by other conditions. Check with a doctor if your child has any of the following:

- Fever with or without an infection.
- Night sweats.
- Shortness of breath.
- Weakness or feeling tired.
- Easy bruising or bleeding.
- Petechiae (flat, pinpoint spots under the skin caused by bleeding).
- Pain in the bones or joints.

- Pain or feeling of fullness below the ribs.
- Painless lumps in the neck, underarm, stomach, groin, or other parts of the body. In childhood AML, these lumps, called leukemia cutis, may be blue or purple.
- Painless lumps that are sometimes around the eyes. These lumps, called chloromas, are sometimes seen in childhood AML and may be blue-green.
- An eczema like skin rash.

The signs and symptoms of TMD may include the following:

- Swelling all over the body.
- Shortness of breath.
- Trouble breathing.
- Weakness or feeling tired.
- Pain below the ribs.

Tests that examine the blood and bone marrow are used to detect (find) and diagnose childhood AML, childhood CML, JMML, and MDS.

The following tests and procedures may be used:

- Physical exam and history
- Complete blood count (CBC) with differential
- Complete blood count (CBC)
- Peripheral blood smear
- Blood chemistry studies
- Chest X-ray
- Biopsy
- Bone marrow aspiration and biopsy
- Tumor biopsy
- Lymph node biopsy
- Cytogenetic analysis

The following test is a type of cytogenetic analysis:

- FISH (fluorescence in situ hybridization)
- Reverse transcription – polymerase chain reaction (RT–PCR) test
- Immunophenotyping
- Molecular testing
- Lumbar puncture

Section 18.2

Lymphoma

This section contains text excerpted from the following sources: Text under the heading "Overview" is excerpted from "Lymphoma—Patient Version," National Cancer Institute (NCI), May 15, 2015; Text beginning with the heading "About Childhood Hodgkin Lymphoma" is excerpted from "Childhood Hodgkin Lymphoma Treatment (PDQ®)—Patient Version," National Cancer Institute (NCI), August 3, 2016; Text under the heading "About Childhood Non-Hodgkin Lymphoma" is excerpted from "Childhood Non-Hodgkin Lymphoma Treatment (PDQ®)—Patient Version," e.g National Cancer Institute (NCI), August 16, 2016.

Overview

Lymphoma is cancer that begins in cells of the lymph system. The lymph system is part of the immune system, which helps the body fight infection and disease. Because lymph tissue is found all through the body, lymphoma can begin almost anywhere.

The two main types of lymphoma are Hodgkin lymphoma and non-Hodgkin lymphoma (NHL). These can occur in both children and adults.

Most people with Hodgkin lymphoma have the classic type. With this type, there are large, abnormal lymphocytes (a type of white blood cell) in the lymph nodes called Reed-Sternberg cells. Hodgkin lymphoma can usually be cured.

There are many different types of NHL that form from different types of white blood cells (B-cells, T-cells, NK cells). Most types of NHL form from B-cells. NHL may be indolent (slow-growing) or aggressive (fast-growing). The most common types of NHL in adults are diffuse large B-cell lymphoma, which is usually aggressive, and follicular lymphoma, which is usually indolent.

Mycosis fungoides and the Sézary syndrome are types of NHL that start in white blood cells in the skin. Primary central nervous system lymphoma is a rare type of NHL that starts in white blood cells in the brain, spinal cord, or eye.

The treatment and the chance of a cure depend on the stage and the type of lymphoma.

About Childhood Hodgkin Lymphoma

Childhood Hodgkin lymphoma is a type of cancer that develops in the lymph system, which is part of the body's immune system. The immune system protects the body from foreign substances, infection, and diseases. The lymph system is made up of the following:

- Lymph: Colorless, watery fluid that carries white blood cells called lymphocytes through the lymph system. Lymphocytes protect the body against infections and the growth of tumors.
- Lymph vessels: A network of thin tubes that collect lymph from different parts of the body and return it to the bloodstream.
- Lymph nodes: Small, bean-shaped structures that filter lymph and store white blood cells that help fight infection and disease. Lymph nodes are located along the network of lymph vessels found throughout the body. Clusters of lymph nodes are found in the neck, underarm, abdomen, pelvis, and groin.
- Spleen: An organ that makes lymphocytes, filters the blood, stores blood cells, and destroys old blood cells. The spleen is on the left side of the abdomen near the stomach.
- Thymus: An organ in which lymphocytes grow and multiply. The thymus is in the chest behind the breastbone.
- Tonsils: Two small masses of lymph tissue at the back of the throat. The tonsils make lymphocytes.
- Bone marrow: The soft, spongy tissue in the center of large bones. Bone marrow makes white blood cells, red blood cells, and platelets.

- Lymph tissue is also found in other parts of the body such as the stomach, thyroid gland, brain, and skin.
- There are two general types of lymphoma: Hodgkin lymphoma and non-Hodgkin lymphoma. Hodgkin lymphoma often occurs in adolescents 15 to 19 years of age. The treatment for children and adolescents is different than treatment for adults.

There Are Two Types of Childhood Hodgkin Lymphoma

The two types of childhood Hodgkin lymphoma are:

- Classical Hodgkin lymphoma.
- Nodular lymphocyte-predominant Hodgkin lymphoma.

Classical Hodgkin lymphoma is divided into four subtypes, based on how the cancer cells look under a microscope:

- Lymphocyte-rich classical Hodgkin lymphoma.
- Nodular sclerosis Hodgkin lymphoma.
- Mixed cellularity Hodgkin lymphoma.
- Lymphocyte-depleted Hodgkin lymphoma.

Anything that increases your risk of getting a disease is called a risk factor. Having a risk factor does not mean that you will get cancer; not having risk factors doesn't mean that you will not get cancer. Talk with your child's doctor if you think your child may be at risk.

Risk factors for childhood Hodgkin lymphoma include the following:

- Being infected with the Epstein-Barr virus.
- Being infected with the human immunodeficiency virus (HIV).
- Having certain diseases of the immune system.
- Having a personal history of mononucleosis ("mono").
- Having a parent or sibling with a personal history of Hodgkin lymphoma.
- Being exposed to common infections in early childhood may decrease the risk of Hodgkin lymphoma in children because of the effect it has on the immune system.

Signs of Childhood Hodgkin Lymphoma

These and other signs and symptoms may be caused by childhood Hodgkin lymphoma or by other conditions. Check with your child's doctor if your child has any of the following:

- Painless, swollen lymph nodes near the collarbone or in the neck, chest, underarm, or groin.
- Fever for no known reason.
- Weight loss for no known reason.
- Night sweats.
- Fatigue.
- Anorexia.
- Itchy skin.
- Pain in the lymph nodes after drinking alcohol.
- Fever, weight loss, and night sweats are called B symptoms.

Tests That Examine the Lymph System Are Used to Detect (Find) and Diagnose Childhood Hodgkin Lymphoma

The following tests and procedures may be used:

- Physical exam and history
- CT scan (CAT scan)
- PET scan (positron emission tomography scan)
- Chest X-ray
- Complete blood count (CBC)
- Sedimentation rate
- Lymph node biopsy

About Childhood Non-Hodgkin Lymphoma

Childhood non-Hodgkin lymphoma is a type of cancer that forms in the lymph system, which is part of the body's immune system. The immune system protects the body from foreign substances, infection, and diseases. The lymph system is made up of the following:

- **Lymph:** Colorless, watery fluid that carries white blood cells called lymphocytes through the lymph system. Lymphocytes protect the body against infections and the growth of tumors. There are three types of lymphocytes:
  - B lymphocytes that make antibodies to help fight infection.
  - T lymphocytes that help B lymphocytes make the antibodies that help fight infection.
  - Natural killer cells that attack cancer cells and viruses.
- **Lymph vessels:** A network of thin tubes that collect lymph from different parts of the body and return it to the bloodstream.
- **Lymph nodes:** Small, bean-shaped structures that filter lymph and store white blood cells that help fight infection and disease. Lymph nodes are located along the network of lymph vessels found throughout the body. Clusters of lymph nodes are found in the neck, underarm, abdomen, pelvis, and groin.
- **Spleen:** An organ that makes lymphocytes, filters the blood, stores blood cells, and destroys old blood cells. The spleen is on the left side of the abdomen near the stomach.
- **Thymus:** An organ in which lymphocytes grow and multiply. The thymus is in the chest behind the breastbone.
- **Tonsils:** Two small masses of lymph tissue at the back of the throat. The tonsils make lymphocytes.
- **Bone marrow:** The soft, spongy tissue in the center of large bones. Bone marrow makes white blood cells, red blood cells, and platelets.

Non-Hodgkin lymphoma can begin in B lymphocytes, T lymphocytes, or natural killer cells. Lymphocytes can also be found in the blood and collect in the lymph nodes, spleen, and thymus.

Lymph tissue is also found in other parts of the body such as the stomach, thyroid gland, brain, and skin.

Non-Hodgkin lymphoma can occur in both adults and children. Treatment for children is different than treatment for adults.

There Are Three Major Types of Childhood Non-Hodgkin Lymphoma

The type of lymphoma is determined by how the cells look under a microscope. The three major types of childhood non-Hodgkin lymphoma are:

Mature B-Cell Non-Hodgkin Lymphoma

Mature B-cell non-Hodgkin lymphomas include:

- **Burkitt and Burkitt-like lymphoma/leukemia:** Burkitt lymphoma and Burkitt leukemia are different forms of the same disease. Burkitt lymphoma/leukemia is an aggressive (fast-growing) disorder of B lymphocytes that is most common in children and young adults. It may form in the abdomen, Waldeyer ring, testicles, bone, bone marrow, skin, or central nervous system (CNS). Burkitt leukemia may start in the lymph nodes as Burkitt lymphoma and then spread to the blood and bone marrow, or it may start in the blood and bone marrow without forming in the lymph nodes first.Both Burkitt leukemia and Burkitt lymphoma have been linked to infection with the Epstein-Barr virus (EBV), although EBV infection is more likely to occur in patients in Africa than in the United States. Burkitt and Burkitt-like lymphoma/leukemia are diagnosed when a sample of tissue is checked and a certain change to the c-myc gene is found.
- **Diffuse large B-cell lymphoma:** Diffuse large B-cell lymphoma is the most common type of non-Hodgkin lymphoma. It is a type of B-cell non-Hodgkin lymphoma that grows quickly in the lymph nodes. The spleen, liver, bone marrow, or other organs are also often affected. Diffuse large B-cell lymphoma occurs more often in adolescents than in children.
- **Primary mediastinal B-cell lymphoma:** A type of lymphoma that develops from B cells in the mediastinum (the area behind the breastbone). It may spread to nearby organs including the lungs and the sac around the heart. It may also spread to lymph nodes and distant organs including the kidneys. In children and adolescents, primary mediastinal B-cell lymphoma occurs more often in older adolescents.

Lymphoblastic Lymphoma

Lymphoblastic lymphoma is a type of lymphoma that mainly affects T-cell lymphocytes. It usually forms in the mediastinum (the area behind the breastbone). This causes trouble breathing, wheezing, trouble swallowing, or swelling of the head and neck. It may spread to lymph nodes, bone, bone marrow, skin, the CNS, abdominal organs, and other areas. Lymphoblastic lymphoma is a lot like acute lymphoblastic leukemia (ALL).

Anaplastic Large Cell Lymphoma

Anaplastic large cell lymphoma is a type of lymphoma that mainly affects T-cell lymphocytes. It usually forms in the lymph nodes, skin, or bone, and sometimes forms in the gastrointestinal tract, lung, tissue that covers the lungs, and muscle. Patients with anaplastic large cell lymphoma have a receptor, called CD30, on the surface of their T cells. In many children, anaplastic large cell lymphoma is marked by changes in the ALK gene that makes a protein called anaplastic lymphoma kinase. A pathologist checks for these cell and gene changes to help diagnose anaplastic large cell lymphoma.

Some Types of Non-Hodgkin Lymphoma Are Rare in Children

Some types of childhood non-Hodgkin lymphoma are less common. These include:

- **Pediatric-type follicular lymphoma:** In children, follicular lymphoma occurs mainly in males. It is more likely to be found in one area and does not spread to other places in the body. It usually forms in the tonsils and lymph nodes in the neck, but may also form in the testicles, kidney, gastrointestinal tract, and salivary gland.
- **Marginal zone lymphoma:** Marginal zone lymphoma is a type of lymphoma that tends to grow and spread slowly and is usually found at an early stage. It may be found in the lymph nodes or in areas outside the lymph nodes. Marginal zone lymphoma found outside the lymph nodes in children is called mucosa-associated lymphoid tissue (MALT) lymphoma and may be linked to *Helicobacter pylori* infection of the gastrointestinal tract and *Chlamydophila psittaci* infection of the conjunctival membrane which lines the eye.
- **Primary central nervous system (CNS) lymphoma:** Primary CNS lymphoma is extremely rare in children.
- **Peripheral T-cell lymphoma:** Peripheral T-cell lymphoma is an aggressive (fast-growing) non-Hodgkin lymphoma that begins in mature T lymphocytes. The T lymphocytes mature in the thymus gland and travel to other parts of the lymph system, such as the lymph nodes, bone marrow, and spleen.

- **Cutaneous T-cell lymphoma:** Cutaneous T-cell lymphoma begins in the skin and can cause the skin to thicken or form a tumor. It is very rare in children, but is more common in adolescents and young adults. There are different types of cutaneous T-cell lymphoma, such as cutaneous anaplastic large cell lymphoma, subcutaneous panniculitis-like T-cell lymphoma, gamma-delta T-cell lymphoma, and mycosis fungoides. Mycosis fungoides rarely occurs in children and adolescents.

Past treatment for cancer and having a weakened immune system affect the risk of having childhood non-hodgkin lymphoma.

Anything that increases your risk of getting a disease is called a risk factor. Having a risk factor does not mean that you will get cancer; not having risk factors doesn't mean that you will not get cancer. Talk with your child's doctor if you think your child may be at risk.

Possible risk factors for childhood non-Hodgkin lymphoma include the following:

- Past treatment for cancer.
- Being infected with the Epstein-Barr virus or human immunodeficiency virus (HIV).
- Having a weakened immune system after a transplant or from medicines given after a transplant.
- Having certain inherited diseases of the immune system

If lymphoma or lymphoproliferative disease is linked to a weakened immune system from certain inherited diseases, HIV infection, a transplant or medicines given after a transplant, the condition is called lymphoproliferative disease associated with immunodeficiency. The different types of lymphoproliferative disease associated with immunodeficiency include:

- Lymphoproliferative disease associated with primary immunodeficiency.
- HIV-associated non-Hodgkin lymphoma.
- Post-transplant lymphoproliferative disease.

Signs of Childhood Non-Hodgkin Lymphoma

These and other signs may be caused by childhood non-Hodgkin lymphoma or by other conditions. Check with a doctor if your child has any of the following:

- Trouble breathing.
- Wheezing.
- Coughing.
- High-pitched breathing sounds.
- Swelling of the head, neck, upper body, or arms.
- Trouble swallowing.
- Painless swelling of the lymph nodes in the neck, underarm, stomach, or groin.
- Painless lump or swelling in a testicle.
- Fever for no known reason.
- Weight loss for no known reason.
- Night sweats.

Tests That Examine the Body and Lymph System Are Used to Detect (Find) and Diagnose Childhood Non-Hodgkin Lymphoma

The following tests and procedures may be used:

- Physical exam and history
- Liver function tests
- CT scan (CAT scan)
- PET scan (positron emission tomography scan)
- MRI (magnetic resonance imaging)
- Lumbar puncture
- Chest X-ray
- Ultrasound exam
- Biopsy

Section 18.3

Neuroblastoma

This section includes text excerpted from "Neuroblastoma Treatment (PDQ®)—Patient Version," National Cancer Institute (NCI), January 20, 2016.

Neuroblastoma is a disease in which malignant (cancer) cells form in nerve tissue of the adrenal gland, neck, chest, or spinal cord.

Neuroblastoma often begins in the nerve tissue of the adrenal glands. There are two adrenal glands, one on top of each kidney in the back of the upper abdomen. The adrenal glands make important hormones that help control heart rate, blood pressure, blood sugar, and the way the body reacts to stress. Neuroblastoma may also begin in the abdomen, in the chest, in nerve tissue near the spine in the neck, or in the spinal cord.

By the time neuroblastoma is diagnosed, the cancer has usually metastasized (spread). Neuroblastoma spreads most often to the lymph nodes, bones, bone marrow, liver, and in infants, skin.

Causes of Neuroblastoma

The gene mutation that increases the risk of neuroblastoma is sometimes inherited (passed from the parent to the child). In patients with this gene mutation, neuroblastoma usually occurs at a younger age and more than one tumor may form in the adrenal medulla.

Signs and Symptoms of Neuroblastoma

The most common signs and symptoms of neuroblastoma are caused by the tumor pressing on nearby tissues as it grows or by cancer spreading to the bone. These and other signs and symptoms may be caused by neuroblastoma or by other conditions.

Check with your child's doctor if your child has any of the following:

- Lump in the abdomen, neck, or chest.

- Bulging eyes.
- Dark circles around the eyes ("black eyes").
- Bone pain.
- Swollen stomach and trouble breathing (in infants).
- Painless, bluish lumps under the skin (in infants).
- Weakness or paralysis (loss of ability to move a body part).

Less common signs and symptoms of neuroblastoma include the following:

- Fever.
- Shortness of breath.
- Feeling tired.
- Easy bruising or bleeding.
- Petechiae (flat, pinpoint spots under the skin caused by bleeding).
- High blood pressure.
- Severe watery diarrhea.
- Jerky muscle movements.
- Uncontrolled eye movement.

Diagnosing Neuroblastoma

The following tests and procedures may be used:

- Physical exam and history
- Neurological exam
- Urine catecholamine studies
- Blood chemistry studies
- Hormone test
- mIBG (metaiodobenzylguanidine) scan
- Bone marrow aspiration and biopsy
- X-ray
- CT scan (CAT scan)

- MRI (magnetic resonance imaging) with gadolinium
- Ultrasound exam

Cells and tissues are removed during a biopsy so they can be viewed under a microscope by a pathologist to check for signs of cancer. The way the biopsy is done depends on where the tumor is in the body. Sometimes the whole tumor is removed at the same time the biopsy is done.

The following tests may be done on the tissue that is removed:

- Cytogenetic analysis
- Light and electron microscopy
- Immunohistochemistry
- MYC-N amplification study

Children who are 6 months old or younger may not need a biopsy or surgery to remove the tumor because the tumor may disappear without treatment.

Section 18.4

Sarcoma and Bone Tumors

This section contains text excerpted from the following sources: Text under the heading "Overview" is excerpted from "Sarcoma," National Cancer Institute (NCI), November 15, 2013; Text beginning with the heading "Ewing Sarcoma" is excerpted from "Ewing Sarcoma Treatment (PDQ®)—Patient Version," National Cancer Institute (NCI), May 18, 2016.

Overview

The term "sarcoma" encompasses a broad family of rare cancers that can affect soft tissue or bone throughout the body, and sometimes both.1 Sarcoma cases constitute about 15 percent of all cancers in children, but are much rarer in adults and make up only about one percent of adult cancer cases.

In 2012, it was estimated that about 11,280 Americans would be diagnosed with soft tissue sarcomas and that approximately one third of those people would not survive. In addition, an estimated 2,890 Americans would be diagnosed with bone sarcomas, and approximately half were not expected to survive.

However, the exact number of people affected is unknown because sarcoma can be misdiagnosed due to being difficult to distinguish from other health problems. Plus, there are often few, if any, symptoms at early stages.

TCGA will be focusing its studies on seven sarcoma subtypes:

- Dedifferentiated liposarcoma
- Desmoid sarcoma
- Malignant peripheral nerve sheath tumor
- Myxofibrosarcoma
- Synovial sarcoma
- Undifferentiated pleomorphic sarcoma.
- Uterine and non-uterine leiomyosarcoma.

Ewing Sarcoma

Ewing sarcoma is a type of tumor that forms in bone or soft tissue.

Ewing sarcoma is a type of tumor that forms from a certain kind of cell in bone or soft tissue. Ewing sarcoma may be found in the bones of the legs, arms, feet, hands, chest, pelvis, spine, or skull. Ewing sarcoma also may be found in the soft tissue of the trunk, arms, legs, head and neck, abdominal cavity, or other areas.

Ewing sarcoma is most common in adolescents and young adults.

Ewing sarcoma has also been called peripheral primitive neuroectodermal tumor, Askin tumor (Ewing sarcoma of the chest wall), extraosseous Ewing sarcoma (Ewing sarcoma in tissue other than bone), and Ewing sarcoma family of tumors.

Signs and Symptoms of Ewing Sarcoma

These and other signs and symptoms may be caused by Ewing sarcoma or by other conditions. Check with your child's doctor if your child has any of the following:

- Pain and/or swelling, usually in the arms, legs, chest, back, or pelvis.

- A lump (which may feel soft and warm) in the arms, legs, chest, or pelvis.
- Fever for no known reason.
- A bone that breaks for no known reason.

Tests That Examine the Bone and Soft Tissue Are Used to Diagnose and Stage Ewing Sarcoma

Procedures that make pictures of the bones and soft tissues and nearby areas help diagnose Ewing sarcoma and show how far the cancer has spread. The process used to find out if cancer cells have spread within and around the bones and soft tissues is called staging.

- In order to plan treatment, it is important to know if the cancer is in the area where it first formed or if it has spread to other parts of the body. Tests and procedures to detect, diagnose, and stage Ewing sarcoma are usually done at the same time.

The following tests and procedures may be used to diagnose or stage Ewing sarcoma:

- Physical exam and history
- MRI (magnetic resonance imaging)
- CT scan (CAT scan)
- PET scan (positron emission tomography scan)
- Bone scan
- Bone marrow aspiration and biopsy
- X-ray
- Complete blood count (CBC)
- Blood chemistry studies

Section 18.5

Wilms Tumor (Nephroblastoma)

This section includes text excerpted from "Wilms Tumor and Other Childhood Kidney Tumors Treatment (PDQ®)—Patient Version," National Cancer Institute (NCI), July 7, 2016.

About Wilms Tumor and Other Childhood Kidney Tumors

Childhood kidney tumors are diseases in which malignant (cancer) cells form in the tissues of the kidney.

There are two kidneys, one on each side of the backbone, above the waist. Tiny tubules in the kidneys filter and clean the blood. They take out waste products and make urine. The urine passes from each kidney through a long tube called a ureter into the bladder. The bladder holds the urine until it passes through the urethra and leaves the body.

There Are Many Types of Childhood Kidney Tumors

Wilms Tumor

In Wilms tumor, one or more tumors may be found in one or both kidneys. Wilms tumor may spread to the lungs, liver, bone, brain, or nearby lymph nodes. Most childhood kidney cancers are Wilms tumors, but in children 15 to 19 years old, renal cell cancer is more common.

Renal Cell Cancer (RCC)

Renal cell cancer is rare in children and adolescents younger than 15 years old. It is much more common in adolescents between 15 and 19 years old. Children and adolescents are more likely to be diagnosed with a large renal cell tumor or cancer that has spread. Renal cell cancers may spread to the lungs, liver, or lymph nodes. Renal cell cancer may also be called renal cell carcinoma.

Rhabdoid Tumor of the Kidney

Rhabdoid tumor of the kidney is a type of kidney cancer that occurs mostly in infants and young children. It is often advanced at the time of diagnosis. Rhabdoid tumor of the kidney grows and spreads quickly, often to the lungs or brain.

Children with a certain gene change are checked regularly to see if a rhabdoid tumor has formed in the kidney or has spread to the brain:

- Children younger than one year old have an ultrasound of the abdomen every two to three months and an ultrasound of the brain every month.
- Children one to four years old have an ultrasound of the abdomen and an MRI of the brain and spine every three months.

Clear Cell Sarcoma of the Kidney

Clear cell sarcoma of the kidney is a type of kidney tumor that may spread to the lung, bone, brain, or soft tissue. When it recurs (comes back) after treatment, it often recurs in the brain.

Congenital Mesoblastic Nephroma

Congenital mesoblastic nephroma is a tumor of the kidney that is often diagnosed during the first year of life. It can usually be cured.

Ewing Sarcoma (Neuroepithelial Tumor) of the Kidney

Ewing sarcoma (neuroepithelial tumor) of the kidney is rare and usually occurs in young adults. These tumors grow and spread to other parts of the body quickly.

Desmoplastic Small Round Cell Tumor of the Kidney

Desmoplastic small round cell tumor of the kidney is a rare soft tissue sarcoma.

Cystic Partially Differentiated Nephroblastoma

Cystic partially differentiated nephroblastoma is a very rare type of Wilms tumor made up of cysts.

Multilocular Cystic Nephroma

Multilocular cystic nephromas are benign tumors made up of cysts. These tumors can occur in one or both kidneys. Children with this type of tumor also may have pleuropulmonary blastomas, so imaging tests that check the lungs for cysts or solid tumors are done. Since multilocular cystic nephroma may be an inherited condition, genetic counseling and genetic testing may be considered.

Primary Renal Synovial Sarcoma

Primary renal synovial sarcoma is a rare tumor of the kidney and is most common in young adults. These tumors grow and spread quickly.

Anaplastic Sarcoma of the Kidney

- Anaplastic sarcoma of the kidney is a rare tumor that is most common in children or adolescents younger than 15 years of age. Anaplastic sarcoma of the kidney often spreads to the lungs, liver, or bones. Imaging tests that check the lungs for cysts or solid tumors may be done based on test results and age of the child. Since anaplastic sarcoma may be an inherited condition, genetic counseling and genetic testing may be considered.

Nephroblastomatosis Is Not Cancer but May Become Wilms Tumor

Sometimes, after the kidneys form in the fetus, abnormal groups of kidney cells remain in one or both kidneys. In nephroblastomatosis (diffuse hyperplastic perilobar nephroblastomatosis), these abnormal groups of cells may grow in many places inside the kidney or make a thick layer around the kidney. When these groups of abnormal cells are found in a kidney that was removed for Wilms tumor, the child has an increased risk of Wilms tumor in the other kidney. Frequent follow-up testing is important at least every 3 months, for at least 7 years after the child is treated.

Tests Are Used to Screen for Wilms Tumor

Screening tests are done in children with an increased risk of Wilms tumor. These tests may help find cancer early and decrease the chance of dying from cancer.

In general, children with an increased risk of Wilms tumor should be screened for Wilms tumor every three months until they are at least 8 years old. An ultrasound test of the abdomen is usually used for screening. Small Wilms tumors may be found early and removed.

Children with Beckwith-Wiedemann syndrome or hemihypertrophy are also screened for liver and adrenal tumors that are linked to these genetic syndromes. A test to check the alpha-fetoprotein (AFP) level in the blood and an ultrasound of the abdomen are done until the child is 4 years old. An ultrasound of the kidneys is done after the child is 4 years old.

Children with aniridia and a certain gene change are screened for Wilms tumor every three months until they are 8 years old. An ultrasound test of the abdomen is used for screening.

Some children develop Wilms tumor in both kidneys. These often appear when Wilms tumor is first diagnosed, but Wilms tumor may also occur in the second kidney after the child is successfully treated for Wilms tumor in one kidney. A second tumor is much more likely to develop in the other kidney when a child's first Wilms tumor is diagnosed before they are one year old or when embryonic cells remain in the kidney. Children with an increased risk of a second Wilms tumor in the other kidney should be screened for Wilms tumor every three months for two to six years. An ultrasound test of the abdomen may be used for screening.

Tests That Examine the Kidney and the Blood Are Used to Detect (Find) and Diagnose Wilms Tumor and Other Childhood Kidney Tumors

The following tests and procedures may be used:

- Physical exam and history
- Complete blood count (CBC)
- Blood chemistry studies
- Renal function test.
- Urinalysis
- Ultrasound exam
- CT scan (CAT scan)
- MRI (magnetic resonance imaging) with gadolinium
- X-ray of the abdomen
- PET-CT scan
- Biopsy

Chapter 19

Cardiovascular Disorders in Children

Chapter Contents

Section 19.1

Arrhythmia

This section includes text excerpted from "Arrhythmia," National Heart, Lung, and Blood Institute (NHLBI), July 1, 2011. Reviewed October 2016.

What Is an Arrhythmia?

An arrhythmia is a problem with the rate or rhythm of the heartbeat. During an arrhythmia, the heart can beat too fast, too slow, or with an irregular rhythm.

A heartbeat that is too fast is called tachycardia. A heartbeat that is too slow is called bradycardia.

Most arrhythmias are harmless, but some can be serious or even life threatening. During an arrhythmia, the heart may not be able to pump enough blood to the body. Lack of blood flow can damage the brain, heart, and other organs.

Outlook

There are many types of arrhythmia. Most arrhythmias are harmless, but some are not. The outlook for a person who has an arrhythmia depends on the type and severity of the arrhythmia.

Even serious arrhythmias often can be successfully treated. Most people who have arrhythmias are able to live normal, healthy lives.

Arrhythmias in Children

Children's heart rates normally decrease as they get older. A newborn's heart beats between 95 to 160 times a minute. A 1-year-old's heart beats between 90 to 150 times a minute, and a 6- to 8-year-old's heart beats between 60 to 110 times a minute.

A baby or child's heart can beat fast or slow for many reasons. Like adults, when children are active, their hearts will beat faster. When they're sleeping, their hearts will beat slower. Their heart rates can speed up and slow down as they breathe in and out. All of these changes are normal.

Some children are born with heart defects that cause arrhythmias. In other children, arrhythmias can develop later in childhood. Doctors use the same tests to diagnose arrhythmias in children and adults.

Treatments for children who have arrhythmias include medicines, defibrillation (electric shock), surgically implanted devices that control the heartbeat, and other procedures that fix abnormal electrical signals in the heart.

What Causes an Arrhythmia?

An arrhythmia can occur if the electrical signals that control the heartbeat are delayed or blocked. This can happen if the special nerve cells that produce electrical signals don't work properly. It also can happen if the electrical signals don't travel normally through the heart.

An arrhythmia also can occur if another part of the heart starts to produce electrical signals. This adds to the signals from the special nerve cells and disrupts the normal heartbeat.

Smoking, heavy alcohol use, use of some drugs (such as cocaine or amphetamines), use of some prescription or over-the-counter medicines, or too much caffeine or nicotine can lead to arrhythmias in some people.

Strong emotional stress or anger can make the heart work harder, raise blood pressure, and release stress hormones. Sometimes these reactions can lead to arrhythmias.

A heart attack or other condition that damages the heart's electrical system also can cause arrhythmias. Examples of such conditions include high blood pressure, coronary heart disease, heart failure, an overactive or underactive thyroid gland (too much or too little thyroid hormone produced), and rheumatic heart disease.

Congenital heart defects can cause some arrhythmias, such as Wolff-Parkinson-White syndrome. The term "congenital" means the defect is present at birth.

Sometimes the cause of arrhythmias is unknown.

What Are the Signs and Symptoms of an Arrhythmia?

Many arrhythmias cause no signs or symptoms. When signs or symptoms are present, the most common ones are:

- Palpitations (feelings that your heart is skipping a beat, fluttering, or beating too hard or fast)
- A slow heartbeat

- An irregular heartbeat
- Feeling pauses between heartbeats

How Are Arrhythmias Diagnosed?

Arrhythmias can be hard to diagnose, especially the types that only cause symptoms every once in a while. Doctors diagnose arrhythmias based on medical and family histories, a physical exam, and the results from tests and procedures.

How Are Arrhythmias Treated?

Common arrhythmia treatments include medicines, medical procedures, and surgery. Your doctor may recommend treatment if your arrhythmia causes serious symptoms, such as dizziness, chest pain, or fainting.

Your doctor also may recommend treatment if the arrhythmia increases your risk for problems such as heart failure, stroke, or sudden cardiac arrest.

Section 19.2

Heart Murmurs

This section includes text excerpted from "Heart Murmur," National Heart, Lung, and Blood Institute (NHLBI), September 20, 2012. Reviewed October 2016.

What Is a Heart Murmur?

A heart murmur is an extra or unusual sound heard during a heartbeat. Murmurs range from very faint to very loud. Sometimes they sound like a whooshing or swishing noise.

Normal heartbeats make a "lub-DUPP" or "lub-DUB" sound. This is the sound of the heart valves closing as blood moves through the heart. Doctors can hear these sounds and heart murmurs using a stethoscope.

The two types of heart murmurs are innocent (harmless) and abnormal.

Innocent heart murmurs aren't caused by heart problems. These murmurs are common in healthy children. Many children will have heart murmurs heard by their doctors at some point in their lives.

People who have abnormal heart murmurs may have signs or symptoms of heart problems. Most abnormal murmurs in children are caused by congenital heart defects. These defects are problems with the heart's structure that are present at birth.

A heart murmur isn't a disease, and most murmurs are harmless. Innocent murmurs don't cause symptoms. Having one doesn't require you to limit your physical activity or do anything else special. Although you may have an innocent murmur throughout your life, you won't need treatment for it.

The outlook and treatment for abnormal heart murmurs depend on the type and severity of the heart problem causing them.

What Causes Heart Murmurs?

Innocent Heart Murmurs

Why some people have innocent heart murmurs and others do not isn't known. Innocent murmurs are simply sounds made by blood flowing through the heart's chambers and valves, or through blood vessels near the heart.

Extra blood flow through the heart also may cause innocent heart murmurs. After childhood, the most common cause of extra blood flow through the heart is pregnancy. This is because during pregnancy, women's bodies make extra blood. Most heart murmurs that occur in pregnant women are innocent.

Abnormal Heart Murmurs

Congenital heart defects or acquired heart valve disease often are the cause of abnormal heart murmurs.

Congenital Heart Defects

Congenital heart defects are the most common cause of abnormal heart murmurs in children. These defects are problems with the heart's structure that are present at birth. They change the normal flow of blood through the heart.

Congenital heart defects can involve the interior walls of the heart, the valves inside the heart, or the arteries and veins that carry blood to and from the heart. Some babies are born with more than one heart defect.

Heart valve problems, septal defects (also called holes in the heart), and diseases of the heart muscle such as hypertrophic cardiomyopathy are common heart defects that cause abnormal heart murmurs.

Examples of valve problems are narrow valves that limit blood flow or leaky valves that don't close properly. Septal defects are holes in the wall that separates the right and left sides of the heart. This wall is called the septum.

A hole in the septum between the heart's two upper chambers is called an atrial septal defect. A hole in the septum between the heart's two lower chambers is called a ventricular septal defect.

Hypertrophic cardiomyopathy (HCM) occurs if heart muscle cells enlarge and cause the walls of the ventricles (usually the left ventricle) to thicken. The thickening may block blood flow out of the ventricle. If a blockage occurs, the ventricle must work hard to pump blood to the body. HCM also can affect the heart's mitral valve, causing blood to leak backward through the valve.

Acquired Heart Valve Disease

Acquired heart valve disease often is the cause of abnormal heart murmurs in adults. This is heart valve disease that develops as the result of another condition.

Many conditions can cause heart valve disease. Examples include heart conditions and other disorders, age-related changes, rheumatic fever, and infections.

Heart conditions and other disorders. Certain conditions can stretch and distort the heart valves, such as:

Damage and scar tissue from a heart attack or injury to the heart.

Advanced high blood pressure and heart failure. These conditions can enlarge the heart or its main arteries.

Age-related changes. As you get older, calcium deposits or other deposits may form on your heart valves. These deposits stiffen and thicken the valve flaps and limit blood flow. This stiffening and thickening of the valve is called sclerosis.

Rheumatic fever. The bacteria that cause strep throat, scarlet fever, and, in some cases, impetigo also can cause rheumatic fever.

This serious illness can develop if you have an untreated or not fully treated streptococcal (strep) infection.

Rheumatic fever can damage and scar the heart valves. The symptoms of this heart valve damage often don't occur until many years after recovery from rheumatic fever.

Today, most people who have strep infections are treated with antibiotics before rheumatic fever develops. It's very important to take all of the antibiotics your doctor prescribes for strep throat, even if you feel better before the medicine is gone.

Infections. Common germs that enter the bloodstream and get carried to the heart can sometimes infect the inner surface of the heart, including the heart valves. This rare but sometimes life-threatening infection is called infective endocarditis, or IE.

IE is more likely to develop in people who already have abnormal blood flow through a heart valve because of heart valve disease. The abnormal blood flow causes blood clots to form on the surface of the valve. The blood clots make it easier for germs to attach to and infect the valve.

IE can worsen existing heart valve disease.

Other Causes

Some heart murmurs occur because of an illness outside of the heart. The heart is normal, but an illness or condition can cause blood flow that's faster than normal. Examples of this type of illness include fever, anemia, and hyperthyroidism.

Anemia is a condition in which the body has a lower than normal number of red blood cells. Hyperthyroidism is a condition in which the body has too much thyroid hormone.

What Are the Signs and Symptoms of a Heart Murmur?

People who have innocent (harmless) heart murmurs don't have any signs or symptoms other than the murmur itself. This is because innocent heart murmurs aren't caused by heart problems.

People who have abnormal heart murmurs may have signs or symptoms of the heart problems causing the murmurs. These signs and symptoms may include:

- Poor eating and failure to grow normally (in infants)
- Shortness of breath, which may occur only with physical exertion

- Excessive sweating with minimal or no exertion
- Chest pain
- Dizziness or fainting
- A bluish color on the skin, especially on the fingertips and lips
- Chronic cough
- Swelling or sudden weight gain
- Enlarged liver
- Enlarged neck veins

Signs and symptoms depend on the problem causing the heart murmur and its severity.

How Is a Heart Murmur Diagnosed?

Doctors use a stethoscope to listen to heart sounds and hear heart murmurs. They may detect heart murmurs during routine checkups or while checking for another condition.

If a congenital heart defect causes a murmur, it's often heard at birth or during infancy. Abnormal heart murmurs caused by other heart problems can be heard in patients of any age.

How Is a Heart Murmur Treated?

A heart murmur isn't a disease. It's an extra or unusual sound heard during the heartbeat. Thus, murmurs themselves don't require treatment. However, if an underlying condition is causing a heart murmur, your doctor may recommend treatment for that condition.

Innocent (Harmless) Heart Murmurs

Healthy children who have innocent (harmless) heart murmurs don't need treatment. Their heart murmurs aren't caused by heart problems or other conditions.

Pregnant women who have innocent heart murmurs due to extra blood volume also don't need treatment. Their heart murmurs should go away after pregnancy.

Abnormal Heart Murmurs

If you or your child has an abnormal heart murmur, your doctor will recommend treatment for the disease or condition causing the murmur.

Some medical conditions, such as anemia or hyperthyroidism, can cause heart murmurs that aren't related to heart disease. Treating these conditions should make the heart murmur go away.

If a congenital heart defect is causing a heart murmur, treatment will depend on the type and severity of the defect. Treatment may include medicines or surgery.

If acquired heart valve disease is causing a heart murmur, treatment usually will depend on the type, amount, and severity of the disease.

Currently, no medicines can cure heart valve disease. However, lifestyle changes and medicines can treat symptoms and help delay complications. Eventually, though, you may need surgery to repair or replace a faulty heart valve.

Section 19.3

Hyperlipidemia (High Cholesterol)

This section includes text excerpted from "HIV and Hyperlipidemia," AIDSinfo, National Institutes of Health (NIH), January 7, 2016.

What Is Hyperlipidemia?

Hyperlipidemia is the medical term for high levels of fat in the blood. Fats in the blood (also called lipids) include cholesterol and triglycerides. The body makes cholesterol and triglycerides. The fats also come from some of the foods we eat.

The body needs cholesterol and triglycerides to function properly but having too much can cause problems. High levels of cholesterol and triglycerides increase the risk of heart disease, gallbladder disease, and pancreatitis (inflammation of the pancreas).

What Are the Symptoms of Hyperlipidemia?

Usually hyperlipidemia has no symptoms. A blood test is used to measure levels of fat in the blood and to detect hyperlipidemia.

Risk Factors for Hyperlipidemia

The following are risk factors for hyperlipidemia:

- Family history of hyperlipidemia
- Other medical conditions, including high blood pressure, diabetes, and an underactive thyroid gland
- A high-fat, high-carbohydrate diet
- Being overweight or obese
- Smoking
- Alcohol use
- Lack of physical activity

Many of these risk factors for hyperlipidemia can be controlled by lifestyle choices. For example, maintaining a healthy weight is one way to reduce the risk of hyperlipidemia.

What Are Other Steps a Person Can Take to Prevent Hyperlipidemia?

Here are additional steps to take to reduce the risk of hyperlipidemia.

- **Eat foods low in saturated fat, trans fat, and cholesterol.** Eat less full-fat dairy products, fatty meats, and desserts high in fat and sugar. Limit foods that are high in cholesterol, such as egg yolks, fatty meats, and organ meat (like liver and kidney). Instead, choose low-fat or fat-free milk, cheese, and yogurt; eat more foods that are high in fiber, like oatmeal, oat bran, beans, and lentils; and eat more vegetables and fruits.
- **Get active.** Get at least 30 minutes of aerobic physical activity on most days of the week. Aerobic activities include walking quickly, biking slowly, and gardening.

What Is the Treatment for Hyperlipidemia?

Lifestyle changes may not be enough to reduce blood fat levels. There are also medicines that can help control blood fat levels. The most common medicines used to reduce cholesterol levels are called statins. Fibrates are a type of medicine used to lower triglycerides.

Section 19.4

Hypertension (High Blood Pressure)

This section contains text excerpted from the following sources: Text under the heading "About High Blood Pressure" is excerpted from "Questions and Answers about High Blood Pressure," National Institute of Diabetes and Digestive and Kidney Diseases (NIDDK), March 1, 2012. Reviewed October 2016; Text under the heading "High Blood Pressure and Children" is excerpted from "High Blood Pressure and Children: What Parents Need to Know," National Institute of Diabetes and Digestive and Kidney Diseases (NIDDK), March 1, 2012. Reviewed October 2016.

About High Blood Pressure

What Is High Blood Pressure?

Blood pressure is the force of blood against the walls of your arteries as it is pumped through your body. When this force stays too high, it becomes a life-threatening condition called hypertension, or high blood pressure. It makes the heart work too hard, causing damage to blood vessels, and can lead to serious health problems like heart disease, stroke, and kidney failure.

A blood pressure of 140/90 mmHg or higher is considered high for most people. In general, lower is better. However, very low blood pressure can sometimes be a cause of concern and should be checked out by a doctor.

Am I at Risk for High Blood Pressure?

Anyone can develop high blood pressure. But there are several factors that increase your risk:

- Being overweight or obese
- Not exercising
- Eating too much salt and sodium
- Not eating enough potassium (found in fruits and vegetables)

- Drinking too much alcohol
- Having diabetes

How Do I Know If I Have High Blood Pressure?

High blood pressure is often called "the silent killer" because it usually has no symptoms.

Some people may not find out they have it until they have complications that affect their heart, brain, or kidneys.

The only way to find out if you have high blood pressure is to have your blood pressure checked regularly by your doctor or healthcare provider. Most doctors will check your blood pressure several times on different days to get repeated readings before deciding whether you have high blood pressure.

How Can I Control or Prevent High Blood Pressure?

High blood pressure can be treated and controlled. Many different types of medicines lower blood pressure. Two types—called ACE inhibitors and ARBs—also protect kidney function. Better yet, high blood pressure can be prevented.

Simple and often small lifestyle changes can help control and prevent high blood pressure:

- Maintain a healthy weight
- Be physically active
- Follow a healthy eating plan
- Reduce salt and sodium in your diet
- Drink alcohol only in moderation
- Quit smoking
- Control your blood sugar if you have diabetes
- Take prescribed medicine as directed

High Blood Pressure and Children

Children Can Have High Blood Pressure

Did you know that children could have high blood pressure? In fact, the number of children with high blood pressure is growing.

The sooner high blood pressure is found in children, the sooner it can be treated.

All Children 3 Years of Age and Older Should Have Their Blood Pressure Checked Regularly

Having high blood pressure may not cause any symptoms. Having your child's blood pressure checked is the only way to know if he or she has high blood pressure. The normal range for blood pressure in children is usually lower than in adults. If the blood pressure is high at three healthcare visits, your child may need further testing.

High Blood Pressure in Children Needs to Be Treated

Untreated high blood pressure can cause kidney disease, heart disease, eye disease, and other serious health problems over time. The longer the high blood pressure goes uncontrolled, the more harm it can cause. Treatment begins with lifestyle changes, such as diet changes, more physical activity, and weight loss. Some children also may need to take blood pressure medicines.

Steps to Keep Your Child's Blood Pressure in the Healthy Range

These tips are good for all children, especially those who have or are at risk for high blood pressure:

- Give your child healthy home cooked food
- Use less canned or pre-prepared food
- Encourage physical activity
- If your child smokes or chews tobacco, talk with his or her doctor about how to help your child quit.
- Make sure that your child takes his or her blood pressure medicine if prescribed.
- You and your family can keep a healthy weight.

What Does It Mean to Eat a Healthy Diet?

Eating for healthy blood pressure means eating:

- less salt and packaged foods that are high in sodium, and
- more fruits and vegetables.

Questions to Ask the Doctor about Your Child's Blood Pressure

- What is my child's blood pressure?
- Is it in the normal range?
- Is my child at risk for high blood pressure?

All children should have their blood pressure checked during their routine physical exams. Those with a family history of high blood pressure and being overweight need to have it checked more often.

Section 19.5

Kawasaki Disease

This section includes text excerpted from "Kawasaki Disease," National Heart, Lung, and Blood Institute (NHLBI), September 20, 2011. Reviewed October 2016.

What Is Kawasaki Disease?

Kawasaki disease is a rare childhood disease. It's a form of a condition called vasculitis. This condition involves inflammation of the blood vessels.

In Kawasaki disease, the walls of the blood vessels throughout the body become inflamed. The disease can affect any type of blood vessel in the body, including the arteries, veins, and capillaries.

Sometimes Kawasaki disease affects the coronary arteries, which carry oxygen-rich blood to the heart. As a result, some children who have Kawasaki disease may develop serious heart problems.

What Causes Kawasaki Disease?

The cause of Kawasaki disease isn't known. The body's response to a virus or infection combined with genetic factors may cause the disease. However, no specific virus or infection has been found, and the role of genetics isn't known.

Kawasaki disease can't be passed from one child to another. Your child won't get it from close contact with a child who has the disease. Also, if your child has the disease, he or she can't pass it to another child.

Who Is at Risk for Kawasaki Disease?

Kawasaki disease affects children of all races and ages and both genders. It occurs most often in children of Asian and Pacific Island descent.

The disease is more likely to affect boys than girls. Most cases occur in children younger than 5 years old. Kawasaki disease is rare in children older than 8.

What Are the Signs and Symptoms of Kawasaki Disease?

One of the main symptoms during the early part of Kawasaki disease, called the acute phase, is fever. The fever lasts longer than 5 days. It remains high even after treatment with standard childhood fever medicines.

Other classic signs of the disease are:

- Swollen lymph nodes in the neck
- A rash on the mid-section of the body and in the genital area
- Red, dry, cracked lips and a red, swollen tongue
- Red, swollen palms of the hands and soles of the feet
- Redness of the eyes

Other Signs and Symptoms

During the acute phase, your child also may be irritable and have a sore throat, joint pain, diarrhea, vomiting, and stomach pain.

Within 2 to 3 weeks of the start of symptoms, the skin on your child's fingers and toes may peel, sometimes in large sheets.

How Is Kawasaki Disease Diagnosed?

Kawasaki disease is diagnosed based on your child's signs and symptoms and the results from tests and procedures.

How Is Kawasaki Disease Treated?

Medicines are the main treatment for Kawasaki disease. Rarely, children whose coronary (heart) arteries are affected may need medical procedures or surgery.

The goals of treatment include:

- Reducing fever and inflammation to improve symptoms
- Preventing the disease from affecting the coronary arteries

Initial Treatment

Kawasaki disease can cause serious health problems. Thus, your child will likely be treated in a hospital, at least for the early part of treatment.

The standard treatment during the disease's acute phase is high-dose aspirin and immune globulin. Immune globulin is a medicine that's injected into a vein.

Most children who receive these treatments improve greatly within 24 hours. For a small number of children, fever remains. These children may need a second round of immune globulin.

At the start of treatment, your child will receive high doses of aspirin. As soon as his or her fever goes away, a low dose of aspirin is given. The low dose helps prevent blood clots, which can form in the inflamed small arteries.

Most children treated for Kawasaki disease fully recover from the acute phase and don't need any further treatment. They should, however, follow a healthy diet and adopt healthy lifestyle habits. Taking these steps can help lower the risk of future heart disease. (Following a healthy lifestyle is advised for all children, not just those who have Kawasaki disease.)

Children who have had immune globulin should wait 11 months before having the measles and chicken pox vaccines. Immune globulin can prevent those vaccines from working well.

Long-Term Care and Treatment

If Kawasaki disease has affected your child's coronary arteries, he or she will need ongoing care and treatment.

It's best if a pediatric cardiologist provides this care to reduce the risk of severe heart problems. A pediatric cardiologist is a doctor who specializes in treating children who have heart problems.

Medicines and Tests

When Kawasaki disease affects the coronary arteries, they may expand and twist. If this happens, your child's doctor may prescribe blood-thinning medicines (for example, warfarin). These medicines help prevent blood clots from forming in the affected coronary arteries.

Blood-thinning medicines usually are stopped after the coronary arteries heal. Healing may occur about 18 months after the acute phase of the disease.

In a small number of children, the coronary arteries don't heal. These children likely will need routine tests, such as:

- Echocardiography. This test uses sound waves to create images of the heart.
- EKG (electrocardiogram). This test detects and records the heart's electrical activity.
- Stress test. This test provides information about how the heart works during physical activity or stress.

Medical Procedures and Surgery

Rarely, a child who has Kawasaki disease may need cardiac catheterization. Doctors use this procedure to diagnose and treat some heart conditions.

A flexible tube called a catheter is put into a blood vessel in the arm, groin (upper thigh), or neck and threaded to the heart. Through the catheter, doctors can perform tests and treatments on the heart.

Very rarely, a child may need to have other procedures or surgery if inflammation narrows his or her coronary arteries and blocks blood flow to the heart.

Percutaneous coronary intervention (PCI), stent placement, or coronary artery bypass grafting (CABG) may be used.

Coronary angioplasty restores blood flow through narrowed or blocked coronary arteries. A thin tube with a balloon on the end is inserted into a blood vessel in the arm or groin. The tube is threaded to the narrowed or blocked coronary artery. Then, the balloon is inflated to widen the artery and restore blood flow.

A stent (small mesh tube) may be placed in the coronary artery during angioplasty. This device helps support the narrowed or weakened artery. A stent can improve blood flow and prevent the artery from bursting.

Rarely, a child may need to have CABG. This surgery is used to treat blocked coronary arteries. During CABG, a healthy artery or vein from another part of the body is connected, or grafted, to the blocked coronary artery.

The grafted artery or vein bypasses (that is, goes around) the blocked part of the coronary artery. This improves blood flow to the heart.

Living with Kawasaki Disease

Most children who have Kawasaki disease recover—usually within weeks of getting symptoms. Further problems are rare. Early treatment reduces the risk of serious problems.

Researchers continue to look for the cause of Kawasaki disease and better ways to diagnose and treat it. They also hope to learn more about long-term health risks, if any, for people who have had the disease.

What to Expect after Treatment

Most children who are treated for Kawasaki disease fully recover from the acute phase. They don't need further treatment.

They should, however, follow a healthy diet and adopt healthy lifestyle habits. Taking these steps can help lower their risk of future heart disease. (Following a healthy lifestyle is advised for all children, not just those who have Kawasaki disease).

Children treated with immune globulin should wait 11 months before having measles and chicken pox vaccines. Immune globulin can prevent these vaccines from working well.

Ongoing Healthcare Needs

If Kawasaki disease has affected your child's coronary arteries, he or she will need ongoing care and treatment. It's best if a pediatric cardiologist provides this care to reduce the risk of severe heart problems. A pediatric cardiologist is a doctor who specializes in treating children who have heart problems.

Support Groups

Joining a support group may help you adjust to caring for a child who has Kawasaki disease. You can see how other parents have coped with the disease. Ask your child's doctor about local support groups or check with an area medical center.

Chapter 20

Diabetes in Children

Diabetes mellitus is a group of diseases characterized by high levels of glucose in the blood resulting from defects in insulin production, insulin action, or both. Diabetes is associated with serious complications, but timely diagnosis and treatment of diabetes can prevent or delay the onset of long-term complications (damage to the cardiovascular system, kidneys, eyes, nerves, blood vessels, skin, gums, and teeth). New management strategies are helping children with diabetes live long and healthy lives.

Diabetes is one of the most common diseases in school-aged children. About 208,000 young people in the United States under age 20 had diabetes in 2012. Both type 1 diabetes and type 2 diabetes are increasing in U.S. children and adolescents.

Type 1 Diabetes

Type 1 diabetes accounts for approximately 5 percent of all diagnosed cases of diabetes, but is the leading cause of diabetes in children of all ages. Type 1 diabetes accounts for almost all diabetes in children less than 10 years of age. Type 1 diabetes is an autoimmune disease in which the immune system destroys the insulin-producing beta cells of the pancreas that help regulate blood glucose levels.

This chapter includes text excerpted from "Overview of Diabetes in Children and Adolescents," National Institute of Diabetes and Digestive and Kidney Diseases (NIDDK), July 2014.

Onset: Type 1 diabetes mostly has an acute onset, with children and adolescents usually able to pinpoint when symptoms began. Onset can occur at any age. Children and adolescents may present with ketoacidosis as the first indication of type 1 diabetes. Others may have post-meal hyperglycemia, or modest fasting hyperglycemia that rapidly progresses to severe hyperglycemia and/or ketoacidosis in the presence of infection or other stress.

Symptoms: The immunologic process that leads to type 1 diabetes can begin years before the symptoms of type 1 diabetes develop. Symptoms become apparent when most of the beta-cell population is destroyed and usually develop over a short period of time. Early symptoms, which are mainly due to hyperglycemia, include increased thirst and urination, constant hunger, weight loss, and blurred vision. Children also may feel very tired. As insulin deficiency worsens, ketones, which are formed from the breakdown of fat, build up in the blood and are excreted in the urine and breath. Increased ketones are associated with shortness of breath and abdominal pain, vomiting, and worsening dehydration. Elevation of blood glucose, acidosis, and dehydration comprise the condition known as diabetic ketoacidosis or DKA. If diabetes is not diagnosed and treated with insulin at this point, the individual can lapse into a life-threatening coma. Often, children with vomiting are mistakenly diagnosed as having gastroenteritis. New-onset diabetes can be differentiated from gastroenteritis by the frequent urination that accompanies continued vomiting, as opposed to decreased urination due to dehydration if the vomiting is caused by gastroenteritis.

Risk Factors: A combination of genetic and environmental factors put people at increased risk for type 1 diabetes. Researchers have identified many factors and continue working so that targeted treatments can be designed to stop the autoimmune process that destroys the pancreatic beta-cells.

Predicting Type 1 Diabetes: As type 1 diabetes is caused by immune destruction of the insulin-producing beta cells in the pancreatic islets, antibodies against islets' proteins are found in children and adolescents months to years 2 before the onset of diabetes. Evidence from several studies suggests that measurement of islet autoantibodies in relatives of those with type 1 diabetes identifies new individuals who are at risk for developing type 1 diabetes. Such testing, coupled with education about symptoms of diabetes and follow-up in an observational clinical study, may allow earlier identification of onset of type 1 diabetes and lessen presentation with ketoacidosis at time of diagnosis.

This testing may be appropriate in those who have relatives with type 1 diabetes, in the context of clinical research studies

Co-morbidities: Children with type 1 diabetes are at risk for the long-term complications of diabetes. Autoimmune diseases such as celiac disease and autoimmune thyroid disease are also associated with type 1 diabetes.

Management: The basic elements of type 1 diabetes management are insulin administration (either by injection or insulin pump), nutrition management, physical activity, blood glucose testing, and the development of strategies to avoid hypoglycemia and hyperglycemia that may lead to DKA. Algorithms are used for insulin dosing based on blood glucose level, food intake, physical activity, and illness, if present.

All people with diabetes are advised to avoid "liquid carbs (carbohydrates)" such as sugar-containing soda, sports or energy drinks, juices (including 100 percent fruit juice), and regular pancake syrup. These liquid carbs raise blood glucose rapidly, contain large amounts of sugars in small volumes, are hard to balance with insulin, and provide little or no nutrition.

Children receiving fixed insulin doses of intermediate- and rapid-acting insulins must have food given at the time of peak action of the insulin. They need a consistent meal plan that aims for a set amount of carb grams at each meal (e.g., 60 grams of carbs at lunch) and snack since they do not adjust their mealtime insulin for the amount of carb intake.

Children receiving a long-acting insulin analogue or using an insulin pump receive a rapid-acting insulin analogue just before meals, with the amount of pre-meal insulin based on carb content of the meal using an insulin to carb ratio and a correction scale for hyperglycemia. Carb counting involves calculating the number of grams of carbohydrate, or choices of carbohydrate, the youth eats. One carb choice equals 15 grams of carbohydrate. Sources of carbs include starches (breads, crackers, cereal, pasta, rice), fruits and vegetables, dried beans and peas, milk, yogurt and sweets. In addition to the amount of insulin needed to cover the carbs (called the carb dosage), extra insulin might be needed if the youth's blood glucose is above the target range before a meal or snack. Further adjustment of insulin or food intake may be made based on anticipation of special circumstances such as increased exercise and intercurrent illness. Children on these regimens are expected to check their blood glucose levels routinely before meals and at bedtime.

Physical activity is a critical element of effective diabetes management. In addition to maintaining cardiovascular fitness and controlling weight, physical activity can help to lower blood glucose levels. To maintain blood glucose levels within the target range during extra physical activity, students will need to adjust their insulin and food intake. They also may need to check their blood glucose levels more frequently to prevent hypoglycemia while engaging in physical activity.

Families need to work with their healthcare team to set target blood glucose levels appropriate for the child. To control diabetes and prevent complications, the American Diabetes Association suggests blood glucose and A1C goals for type 1 diabetes by age group.

Type 2 Diabetes

Type 2 diabetes used to occur mainly in adults who were overweight and older than 40 years. Now, as more children and adolescents in the United States become overweight or obese and inactive, type 2 diabetes is occurring more often in young people aged 10 or older. Most children and adolescents diagnosed with type 2 diabetes are also insulin resistant, and have a family history of type 2 diabetes. Type 2 diabetes is more common in certain racial and ethnic groups such as African Americans, American Indians, Hispanic/Latino Americans, and some Asian and Pacific Islander Americans.

The increased incidence of type 2 diabetes in youth is a first consequence of the obesity epidemic among young people, and is a significant and growing public health problem.

Results from the 2007–2008 National Health and Nutrition Examination Survey (NHANES), using measured heights and weights, indicate that an estimated 16 to 17 percent of children and adolescents ages 2 to 19 years had a BMI greater than or equal to the 95th percentile of the age- and sex-specific BMI—about double the number of two decades ago.

Onset: The first stage in the development of type 2 diabetes is often insulin resistance, requiring increasing amounts of insulin to be produced by the pancreas to control blood glucose levels. Initially, the pancreas responds by producing more insulin, but after several years, insulin production may decrease and diabetes develops. Type 2 diabetes usually develops slowly and insidiously.

Symptoms: Some children or adolescents with type 2 diabetes may show no symptoms at all. In others, symptoms may be similar to those of type 1 diabetes. A youth may feel very tired, thirsty, or nauseated and have to urinate often. Other symptoms may include weight loss, blurred vision, frequent infections, and slow healing of wounds or sores. Some youth may present with vaginal yeast infection or burning on urination due to yeast infection. Some may have extreme elevation of the blood glucose level associated with severe dehydration and coma. Because symptoms are varied, it is important for healthcare providers to identify and test youth who are at high risk for the disease.

Signs of Diabetes: Physical signs of insulin resistance include acanthosis nigricans, where the skin around the neck or in the armpits appears dark and thick, and feels velvety. Girls can have polycystic ovary syndrome with infrequent or absent periods, and excess hair and acne. Microalbuminuria and cardiovascular risk factors such as abnormal cholesterol and high blood pressure may be present at the time of diagnosis.

Type 2 Diabetes Risk Factors and Testing Criteria.

Overweight (BMI >85th percentile for age and gender; weight for height >85th percentile; or weight >120 percent of ideal for height

PLUS

Any two of the following risk factors

- family history of type 2 diabetes in first- or second-degree relative
- race/ethnicity—American Indian, African American, Hispanic/Latino, Asian American, or Pacific Islander
- signs of insulin resistance or conditions associated with insulin resistance (acanthosis nigricans, hypertension, dyslipidemia, polycystic ovarian syndrome, or small-for-gestational-age birth weight)
- maternal history of diabetes or GDM during the child's gestation

Age to begin testing—10 years old or at onset of puberty if puberty occurs earlier

Frequency of testing—every 3 years

Tests to use—fasting plasma glucose, A1C, 2-h oral glucose tolerance test

Clinical judgment should be used to perform testing in children and adolescents who do not meet the above criteria.

Co-morbidities: Children with type 2 diabetes also are at risk for the long-term complications of diabetes and the comorbidities associated with insulin resistance (lipid abnormalities and hypertension). Recent studies show that the onset of complications and co-morbidities and the speed of progression is particularly aggressive in youth with type 2 diabetes.

Management: The cornerstone of diabetes management for children with type 2 diabetes is healthy eating with portion control, and increased physical activity. Metformin should also be initiated at the time of diagnosis of type 2 diabetes. However, research shows that approximately half of youth with type 2 diabetes will be unable to maintain A1C less than 8 percent on metformin alone, with or without lifestyle change.

If metformin is not sufficient to normalize blood glucose levels, the addition of insulin may be needed. While there are numerous other oral medications for use in adults, they are not approved in children. Insulin may be taken by injection or via a subcutaneous pump.

Management Considerations for All Children with Diabetes

There is no singlc approach to manage diabetes that fits all children. Blood glucose targets, frequency of blood glucose testing, type, dose and frequency of insulin, use of insulin injections with a syringe or a pen or pump, use of oral glucose-lowering medication and details of nutrition management all may vary among individuals. The family and diabetes care team determine the regimen that best suits each child's individual characteristics and circumstances.

Hypoglycemia: Diabetes treatment can sometimes cause hypoglycemia (low blood glucose levels). Taking too much insulin, missing a meal or snack, strenuous exercise, or illness may cause hypoglycemia. In addition, hypoglycemia can occur with no apparent cause. A child can become irritable, shaky, or confused. When blood glucose levels fall very low, loss of consciousness or seizures may develop.

When hypoglycemia is recognized, the child should drink or eat 15 grams of a glucose-containing carbohydrate source to quickly raise the blood glucose to normal levels. Examples of 15 grams of carbohydrate include 3 or 4 glucose tablets, or 4 ounces of fruit juice (not low-calorie or reduced sugar). The blood glucose should be rechecked in 10–15 minutes and re-treated with carbohydrate if hypoglycemia persists. Once the blood glucose returns to normal, the child can eat a meal or snack to prevent recurrence of hypoglycemia. If the child is unable to eat or drink, glucagon should be administered. Frequent hypoglycemia or a single episode of severe hypoglycemia warrants review of treatment plan (medicine, diet, and activity) to avoid recurrent episodes.

Glycemic goals may need to be modified to take into account the fact that most children younger than 6 or 7 years of age have a form of "hypoglycemic unawareness." They lack the cognitive capacity to recognize and respond to hypoglycemic symptoms and may be at greater risk for hypoglycemia. Children under 5 years of age may be at risk for permanent cognitive impairment after episodes of severe hypoglycemia.

Hyperglycemia: Causes of hyperglycemia include forgetting to take medications on time, eating too much, getting too little exercise, and stress. Some episodes of hyperglycemia may occur without an apparent reason. Being ill also can raise blood glucose levels. Over time, hyperglycemia can cause damage to the eyes, kidneys, nerves, blood vessels, gums, and teeth. Neurocognitive complications of hyperglycemia have also been documented.

Helping Children Manage Diabetes

The healthcare professional team, in partnership with the young person with diabetes and parents or other caregivers, needs to develop a personal diabetes management plan and daily schedule. The plan helps the child or teen to follow a healthy meal plan, get regular physical activity, check blood glucose levels, take insulin or oral medication as prescribed, and manage hyperglycemia and hypoglycemia.

Follow a healthy meal plan: Young people with diabetes need to follow a meal plan developed by a registered dietitian, diabetes educator, or physician. For children with diabetes, the meal plan should outline appropriate changes in eating habits that ensure proper nutrition for growth and reduce or prevent obesity. A meal plan also helps keep blood glucose levels in the target range.

Children or adolescents and their families can learn how different types of food—especially carbohydrates such as breads, pasta, and rice—can affect blood glucose levels. Portion sizes, the right amount of calories for the child's age and activity level, and ideas for healthy food choices at meal and snack time also should be discussed, including reduction in soda and juice intake. Family support for following the meal plan and setting up regular meal times are keys to success, especially if the child or teen is taking insulin.

Get regular physical activity: Children with diabetes need regular physical activity, ideally a total of 60 minutes each day. Physical activity helps to lower blood glucose levels and increase insulin sensitivity. Physical activity is also a good way to help children control their weight. In children with type 1 diabetes, the most common problem encountered during physical activity is hypoglycemia. If possible, a child or a teen should check blood glucose levels before beginning a game or a sport. If blood glucose levels are too low, the child should not be physically active until the low blood glucose level has been treated.

Check blood glucose levels regularly: Young people with diabetes should know the acceptable range for their blood glucose. Children, particularly those using insulin, should check blood glucose values regularly with a blood glucose meter, preferably one with a built-in memory. A healthcare team member can teach the child or teen how to use a blood glucose meter properly and how often to use it. Children should keep a journal or other records such as downloaded computer files of their glucose meter results to discuss with their healthcare team. This information helps providers make any needed changes to the child's or teen's personal diabetes plan.

Continuous Glucose Monitoring Systems: Continuous glucose monitoring systems are available for young people and adults with type 1 diabetes. All continuous glucose sensing systems have the same basic components: a sensor that is placed underneath the skin to measure interstitial glucose (the glucose found in the fluid between cells), a small transmitter worn on the body that connects to the sensor, and a hand-held cell-phone sized receiver that displays the current glucose levels and trends. Some systems integrate the receiver into an insulin pump, thereby reducing the number of extra components that need to be carried.

By having more glucose values available, users are able to see trends and better understand the effects of different foods, exercise, stress, and illness. Receivers sound an alarm when the person's glucose level drops below or goes above a certain pre-set level and in some systems when the projected glucose level will be high or low in 10 or 20 minutes, giving users a chance to prevent high or low blood glucose with early treatment.

Take all diabetes medication as prescribed. Parents, caregivers, school nurses, and others can help a child or teen learn how to take medications as prescribed. For type 1 diabetes, a child or teen takes insulin at prescribed times each day via multiple injections or an insulin pump. Some young people with type 2 diabetes need oral medication or insulin or both. In any case, it is important to stress that all medication should be balanced with food and activity every day.

Special Issues

Care of children and teens with diabetes requires integration of diabetes management with the complicated physical and emotional growth needs of children, adolescents, and their families, as well as consideration of teens' emerging autonomy and independence.

Diabetes presents unique issues for young people with the disease. Simple things, such as going to a birthday party, playing sports, or staying overnight with friends, need careful planning. Checking blood glucose, making correct food choices, and taking insulin or oral medication can make school-age children feel "different" from their classmates and this can be particularly bothersome for teens.

For any child or teen with diabetes, learning to cope with the disease is a big task. Dealing with a chronic illness such as diabetes may cause emotional and behavioral challenges, sometimes leading to depression. Talking to a social worker or psychologist may help young people and their families learn to adjust to the lifestyle changes needed to stay healthy.

Family Support.

Managing diabetes in children and adolescents is most effective when the entire family gets involved. Diabetes education should involve family members. Families can be encouraged to share concerns with physicians, diabetes educators, dietitians, and other healthcare team members to get their help in the day-to-day management of diabetes. Extended family members, teachers, school nurses, counselors, coaches, day care providers, and others in the community can provide information, support, guidance, and help with coping skills.

These individuals also may be knowledgeable about resources for health education, financial services, social services, mental health counseling, transportation, and home visits. Diabetes is stressful for both the children and their families. Parents should be alert for signs of depression or eating disorders or insulin omission to lose weight and seek appropriate treatment. While all parents should talk to their children about avoiding tobacco, alcohol, and other drugs, this is particularly important for children with diabetes. Smoking and diabetes each independently increase the risk of cardiovascular disease and people with diabetes who smoke have a greatly increased risk of heart disease and circulatory problems. Binge drinking can cause hyperglycemia acutely, followed by an increased risk of hypoglycemia. The symptoms of intoxication are very similar to the symptoms of hypoglycemia, and thus, may result in delay of treatment of hypoglycemia with potentially disastrous consequences.

Transition to Independence: Children with diabetes —depending on their age and level of maturity —will learn to take over much of their care. Most school-age children can recognize symptoms of hypoglycemia and monitor blood glucose levels. They also participate in nutrition decisions. They often can give their own insulin injections but may not be able to draw up the dose accurately in a syringe until a developmental age of 11 to 12 years.

Adolescents often have the motor and cognitive skills to perform all diabetes-related tasks and determine insulin doses based on blood glucose levels and food intake. This is a time, however, when peer acceptance is important, risk-taking behaviors common, and rebellion against authority is part of teens' search for independence. Thus, adolescents must be supervised in their diabetes tasks and allowed gradual independence with the understanding that the independence will be continued only if they adhere to the diabetes regimen and succeed in maintaining reasonable metabolic control. During mid-adolescence, the family and healthcare team should stress to teens the importance of checking blood glucose levels prior to driving a car to avoid hypoglycemia while driving.

Written Plans

Written plans outlining each student's diabetes management help students, their families, school staff, and the student's healthcare providers know what is expected of them. These expectations should be laid out in written documents, such as

- A Diabetes Medical Management Plan, developed by the student's personal healthcare team and family
- An Individualized Health Care Plan (or nursing care plan), developed by the school nurse presenting how the diabetes medical management plan will be implemented in the school

- Emergency Care Plans, which describe how to recognize hypoglycemia and hyperglycemia and what to do as soon as signs or symptoms of these conditions are observed
- Education plans, such as the Section 504 Plan, other Education Plan, or an Individualized Education Program (IEP) generated by the 504 or IEP teams to address each student's needs for services to manage their diabetes effectively in school

The school nurse is the most appropriate person to coordinate care for students with diabetes. Each student with diabetes should have a written Individualized Health Care Plan, developed by the school nurse, incorporating physician orders, parent requests, and tailored to the specific developmental, physical, cognitive, and skill ability of the child. The nurse will conduct a nursing assessment of the student and develop the plan, taking into consideration the child's cognitive, emotional, and physical status as well as the medical orders contained in the Diabetes Medical Management Plan. A team approach to developing the plan, involving the student, parent, healthcare provider, key school personnel, and school nurse, is the most effective way to ensure safe and effective diabetes management during the school day.

The Individualized Health Care Plan should also identify school personnel needed to provide care to an individual student, under the direction of the school nurse, when allowed by state nurse practice laws. The school nurse is responsible for training, monitoring, and supervising these school personnel. The school nurse will promote and encourage independence and self-care consistent with the student's ability, skill, maturity, and developmental level.

Camps and Support Groups.

Local peer groups and camps for children and teens with diabetes can provide positive role models and group activities. Peer encouragement often helps children perform diabetes-related tasks that they had been afraid to do previously and encourages independence in diabetes management. Talking with other children who have diabetes helps young people feel less isolated and less alone in having to deal with the demands of diabetes. They have the opportunity to discuss issues they share in common that others in their peer group can't understand, and they can share solutions to problems that they have encountered. Often, these programs challenge children physically and teach them how to deal with increased exercise, reinforcing the fact that diabetes should not limit them in their ability to perform strenuous physical activity.

Chapter 21

Ear, Nose, and Throat Disorders in Children

Chapter Contents

Section 21.1

Ear Infection (Otitis Media)

This section includes text excerpted from "Ear Infections in Children," National Institute on Deafness and Other Communication Disorders (NIDCD), July 13, 2015.

What Is An Ear Infection?

An ear infection is an inflammation of the middle ear, usually caused by bacteria, that occurs when fluid builds up behind the eardrum. Anyone can get an ear infection, but children get them more often than adults. Five out of six children will have at least one ear infection by their third birthday. In fact, ear infections are the most common reason parents bring their child to a doctor. The scientific name for an ear infection is otitis media (OM).

What Are The Symptoms of An Ear Infection?

There are three main types of ear infections. Each has a different combination of symptoms.

- **Acute otitis media (AOM)** is the most common ear infection. Parts of the middle ear are infected and swollen and fluid is trapped behind the eardrum. This causes pain in the ear—commonly called an earache. Your child might also have a fever.
- **Otitis media with effusion (OME)** sometimes happens after an ear infection has run its course and fluid stays trapped behind the eardrum. A child with OME may have no symptoms, but a doctor will be able to see the fluid behind the eardrum with a special instrument.
- **Chronic otitis media with effusion (COME)** happens when fluid remains in the middle ear for a long time or returns over and over again, even though there is no infection. COME makes it harder for children to fight new infections and also can affect their hearing.

How Can I Tell If My Child Has an Ear Infection?

Most ear infections happen to children before they've learned how to talk. If your child isn't old enough to say "My ear hurts," here are a few things to look for:

- Tugging or pulling at the ear(s)
- Fussiness and crying
- Trouble sleeping
- Fever (especially in infants and younger children)
- Fluid draining from the ear
- Clumsiness or problems with balance
- Trouble hearing or responding to quiet sounds

What Causes an Ear Infection?

An ear infection usually is caused by bacteria and often begins after a child has a sore throat, cold, or other upper respiratory infection. If the upper respiratory infection is bacterial, these same bacteria may spread to the middle ear; if the upper respiratory infection is caused by a virus, such as a cold, bacteria may be drawn to the microbe-friendly environment and move into the middle ear as a secondary infection. Because of the infection, fluid builds up behind the eardrum.

The ear has three major parts: the outer ear, the middle ear, and the inner ear. The outer ear, also called the pinna, includes everything we see on the outside—the curved flap of the ear leading down to the earlobe—but it also includes the ear canal, which begins at the opening to the ear and extends to the eardrum. The eardrum is a membrane that separates the outer ear from the middle ear.

The middle ear—which is where ear infections occur—is located between the eardrum and the inner ear. Within the middle ear are three tiny bones called the malleus, incus, and stapes that transmit sound vibrations from the eardrum to the inner ear. The bones of the middle ear are surrounded by air.

The inner ear contains the labyrinth, which help us keep our balance. The cochlea, a part of the labyrinth, is a snail-shaped organ that converts sound vibrations from the middle ear into electrical signals. The auditory nerve carries these signals from the cochlea to the brain.

Other nearby parts of the ear also can be involved in ear infections. The eustachian tube is a small passageway that connects the upper part of the throat to the middle ear. Its job is to supply fresh air to the middle ear, drain fluid, and keep air pressure at a steady level between the nose and the ear.

Adenoids are small pads of tissue located behind the back of the nose, above the throat, and near the eustachian tubes. Adenoids are mostly made up of immune system cells. They fight off infection by trapping bacteria that enter through the mouth.

How Does a Doctor Diagnose a Middle Ear Infection?

The first thing a doctor will do is ask you about your child's health. Has your child had a head cold or sore throat recently? Is he having trouble sleeping? Is she pulling at her ears? If an ear infection seems likely, the simplest way for a doctor to tell is to use a lighted instrument, called an otoscope, to look at the eardrum. A red, bulging eardrum indicates an infection.

A doctor also may use a pneumatic otoscope, which blows a puff of air into the ear canal, to check for fluid behind the eardrum. A normal eardrum will move back and forth more easily than an eardrum with fluid behind it.

Tympanometry, which uses sound tones and air pressure, is a diagnostic test a doctor might use if the diagnosis still isn't clear. A tympanometer is a small, soft plug that contains a tiny microphone and speaker as well as a device that varies air pressure in the ear. It measures how flexible the eardrum is at different pressures.

How Is an Acute Middle Ear Infection Treated?

Many doctors will prescribe an antibiotic, such as amoxicillin, to be taken over seven to 10 days. Your doctor also may recommend over-the-counter pain relievers such as acetaminophen or ibuprofen, or eardrops, to help with fever and pain. (Because aspirin is considered a major preventable risk factor for Reye syndrome, a child who has a fever or other flu-like symptoms should not be given aspirin unless instructed to by your doctor.)

If your doctor isn't able to make a definite diagnosis of OM and your child doesn't have severe ear pain or a fever, your doctor might ask you to wait a day or two to see if the earache goes away. The American Academy of Pediatrics issued guidelines in 2013 (link is external) that encourage doctors to observe and closely follow these children with ear infections that can't be definitively diagnosed, especially those between the ages of 6 months to 2 years. If there's no improvement within 48 to 72 hours from when symptoms began, the guidelines recommend doctors start antibiotic therapy. Sometimes ear pain isn't caused by infection, and some ear infections may get better without antibiotics. Using antibiotics cautiously and with good reason helps prevent the development of bacteria that become resistant to antibiotics.

If your doctor prescribes an antibiotic, it's important to make sure your child takes it exactly as prescribed and for the full amount of time. Even though your child may seem better in a few days, the infection still hasn't completely cleared from the ear. Stopping the medicine too soon could allow the infection to come back. It's also important to return for your child's follow-up visit, so that the doctor can check if the infection is gone.

How Long Will It Take My Child to Get Better?

Your child should start feeling better within a few days after visiting the doctor. If it's been several days and your child still seems sick, call your doctor. Your child might need a different antibiotic. Once the infection clears, fluid may still remain in the middle ear but usually disappears within three to six weeks.

What Happens If My Child Keeps Getting Ear Infections?

To keep a middle ear infection from coming back, it helps to limit some of the factors that might put your child at risk, such as not being around people who smoke and not going to bed with a bottle. In spite of these precautions, some children may continue to have middle ear infections, sometimes as many as five or six a year. Your doctor may want to wait for several months to see if things get better on their own but, if the infections keep coming back and antibiotics aren't helping, many doctors will recommend a surgical procedure that places a small ventilation tube in the eardrum to improve air flow and prevent fluid backup in the middle ear. The most commonly used tubes stay in place for six to nine months and require follow-up visits until they fall out.

If placement of the tubes still doesn't prevent infections, a doctor may consider removing the adenoids to prevent infection from spreading to the eustachian tubes.

Can Ear Infections Be Prevented?

Currently, the best way to prevent ear infections is to reduce the risk factors associated with them. Here are some things you might want to do to lower your child's risk for ear infections.

- Vaccinate your child against the flu. Make sure your child gets the influenza, or flu, vaccine every year.
- It is recommended that you vaccinate your child with the 13-valent pneumococcal conjugate vaccine (PCV13). The PCV13 protects against more types of infection-causing bacteria than the previous vaccine, the PCV7. If your child already has begun PCV7 vaccination, consult your physician about how to transition to PCV13. The Centers for Disease Control and Prevention (CDC) recommends that children under age 2 be vaccinated, starting at 2 months of age. Studies have shown that vaccinated children get far fewer ear infections than children who aren't vaccinated. The vaccine is strongly recommended for children in daycare.
- Wash hands frequently. Washing hands prevents the spread of germs and can help keep your child from catching a cold or the flu.
- Avoid exposing your baby to cigarette smoke. Studies have shown that babies who are around smokers have more ear infections.
- Never put your baby down for a nap, or for the night, with a bottle.
- Don't allow sick children to spend time together. As much as possible, limit your child's exposure to other children when your child or your child's playmates are sick.

Section 21.2

Enlarged Adenoids

This section includes text excerpted from documents published by four public domain sources. Text under headings marked 1 are excerpted from "Ear Infections in Children," National Institute on Deafness and Other Communication Disorders (NIDCD), March 2013; text under the heading marked 2 is excerpted from "Tonsils and Adenoids," MedlinePlus, U.S. Department of Health and Human Services (HHS), August 28, 2014; text under the heading marked 3 is excerpted from "Tonsil Surgery Improves Some Behaviors in Children with Sleep Apnea Syndrome," National Heart, Lung, and Blood Institute (NHLBI), May 21, 2013; text under the heading marked 4 is excerpted from "Routine Goes Awry," Agency for Healthcare Research and Quality (AHRQ), U.S. Department of Health and Human Services (HHS), June 2011. Reviewed October 2016.

What Are Adenoids?[1]

Adenoids are small pads of tissue located behind the back of the nose, above the throat, and near the eustachian tubes. Adenoids are mostly made up of immune system cells. They fight off infection by trapping bacteria that enter through the mouth.

Tonsils and Adenoids[2]

Your tonsils and adenoids are part of your lymphatic system. Your tonsils are in the back of your throat. Your adenoids are higher up, behind your nose. Both help protect you from infection by trapping germs coming in through your mouth and nose.

Sometimes your tonsils and adenoids become infected. Tonsillitis makes your tonsils sore and swollen and causes a sore throat. Enlarged adenoids can be sore, make it hard to breathe and cause ear problems.

The first treatment for infected tonsils and adenoids is antibiotics. If you have frequent infections or trouble breathing, you may need surgery. Surgery to remove the tonsils is tonsillectomy. Surgery to remove adenoids is adenoidectomy.

Adenoids and Middle Ear Infections[1]

As part of the immune system, the adenoids respond to bacteria passing through the nose and mouth. Sometimes bacteria get trapped in the adenoids, causing a chronic infection that can then pass on to the eustachian tubes and the middle ear.

To keep a middle ear infection from coming back, it helps to limit some of the factors that might put your child at risk, such as not being around people who smoke and not going to bed with a bottle. In spite of these precautions, some children may continue to have middle ear infections, sometimes as many as five or six a year. Your doctor may want to wait for several months to see if things get better on their own but, if the infections keep coming back and antibiotics aren't helping, many doctors will recommend a surgical procedure that places a small ventilation tube in the eardrum to improve airflow and prevent fluid backup in the middle ear. The most commonly used tubes stay in place for six to nine months and require follow-up visits until they fall out.

If placement of the tubes still doesn't prevent infections, a doctor may consider removing the adenoids to prevent infection from spreading to the eustachian tubes.

Adenoids and Sleep Apnea[3]

Children with sleep apnea syndrome who have their tonsils and adenoids removed sleep better, are less restless and impulsive, and report a generally better quality of life, finds a new study funded by the National Institutes of Health. However, the study found cognitive abilities did not improve compared with children who did not have surgery, and researchers say the findings don't mean surgery is an automatic first choice.

Obstructive sleep apnea syndrome is a common disorder in which the airway becomes blocked during sleep, causing shallow breathing or breathing pauses. The sleep disturbances that result can lead to many issues in children, including learning difficulties and behavioral problems.

Enlarged or swollen tonsils are a major risk factor for pediatric sleep apnea syndrome, and surgery to remove them and the nearby adenoid can help open up blocked airways. Over 500,000 adeno tonsillectomies are performed annually on children, primarily for sleep apnea. However, the extent that surgery can improve cognition and behavior previously had not been rigorously studied.

Potential Complications and Outcomes from Surgery[4]

Adenotonsillectomy, like all surgeries, is associated with potential risks and complications. The most commonly cited preoperative risk is bleeding, which occurs in up to 3% of patients. The highest risk of return to the operating room to control hemorrhage occurs one week postoperatively. Multiple instruments and techniques have been used to remove tonsils over the years ranging from sharp "cold" dissection to monopolar electrocautery. However, there are no evidence-based reviews demonstrating superior recovery or bleeding rates by any single method. Therefore, surgical technique continues to differ based on individual surgeon preference and experience.

Dehydration is another potential complication after adenotonsillectomy related to inadequate oral intake from poorly controlled postoperative throat pain. Airway obstruction is a much less common complication but is more likely to occur in certain populations of children, including those with neurologic delay, craniofacial abnormalities, lower airway disease (i.e., asthma), children younger than 3 years, and those with moderate or severe sleep disordered breathing (SDB) documented by preoperative sleep study. Though death is rare from the procedure, mortality rates from tonsillectomy are quoted at a rate of 1 in 16,000 to 1 in 35,000 procedures.

Other complications to note include temporary ear pain (due to referred throat pain), halitosis due to moist scabs in tonsil beds, temporary (rarely permanent) velopharyngeal insufficiency (VPI) that may manifest as hypernasal voice or leakage of food or liquid from the nose during oral intake, and voice changes due to changes in the resonance of the oropharynx. The majority of these complications will resolve with time, but not all; it is important to describe them and their self-limited time course during pre- and perioperative counseling sessions to parents and family members.

Section 21.3

Hearing Loss

This section contains text excerpted from the following sources: Text under the heading "Statistics on Hearing Loss," is excerpted from "Quick Statistics about Hearing," National Institute on Deafness and Other Communication Disorders (NIDCD), June 17, 2016; Text beginning with the heading "What Is Hearing Loss?" is excerpted from "Hearing Loss in Children," Centers for Disease Control and Prevention (CDC), October 23, 2015.

Statistics on Hearing Loss

- About 2 to 3 out of every 1,000 children in the United States are born with a detectable level of hearing loss in one or both ears.
- More than 90 percent of deaf children are born to hearing parents.
- Approximately 15% of American adults (37.5 million) aged 18 and over report some trouble hearing.
- Men are more likely than women to report having hearing loss.
- One in eight people in the United States (13 percent, or 30 million) aged 12 years or older has hearing loss in both ears, based on standard hearing examinations.
- About 2 percent of adults aged 45 to 54 have disabling hearing loss. The rate increases to 8.5 percent for adults aged 55 to 64. Nearly 25 percent of those aged 65 to 74 and 50 percent of those who are 75 and older have disabling hearing loss.
- The National Institute on Deafness and Other Communication Disorders (NIDCD) estimates that approximately 15 percent of Americans (26 million people) between the ages of 20 and 69 have high frequency hearing loss due to exposure to noise at work or during leisure activities.
- Roughly 10 percent of the U.S. adult population, or about 25 million Americans, has experienced tinnitus lasting at least five minutes in the past year.

- 28.8 million U.S. adults could benefit from using hearing aids.
- Among adults aged 70 and older with hearing loss who could benefit from hearing aids, fewer than one in three (30 percent) has ever used them. Even fewer adults aged 20 to 69 (approximately 16 percent) who could benefit from wearing hearing aids have ever used them.
- As of December 2012, approximately 324,200 cochlear implants have been implanted worldwide. In the United States, roughly 58,000 devices have been implanted in adults and 38,000 in children.
- Five out of 6 children experience ear infection (otitis media) by the time they are 3 years old.

What Is Hearing Loss?

A hearing loss can happen when any part of the ear is not working in the usual way. This includes the outer ear, middle ear, inner ear, hearing (acoustic) nerve, and auditory system.

Signs and Symptoms

The signs and symptoms of hearing loss are different for each child. If you think that your child might have hearing loss, ask the child's doctor for a hearing screening as soon as possible. Don't wait!

Even if a child has passed a hearing screening before, it is important to look out for the following signs.

Signs in Babies

- Does not startle at loud noises.
- Does not turn to the source of a sound after 6 months of age.
- Does not say single words, such as "dada" or "mama" by 1 year of age.
- Turns head when he or she sees you but not if you only call out his or her name. This sometimes is mistaken for not paying attention or just ignoring, but could be the result of a partial or complete hearing loss.
- Seems to hear some sounds but not others.

Signs in Children

- Speech is delayed.
- Speech is not clear.
- Does not follow directions. This sometimes is mistaken for not paying attention or just ignoring, but could be the result of a partial or complete hearing loss.
- Often says, "Huh?"
- Turns the TV volume up too high.

Babies and children should reach milestones in how they play, learn, communicate and act. A delay in any of these milestones could be a sign of hearing loss or other developmental problem.

Screening and Diagnosis

Hearing screening can tell if a child might have hearing loss. Hearing screening is easy and is not painful. In fact, babies are often asleep while being screened. It takes a very short time—usually only a few minutes.

Babies

All babies should have a hearing screening no later than 1 month of age. Most babies have their hearing screened while still in the hospital. If a baby does not pass a hearing screening, it's very important to get a full hearing test as soon as possible, but no later than 3 months of age.

Children

Children should have their hearing tested before they enter school or any time there is a concern about the child's hearing. Children who do not pass the hearing screening need to get a full hearing test as soon as possible.

Treatments and Intervention Services

No single treatment or intervention is the answer for every person or family. Good treatment plans will include close monitoring, follow-ups and any changes needed along the way. There are many different types of communication options for children with hearing loss and for their families. Some of these options include:

- Learning other ways to communicate, such as sign language
- Technology to help with communication, such as hearing aids and cochlear implants
- Medicine and surgery to correct some types of hearing loss
- Family support services

Causes and Risk Factors

Hearing loss can happen any time during life—from before birth to adulthood.

Following are some of the things that can increase the chance that a child will have hearing loss:

- A genetic cause: About 1 out of 2 cases of hearing loss in babies is due to genetic causes. Some babies with a genetic cause for their hearing loss might have family members who also have a hearing loss. About 1 out of 3 babies with genetic hearing loss have a "syndrome." This means they have other conditions in addition to the hearing loss, such as Down syndrome or Usher syndrome.
- 1 out of 4 cases of hearing loss in babies is due to maternal infections during pregnancy, complications after birth, and head trauma. For example, the child:
- Was exposed to infection, such as cytomegalovirus (CMV) infection, before birth
- Spent 5 days or more in a hospital neonatal intensive care unit (NICU) or had complications while in the NICU
- Needed a special procedure like a blood transfusion to treat bad jaundice
- Has head, face or ears shaped or formed in a different way than usual
- Has a condition like a neurological disorder that may be associated with hearing loss
- Had an infection around the brain and spinal cord called meningitis

- Received a bad injury to the head that required a hospital stay
- For about 1 out of 4 babies born with hearing loss, the cause is unknown.

Prevention

Following are tips for parents to help prevent hearing loss in their children:

- Have a healthy pregnancy.
- Learn how to prevent cytomegalovirus (CMV) infection during pregnancy.
- Make sure your child gets all the regular childhood vaccines.
- Keep your child away from high noise levels, such as from very loud toys.

Section 21.4

Hoarseness

This section includes text excerpted from "Hoarseness," National Institute on Deafness and Other Communication Disorders (NIDCD), March 23, 2016.

What Is Hoarseness?

If you are hoarse, your voice will sound breathy, raspy, or strained, or will be softer in volume or lower in pitch. Your throat might feel scratchy. Hoarseness is often a symptom of problems in the vocal folds of the larynx.

How Does Our Voice Work?

The sound of our voice is produced by vibration of the vocal folds, which are two bands of smooth muscle tissue that are positioned opposite each other in the larynx. The larynx is located between the base of the tongue and the top of the trachea, which is the passageway to the lungs.

When we're not speaking, the vocal folds are open so that we can breathe. When it's time to speak, however, the brain orchestrates a series of events. The vocal folds snap together while air from the lungs blows past, making them vibrate. The vibrations produce sound waves that travel through the throat, nose, and mouth, which act as resonating cavities to modulate the sound. The quality of our voice—its pitch, volume, and tone—is determined by the size and shape of the vocal folds and the resonating cavities. This is why people's voices sound so different.

Individual variations in our voices are the result of how much tension we put on our vocal folds. For example, relaxing the vocal folds makes a voice deeper; tensing them makes a voice higher.

If My Voice Is Hoarse, When Should I See My Doctor?

You should see your doctor if your voice has been hoarse for more than three weeks, especially if you haven't had a cold or the flu. You should also see a doctor if you are coughing up blood or if you have difficulty swallowing, feel a lump in your neck, experience pain when speaking or swallowing, have difficulty breathing, or lose your voice completely for more than a few days.

How Will My Doctor Diagnose What Is Wrong?

Your doctor will ask you about your health history and how long you've been hoarse. Depending on your symptoms and general health, your doctor may send you to an otolaryngologist (a doctor who specializes in diseases of the ears, nose, and throat). An otolaryngologist will usually use an endoscope (a flexible, lighted tube designed for looking at the larynx) to get a better view of the vocal folds. In some cases, your doctor might recommend special tests to evaluate voice irregularities or vocal airflow.

What Are Some of the Disorders That Cause Hoarseness and How Are They Treated?

Your doctor will ask you about your health history and how long you've been hoarse. Depending on your symptoms and general health, your doctor may send you to an otolaryngologist (a doctor who specializes in diseases of the ears, nose, and throat). An otolaryngologist will usually use an endoscope (a flexible, lighted tube designed for looking at the larynx) to get a better view of the vocal folds. In some cases, your doctor might recommend special tests to evaluate voice irregularities or vocal airflow.

Hoarseness can have several possible causes and treatments, as described below:

Laryngitis. Laryngitis is one of the most common causes of hoarseness. It can be due to temporary swelling of the vocal folds from a cold, an upper respiratory infection, or allergies. Your doctor will treat laryngitis according to its cause. If it's due to a cold or upper respiratory infection, your doctor might recommend rest, fluids, and nonprescription pain relievers. Allergies might be treated similarly, with the addition of over-the-counter allergy medicines.

Misusing or overusing your voice. Cheering at sporting events, speaking loudly in noisy situations, talking for too long without resting your voice, singing loudly, or speaking with a voice that's too high or too low can cause temporary hoarseness. Resting, reducing voice use, and drinking lots of water should help relieve hoarseness from misuse or overuse. Sometimes people whose jobs depend on their voices—such as teachers, singers, or public speakers—develop hoarseness that won't go away. If you use your voice for a living and you regularly experience hoarseness, your doctor might suggest seeing a speech-language pathologist for voice therapy. In voice therapy, you'll be given vocal exercises and tips for avoiding hoarseness by changing the ways in which you use your voice.

Gastroesophageal reflux (GERD). GERD—commonly called heartburn—can cause hoarseness when stomach acid rises up the throat and irritates the tissues. Usually hoarseness caused by GERD is worse in the morning and improves throughout the day. In some people, the stomach acid rises all the way up to the throat and larynx and irritates the vocal folds. This is called laryngopharyngeal reflux (LPR). LPR can happen during the day or night. Some people will have no heartburn with LPR, but they may feel as if they constantly have to cough to clear their throat and they may become hoarse. GERD and LPR are treated with dietary modifications and medications that reduce stomach acid.

Vocal nodules, polyps, and cysts. Vocal nodules, polyps, and cysts are benign (noncancerous) growths within or along the vocal folds. Vocal nodules are sometimes called "singer's nodes" because they are a frequent problem among professional singers. They form in pairs on opposite sides of the vocal folds as the result of too much pressure or friction, much like the way a callus forms on the foot from a shoe that's too tight. A vocal polyp typically occurs only on one side of the vocal fold. A vocal cyst is a hard mass of tissue encased in a membrane sac inside the vocal fold. The most common treatments for nodules, polyps, and cysts are voice rest, voice therapy, and surgery to remove the tissue.

Vocal fold hemorrhage. Vocal fold hemorrhage occurs when a blood vessel on the surface of the vocal fold ruptures and the tissues fill with blood. If you lose your voice suddenly during strenuous vocal use (such as yelling), you may have a vocal fold hemorrhage. Sometimes a vocal fold hemorrhage will cause hoarseness to develop quickly over a short amount of time and only affect your singing but not your speaking voice. Vocal fold hemorrhage must be treated immediately with total voice rest and a trip to the doctor.

Vocal fold paralysis. Vocal fold paralysis is a voice disorder that occurs when one or both of the vocal folds don't open or close properly. It can be caused by injury to the head, neck or chest; lung or thyroid cancer; tumors of the skull base, neck, or chest; or infection (for example, Lyme disease). People with certain neurologic conditions such as multiple sclerosis or Parkinson disease or who have sustained a stroke may experience vocal fold paralysis. In many cases, however, the cause is unknown. Vocal fold paralysis is treated with voice therapy and, in some cases, surgery.

Neurological diseases and disorders. Neurological conditions that affect areas of the brain that control muscles in the throat or larynx can also cause hoarseness. Hoarseness is sometimes a symptom of Parkinson disease or a stroke. Spasmodic dysphonia is a rare neurological disease that causes hoarseness and can also affect breathing. Treatment in these cases will depend upon the type of disease or disorder.

Section 21.5

Nosebleeds

A nosebleed, also known as epistaxis, is a common condition that occurs when one of the small, delicate blood vessels inside the nose bursts open. Many children under the age of 10 are prone to nosebleeds. Although blood streaming from the nose can seem alarming, nosebleeds are usually harmless and easy to manage at home with simple first-aid techniques.

Blood vessels on the nasal septum—the tissue that separates the nostrils—are responsible for most nosebleeds. Those that occur in the front part of the nose are known as anterior nosebleeds, and they are the most common among children and the easiest to stop. Posterior nosebleeds, on the other hand, occur deep inside the nasal cavity. They usually affect older adults, people with high blood pressure, and people who have experienced facial injuries.

Causes of Nosebleeds

Irritation of the membranes lining the inside of the nose is the cause of most nosebleeds. Breathing cold, dry, or overheated air can cause irritation of nasal membranes, as can the accumulation of mucus from allergies, colds, sinus infections, or the flu. Medications used to dry out the sinuses, such as decongestants or antihistamines, can also cause irritation of the nasal membranes. Irritation causes crusts to form inside the nose, which can bleed when they are removed by blowing or picking the nose.

Injuries or bumps to the nose can also cause surface capillaries to burst and create nosebleeds. Children may also get nosebleeds by inserting foreign objects into their nose. In rare cases, repeated nosebleeds may be symptomatic of an underlying disorder, such as high blood pressure, hemophilia, or a tumor in the nose or sinuses.

First Aid at Home

The first step in treating a nosebleed is to remain calm and reassuring. Children often become upset at the sight or taste of blood, and it is important to let them know that everything will be fine. The next step is to stop the bleeding by applying pressure to the soft part of the nose. With the child sitting down and leaning forward slightly, use the fingers, a tissue, or a soft cloth to hold the nostrils closed for 10 minutes. Do not release the pressure to check whether the bleeding has stopped until the full time has passed. Encourage the child to spit out any blood in the mouth, as swallowing blood can cause vomiting and make the nosebleed worse. It may also be helpful to apply an icepack or cold compress to the bridge of the nose. If the bleeding has not stopped after 10 minutes, repeat the above procedures for 10 more minutes.

Once the bleeding stops, it is important to have the child pursue quiet activities for a few hours instead of running around. The child should also avoid taking hot baths or showers and drinking hot liquids for the next 24 hours to prevent dilation of blood vessels in the nose. Finally, the child should not be allowed to sniff, blow, or pick their nose for at least 24 hours following a nosebleed.

Medical Treatment

In most cases, nosebleeds can be treated successfully at home. It may be necessary to seek medical treatment, however, under the following conditions:

- the bleeding continues for more than 20 minutes
- the nosebleed accompanies a head injury
- the nose may have been fractured by a fall or blow to the face
- a foreign object may have been inserted into the nose
- the child tends to bruise easily or bleed profusely from minor wounds
- the child has recently begun taking a new medication

For a persistent nosebleed, the doctor is likely to apply a medicated cream or ointment to the inside of the nose to help stop the bleeding. The doctor may also use heat, electric current, or silver nitrate sticks to cauterize the blood vessel and stop the bleeding. Finally, the doctor may pack the child's nose with gauze, which should remain in place for 24 to 48 hours. Once the bleeding has stopped, the doctor can take steps to address any underlying causes of the nosebleed. The doctor may remove a foreign object from the nose, for instance, or reset a broken nose. If nosebleeds are related to medication, a change in prescription may be recommended.

Although it is rare, frequent, severe nosebleeds can create enough blood loss to cause anemia in children. Doctors may perform blood tests to determine whether haemoglobin levels are low. They may also check for signs of low blood pressure due to blood loss. Children who have frequent nosebleeds may also be referred to an ear, nose, and throat (ENT) specialist for further testing, such as nasal endoscopy or computerized tomography (CT) scan of the nose and sinuses.

Preventing Nosebleeds

To prevent nosebleeds caused by dry air, it may be helpful to use a vaporizer at home to add moisture. In addition, using a saline nasal spray, water-based lubricating gel, or antibiotic ointment can help prevent nasal membranes from drying out. Cutting children's fingernails can help discourage nose-picking. Finally, wearing appropriate protective headgear during sports and activities can help prevent head and facial injuries that cause nosebleeds.

References

1. Jothi, Sumana. "Nosebleed," MedlinePlus, August 5, 2015.
2. "Nosebleeds," KidsHealth, 2016.
3. "Nosebleeds," Royal Children's Hospital Melbourne, August 2015.

Section 21.6

Obstructive Sleep Apnea

This section includes text excerpted from "What Is Sleep Apnea?" National Heart, Lung, and Blood Institute (NHLBI), July 10, 2012. Reviewed October 2016.

What Is Sleep Apnea?

Sleep apnea is a common disorder in which you have one or more pauses in breathing or shallow breaths while you sleep.

Breathing pauses can last from a few seconds to minutes. They may occur 30 times or more an hour. Typically, normal breathing then starts again, sometimes with a loud snort or choking sound.

Sleep apnea usually is a chronic (ongoing) condition that disrupts your sleep. When your breathing pauses or becomes shallow, you'll often move out of deep sleep and into light sleep.

As a result, the quality of your sleep is poor, which makes you tired during the day. Sleep apnea is a leading cause of excessive daytime sleepiness.

What Causes Sleep Apnea?

When you're awake, throat muscles help keep your airway stiff and open so air can flow into your lungs. When you sleep, these muscles relax, which narrows your throat.

Normally, this narrowing doesn't prevent air from flowing into and out of your lungs. But if you have sleep apnea, your airway can become partially or fully blocked because:

- Your throat muscles and tongue relax more than normal.
- Your tongue and tonsils (tissue masses in the back of your mouth) are large compared with the opening into your windpipe.
- You're overweight. The extra soft fat tissue can thicken the wall of the windpipe. This narrows the inside of the windpipe, which makes it harder to keep open.

- The shape of your head and neck (bony structure) may cause a smaller airway size in the mouth and throat area.
- The aging process limits your brain signals' ability to keep your throat muscles stiff during sleep. Thus, your airway is more likely to narrow or collapse.

Not enough air flows into your lungs if your airway is partially or fully blocked during sleep. As a result, loud snoring and a drop in your blood oxygen level can occur.

If the oxygen drops to a dangerous level, it triggers your brain to disturb your sleep. This helps tighten the upper airway muscles and open your windpipe. Normal breathing then starts again, often with a loud snort or choking sound.

Frequent drops in your blood oxygen level and reduced sleep quality can trigger the release of stress hormones. These hormones raise your heart rate and increase your risk for high blood pressure, heart attack, stroke, and arrhythmias (irregular heartbeats). The hormones also can raise your risk for, or worsen, heart failure.

Untreated sleep apnea also can lead to changes in how your body uses energy. These changes increase your risk for obesity and diabetes.

Who Is at Risk for Sleep Apnea?

Obstructive sleep apnea is a common condition. About half of the people who have this condition are overweight.

Men are more likely than women to have sleep apnea. Although the condition can occur at any age, the risk increases as you get older. A family history of sleep apnea also increases your risk for the condition.

People who have small airways in their noses, throats, or mouths are more likely to have sleep apnea. Small airways might be due to the shape of these structures or allergies or other conditions that cause congestion.

Small children might have enlarged tonsil tissues in their throats. Enlarged tonsil tissues raise a child's risk for sleep apnea. Overweight children also might be at increased risk for sleep apnea.

About half of the people who have sleep apnea also have high blood pressure. Sleep apnea also is linked to smoking, metabolic syndrome, diabetes, and risk factors for stroke and heart failure.

Race and ethnicity might play a role in the risk of developing sleep apnea. However, more research is needed.

What Are the Signs and Symptoms of Sleep Apnea?

Major Signs and Symptoms

One of the most common signs of obstructive sleep apnea is loud and chronic (ongoing) snoring. Pauses may occur in the snoring. Choking or gasping may follow the pauses.

The snoring usually is loudest when you sleep on your back; it might be less noisy when you turn on your side. You might not snore every night. Over time, however, the snoring can happen more often and get louder.

You're asleep when the snoring or gasping happens. You likely won't know that you're having problems breathing or be able to judge how severe the problem is. A family member or bed partner often will notice these problems before you do.

Not everyone who snores has sleep apnea.

Another common sign of sleep apnea is fighting sleepiness during the day, at work, or while driving. You may find yourself rapidly falling asleep during the quiet moments of the day when you're not active. Even if you don't have daytime sleepiness, talk with your doctor if you have problems breathing during sleep.

Other Signs and Symptoms

Others signs and symptoms of sleep apnea include:

- Morning headaches
- Memory or learning problems and not being able to concentrate
- Feeling irritable, depressed, or having mood swings or personality changes
- Waking up frequently to urinate
- Dry mouth or sore throat when you wake up

In children, sleep apnea can cause hyperactivity, poor school performance, and angry or hostile behavior. Children who have sleep apnea also may breathe through their mouths instead of their noses during the day.

How Is Sleep Apnea Diagnosed?

Doctors diagnose sleep apnea based on medical and family histories, a physical exam, and sleep study results. Your primary care doctor may evaluate your symptoms first. He or she will then decide whether you need to see a sleep specialist.

Sleep specialists are doctors who diagnose and treat people who have sleep problems. Examples of such doctors include lung and nerve specialists and ear, nose, and throat specialists. Other types of doctors also can be sleep specialists.

How Is Sleep Apnea Treated?

Sleep apnea is treated with lifestyle changes, mouthpieces, breathing devices, and surgery. Medicines typically aren't used to treat the condition.

The goals of treating sleep apnea are to:

- Restore regular breathing during sleep
- Relieve symptoms such as loud snoring and daytime sleepiness

Treatment may improve other medical problems linked to sleep apnea, such as high blood pressure. Treatment also can reduce your risk for heart disease, stroke, and diabetes.

If you have sleep apnea, talk with your doctor or sleep specialist about the treatment options that will work best for you.

Lifestyle changes and/or mouthpieces may relieve mild sleep apnea. People who have moderate or severe sleep apnea may need breathing devices or surgery.

Section 21.7

Perforated Eardrum

A perforated eardrum—also called a ruptured eardrum or perforated tympanic membrane—is a tear in the thin membrane that separates the outer ear from the middle ear. The function of this cone-shaped membrane is to transmit sound waves gathered by the outer ear to the ossicles (three small bones) in the middle ear and then to the oval window, the port to the fluid-filled inner ear. Structures in the inner ear stimulate auditory nerves, which then transmit impulses that the brain interprets as sound.

Perforated eardrums generally result in some degree of hearing loss, and in rare cases this could be permanent. Much of the time, the tear will heal on its own in a few weeks, but in more serious instances, surgery or another type of medical intervention may be necessary. And until the perforation heals or is repaired, the normally sterile middle ear is subject to infection.

Causes

There are numerous potential causes for a perforated eardrum, some pathological (caused by disease) and some traumatic (caused by injury). These can include:

- middle ear infections
- damage from foreign objects, such as cotton swabs, inserted into the ear
- injury to the ear from a powerful slap or other impact
- barotrauma, damage caused by a change in pressure, as with air travel or scuba diving
- very loud noise, like as a gunshot or explosion, close to the ear
- severe head trauma, such as a skull fracture

Symptoms

The primary symptom of a perforated eardrum is pain, which might initially seem like a common earache but then increases in severity. It can be extremely sharp and sudden, dull and steady, or intermittent. Other symptoms may include:

- partial or complete hearing loss in the affected ear
- ringing or buzzing in the ear
- drainage from the ear, which may be pus, blood, or clear liquid
- facial weakness
- dizziness
- repeated ear infections

Diagnosis

A physician—either a family doctor or an ear, nose, and throat specialist (ENT)—will generally begin by taking a medical history of the patient and his or her family. This will likely be followed by a series of questions about symptoms of the ailment and any medications taken by the patient.

The physical examination is done with an otoscope, a specialized instrument with a light that will allow the doctor to see into the ear and determine whether or not the eardrum has been ruptured.

Other tests that may be performed include:

- audiology test
- tuning-fork test
- tympanometry
- laboratory tests of fluid draining from the ear, if any

Treatment

Many ear infections heal on their own over the course of a few weeks, or at most a few months. In such cases, the doctor may prescribe antibiotics, either pills or ear drops, to help prevent infection, as well as pain medicine, usually over-the-counter medications like acetaminophen or ibuprofen. Warm compresses might also be recommended to relieve discomfort.

If the perforation doesn't begin to heal on its own, and if the hole isn't too large, the ENT may apply a special patch to the eardrum. This is done with a very thin, medicated material that both protects the wound and encourages healing of the membrane. The procedure takes only 15 to 30 minutes and can usually be done in the doctor's office using a local anesthetic.

If the eardrum doesn't heal on its own, and the rupture is too large for a patch, a surgical repair called a tympanoplasty might be required. In this procedure, the surgeon makes the repair through the ear canal itself or through an incision behind the ear. After cleaning and preparing the damaged area, the surgeon will take a small piece of tissue from elsewhere on the body and graft it onto the eardrum to seal the perforation.

Tympanoplasty is generally performed in a hospital with the patient under general anesthetic. It usually lasts up to one hour if the procedure is done through the ear canal, or up to three hours if an incision behind the ear is required.

In cases in which the ossicles—the tiny bones in the middle ear—have been damaged by injury or infection, an ossiculoplasty might need to be performed. This procedure, which is also done in a hospital under general anesthetic, involves the replacement of the damaged bones with bones from a donor or with an artificial substitute.

Complications

Most perforated eardrums heal well with simple treatment, and even patients with more extensive ruptures can achieve a good result with proper medical attention. However, left untreated, a punctured eardrum can lead to potentially serious complications, including:

- fever
- severe pain
- dizziness
- hearing loss, usually temporary but possibly permanent
- middle ear infections, caused by bacteria entering through the opening
- damage to the bones of the middle ear
- middle ear cholesteatoma, a cyst composed of skin cells and other debris
- in rare cases, infection may spread to the brain

Prevention

One of the most effective ways to prevent a perforated eardrum is to keep foreign objects out of the ear. And if an object does become lodged in the ear canal, it's best to have it removed by a medical professional. Another important prevention method is to get treatment for ear infections before they become serious enough to damage the eardrum.

A few other ways to prevent ruptured eardrums include:

- keep ears dry to help avoid infection
- if susceptible to ear infections, wear earplugs when swimming or bathing
- protect ears while flying (yawn or chew gum to equalize pressure)

- avoid flying with a cold or sinus infection
- wear earplugs or earmuffs to protect against loud noises

References

1. Derrer, David T., MD. "Ruptured Eardrum: Symptoms and Treatments," WebMD, August 17, 2014.
2. "Eardrum Rupture," Healthline.com, August 25, 2016.
3. Kacker, Ashutosh, MD, BS. "Ruptured Eardrum," MedLine-Plus.gov, May 18, 2014.
4. "Ruptured Eardrum," Mount Sinai Hospital, August 10, 2015.
5. "Ruptured Eardrum (Perforated Eardrum)," Mayo Clinic, January 4, 2014.

Section 21.8

Sinusitis

This section includes text excerpted from "Sinus Infection (Sinusitis)," Centers for Disease Control and Prevention (CDC), April 17, 2015.

What Are Sinus Infections?

Sinus infections occur when fluid is trapped or blocked in the sinuses, allowing germs to grow. Sinus infections are usually (9 out of 10 cases in adults; 5–7 out of 10 cases in children) caused by a virus. They are less commonly (1 out of 10 cases in adults; 3–5 out of 10 cases in children) caused by bacteria.

Other conditions can cause symptoms similar to a sinus infection, including:

- Allergies
- Pollutants (airborne chemicals or irritants)
- Fungal infections

Risk Factors

Several conditions can increase your risk of getting a sinus infection:

- A previous respiratory tract infection, such as the common cold
- Structural problems within the sinuses
- A weak immune system or taking drugs that weaken the immune system
- Nasal polyps
- Allergies

In children, the following are also risk factors for a sinus infection:

- Going to daycare
- Using a pacifier
- Drinking a bottle while laying down
- Being exposed to secondhand smoke

Signs and Symptoms

Common signs and symptoms of a sinus infection include:

- Headache
- Stuffy or runny nose
- Loss of the sense of smell
- Facial pain or pressure
- Postnasal drip (mucus drips down the throat from the nose)
- Sore throat
- Fever
- Coughing
- Fatigue (being tired)
- Bad breath

When to Seek Medical Care

See a healthcare professional if you or your child has any of the following:

- Temperature higher than 100.4°F

- Symptoms that are getting worse or lasting more than 10 days
- Multiple sinus infections in the past year
- Symptoms that are not relieved with over-the-counter medicines

If your child is younger than three months of age and has a fever, it's important to call your healthcare professional right away.

You may have chronic sinusitis if your sinus infection lasts more than 8 weeks or if you have more than 4 sinus infections each year. If you are diagnosed with chronic sinusitis, or believe you may have chronic sinusitis, you should visit your healthcare professional for evaluation. Chronic sinusitis can be caused by nasal growths, allergies, or respiratory tract infections (viral, bacterial, or fungal).

Diagnosis and Treatment

A sinus infection (sinusitis) does not typically need to be treated with antibiotics in order to get better. If you or your child is diagnosed with a sinus infection, your healthcare professional can decide if antibiotics are needed.

Your healthcare professional will determine if you or your child has a sinus infection by asking about symptoms and doing a physical examination. Sometimes they will also swab the inside of your nose.

Antibiotics may be needed if the sinus infection is likely to be caused by bacteria. Antibiotics will not help a sinus infection caused by a virus or an irritation in the air (like secondhand smoke). These infections will almost always get better on their own. Antibiotic treatment in these cases may even cause harm in both children and adults.

If symptoms continue for more than 10 days, schedule a follow-up appointment with your healthcare professional for re-evaluation.

Symptom Relief

Rest, over-the-counter medicines and other self-care methods may help you or your child feel better.

Prevention

There are several steps you can take to help prevent a sinus infection, including:

- Practice good hand hygiene

- Keep you and your child up to date with recommended immunizations
- Avoid close contact with people who have colds or other upper respiratory infections
- Avoid smoking and exposure to secondhand smoke
- Use a clean humidifier to moisten the air at home

Section 21.9

Stridor

Stridor is a harsh, high-pitched whistling or wheezing sound that occurs while breathing. It is typically the result of a partial blockage of airflow through the throat, windpipe, or voice box. Children are particularly at risk of developing stridor because their airways are narrower and softer than those of adults. Stridor has many possible causes, several of which are easily treated or naturally outgrown. In some cases, however, stridor can be symptomatic of a serious or potentially life-threatening disorder. Stridor and other symptoms of airway blockage should thus be considered reasons to seek immediate medical attention.

Causes of Stridor

Stridor can be caused by a variety of health conditions. Some of the most common causes include the following:

- food or other objects obstructing the airway
- anaphylaxis from a severe allergic reaction
- inflammation of the throat or windpipe caused by viral or bacterial infections, such as croup, bronchitis, tonsillitis, or epiglottitis

- irritation from phlegm or laryngitis
- trauma to the airway from neck fractures, neck surgery, prolonged use of a breathing tube, or inhalation of smoke or harmful chemicals
- trauma to the throat from swallowing harmful substances
- cancer, tumors, or abscesses in the throat, windpipe, or vocal cords
- paralysis of the vocal cords
- congenital conditions such as subglottic stenosis (a narrow voice box), subglottic hemangioma (a mass of blood vessels obstructing the airway), or vascular rings (an artery or vein compressing the windpipe)

Among infants, the cause of up to 75 inspiratory percent of stridor cases is laryngomalacia, a condition in which soft tissues obstruct the airway. Laryngomalacia typically manifests shortly after birth, peaks around the age of six months, and gradually disappears around the age of two as the child's airway hardens. Stridor symptoms caused by laryngomalacia, such as squeaking or rattling sounds while breathing, are usually most noticeable when babies lie on their backs. Other common indicators of laryngomalacia in infants include difficulty breathing, hoarse crying, trouble nursing, and poor weight gain.

Diagnosis and Treatment

It is important to note that unexplained stridor can be a sign of an emergency. If a child has difficulty breathing, and especially if there is a blue tint in the child's lips, skin, or nails, caregivers should seek medical attention immediately. In such cases, the doctor will take action to reopen the child's airway to allow them to breathe properly. The doctor may perform the Heimlich maneuver if a foreign object is blocking the airway, or may administer medication if the patient is experiencing anaphylaxis. In some cases, a breathing tube may be needed to support respiration until the patient is stabilized.

In many cases, however, stridor is caused by a medical condition that can be diagnosed and treated effectively. For non-emergency situations, the doctor will conduct a physical examination and take a complete medical history to find the underlying cause of the stridor. For instance, the doctor is likely to ask about when the breathing problem started, and the exact nature of the abnormal sounds. To determine whether an infection may be involved, the doctor may inquire about recent illnesses and the presence of other symptoms, such as a runny nose, cough, or sore throat. The doctor will also observe and listen to the child's breathing and look for additional symptoms, such as swelling in the face or neck or a bluish tint to the skin.

The process of diagnosing the underlying cause of stridor may also involve medical tests, including the following:

- X-rays or computerized tomography (CT)
- bronchoscopy or laryngoscopy
- arterial blood gas analysis
- sputum culture

Treatment of stridor depends on the diagnosis of the underlying cause, as well as the severity of the condition and the child's overall health. Some cases only require monitoring until the symptoms go away on their own. In other cases, medications may be prescribed to treat infections or reduce inflammation in the airway. Referral to an ear, nose, and throat specialist may be indicated in some situations, while severe cases of stridor may require surgery to correct.

References

1. Kaneshiro, Neil K. "Stridor," MedlinePlus, 2016.
2. Leung, Alexander K. C., and Helen Cho. "Diagnosis of Stridor in Children," American Family Physician, November 15, 1999.
3. Phillips, Natalie. "What Causes Stridor?" Healthline, 2016.

Section 21.10

Swimmer's Ear (Otitis Externa)

This section includes text excerpted from "Facts About "Swimmer's Ear," Centers for Disease Control and Prevention (CDC), June 9, 2013.

What Is Swimmer's Ear?

Swimmer's ear (also known as otitis externa) is an infection of the outer ear canal. Symptoms of swimmer's ear usually appear within a few days of swimming and include:

- Itchiness inside the ear.
- Redness and swelling of the ear.
- Pain when the infected ear is tugged or when pressure is placed on the ear.
- Pus draining from the infected ear.

Although all age groups are affected by swimmer's ear, it is more common in children and can be extremely painful.

How Is Swimmer's Ear Spread in the Places We Swim?

Swimmer's ear can occur when water stays in the ear canal for long periods of time, providing the perfect environment for germs to grow and infect the skin. Germs found in pools and other places we swim are one of the most common causes of swimmer's ear.

Swimmer's ear cannot be spread from one person to another.

If you think you have swimmer's ear, consult your healthcare provider. Swimmer's ear can be treated with antibiotic ear drops.

Is There a Difference between a Childhood Middle Ear Infection and Swimmer's Ear?

Yes. Swimmer's ear is not the same as the common childhood middle ear infection. If you can wiggle the outer ear without pain or discomfort then your ear condition is probably not swimmer's ear.

How Do I Protect Myself and My Family?

To reduce the risk of swimmer's ear:
Do keep your ears as dry as possible.

- Use a bathing cap, ear plugs, or custom-fitted swim molds when swimming.

Do dry your ears thoroughly after swimming or showering.

- Use a towel to dry your ears well.
- Tilt your head to hold each ear facing down to allow water to escape the ear canal.
- Pull your earlobe in different directions while the ear is faced down to help water drain out.
- If there is still water left in ears, consider using a hair dryer to move air within the ear canal.
- Put the dryer on the lowest heat and speed/fan setting; hold it several inches from the ear.

Don't put objects in the ear canal (including cotton-tip swabs, pencils, paperclips, or fingers).

Don't try to remove ear wax. Ear wax helps protect your ear canal from infection.

- If you think that the ear canal is blocked by ear wax, consult your healthcare provider.

Consult your healthcare provider about using ear drops after swimming.

- Drops should not be used by people with ear tubes, damaged ear drums, outer ear infections, or ear drainage (pus or liquid coming from the ear).

Consult your healthcare provider if you have ear pain, discomfort, or drainage from your ears.

Ask your pool/hot tub operator if disinfectant and pH levels are checked at least twice per day—hot tubs and pools with proper disinfectant and pH levels are less likely to spread germs.

Use pool test strips to check the pool or hot tub (or spa) yourself for adequate disinfectant and pH levels.

Section 21.11

Tonsillitis

Tonsillitis is an inflammation of the tonsils, two oval-shaped masses of tissue at the back of the throat that help protect the body from disease. They do this in several ways, including filtering out germs that enter through the mouth and producing antibodies that fight infection. The condition is most prevalent in children and teenagers, since adult immune systems have usually developed enough that the tonsils are less important in fighting disease.

Causes

Tonsillitis can be caused by a bacterial infection, such as streptococcus (strep). But it is most often the result of infection by viruses, including:

- adenovirus
- coronavirus
- cytomegalovirus
- enterovirus
- Epstein-Barr virus
- herpes simplex virus
- Human immunodeficiency virus (HIV)
- influenza
- parainfluenza
- respiratory syncytial virus
- rhinovirus

Symptoms

The most prevalent symptoms of tonsillitis are a very sore throat and redness and swelling of the tonsils. Other common symptoms include:

- white or yellow coating on the tonsils
- jaw and neck pain caused by swollen lymph nodes

- headache
- earache
- high temperature (above 100.4F)
- cough
- difficulty swallowing
- loss of voice or scratchy voice
- stiff neck
- tiredness
- bad breath

In addition, to these signs of tonsillitis, very young children may experience nausea, vomiting, and stomachaches, as well as unusual fussiness and excessive drooling as a result of painful swallowing.

Diagnosis

To diagnose tonsillitis, a physician will typically begin with a physical examination, which includes listening to the child's chest with a stethoscope, feeling for swollen lymph nodes, and checking the throat, ears, and nose with a lighted instrument. The doctor may also look for a rash (scarlatina), which can be a sign of a strep infection, and feel the upper abdomen to check for an enlarged spleen, a sign of mononucleosis, which can also cause inflammation of the tonsils.

Because the condition my result from either a viral or bacterial infection, tests are needed to determine the cause before treatment can proceed. To check for bacterial infection, the physician will take a throat culture using a cotton swab. This can be used to perform a rapid strep test in the doctor's office, although a more thorough analysis will be performed when the culture is sent to a lab for confirmation.

If the strep test is negative, the physician may order a complete blood count (CBC), which involves drawing a small amount of blood and sending it to a lab for testing. A CBC is used to provide a numerical measure of the physical characteristics of the blood, including red blood cells, white blood cells, and plasma. Although it is not a definitive test for tonsillitis, it is a good indicator of immune system function and the overall health of the patient, and it may help the doctor arrive at a diagnosis.

Treatment

The treatment for tonsillitis depends on its cause. Bacterial infections will generally be treated with antibiotics, such as penicillin or amoxicillin, which may be given by injection at the doctor's office or prescribed as pills or a liquid. But a viral infection will not respond to antibiotics, so unless tests reveal a problem with the immune system, the body should be able to recover on its own with just home care.

At one time, removal of the tonsils—a surgical procedure called a tonsillectomy—was a very common treatment. Today, however, tonsillectomies are generally only performed when patients experience chronic (persistent or recurring) tonsillitis, when the condition fails to respond to conventional treatment, or when complications occur.

If surgery is necessary, it will be done in a hospital under general anesthesia. Some surgeons use a scalpel to remove the tonsils, while others prefer different instruments, such as lasers, ultrasonic (highly focused sound) devices, or electrocautery (high temperature) instruments. The surgery usually takes less than an hour, and recovery should take fewer than two weeks.

Home Care

Whether the diagnosis is bacterial or viral, proper home care for tonsillitis is vital for a speedy and full recovery, which can be expected to take seven to ten days. The physician is likely to recommend:

- Rest. Plenty of sleep is needed to help the immune system do its job.
- Fluids. Water, broth, decaf tea, and other liquids will moisten the throat and prevent dehydration.
- Soothing beverages. Cool liquids or frozen fruit bars will help ease a sore throat.
- Nutrition. Begin with soft foods, such as applesauce, pudding, smoothies, and yogurt, and then add other items as the pain subsides.
- Saltwater gargle. A solution of one teaspoon of salt in an eight-ounce glass of water gargled several times per day can help ease pain.
- Pain medication. Over-the-counter pain relievers such, as acetaminophen or ibuprofen, are fine, but do not give aspirin to children unless directed by a physician.

- Moist air. Use a cool-mist vaporizer to eliminate dry air that can cause further irritation.
- Lozenges. Children over the age of four can get relief by sucking on lozenges containing anesthetics, such as benzocaine.

Complications

If the doctor's instructions regarding medications and home care are followed, tonsillitis rarely results in serious complications. But as with any medical condition, some complications are possible, including:

- dehydration and kidney failure, resulting from difficulty swallowing
- blocked airway, due to inflammation in the throat
- abscess in the tonsil area (called a peritonsillar abscess)
- tonsillar cellulitis, infection that spreads to other parts of the body
- sleep apnea, due to chronic tonsillitis
- middle ear infection
- pharyngitis, or inflammation of the pharynx, caused by infection

In addition, if the tonsillitis is caused by strep, leaving the condition untreated or discontinuing antibiotics too soon could result in serious complications, such as kidney disease, rheumatic fever, scarlet fever, and toxic shock syndrome.

Prevention

Tonsillitis can be highly contagious, so the first step in prevention is to keep the child away from other individuals who have an active infection. Other preventative measures include:

- washing hands often, especially before eating and after coughing, sneezing, or using the toilet
- using hand sanitizer frequently
- teaching children not to take food from other people's plates
- not sharing eating utensils, drinking glasses, or water bottles
- washing eating utensils in hot, soapy water

- cleaning toys often
- replacing toothbrushes on a regular basis
- eating a well-balanced diet to maintain immune system health
- washing and disinfecting home surfaces, particularly those in the kitchen and bathroom

References

1. Kaneshiro, Neil K., MD, MHA. “Tonsillitis,” MedLinePlus.gov., November 20, 2014.
2. Pietrangelo, Ann, and Rachel Nall, RN, BSN, CCRN. “Tonsillitis,” Healthline.com, April 18, 2016.
3. “Tonsillitis,” KidsHealth.org, January 2016.
4. “Tonsillitis,” Mayo Clinic, July 17, 2015.
5. “Tonsillitis,” NHS Choices, December 29, 2015.
6. “Tonsillitis: Symptoms, Causes, and Treatments,” WebMD, September 25, 2014.

Chapter 22

Endocrine and Growth Disorders in Children

Chapter Contents

Section 22.1

Adrenal Gland Disorders and Addison Disease

This section includes text excerpted from "Adrenal Insufficiency and Addison Disease," National Institute of Diabetes and Digestive and Kidney Diseases (NIDDK), May 2014.

What Is Adrenal Insufficiency?

Adrenal insufficiency is an endocrine, or hormonal, disorder that occurs when the adrenal glands do not produce enough of certain hormones. The adrenal glands are located just above the kidneys.

Adrenal insufficiency can be primary or secondary. Addison disease, the common term for primary adrenal insufficiency, occurs when the adrenal glands are damaged and cannot produce enough of the adrenal hormone cortisol. The adrenal hormone aldosterone may also be lacking. Addison disease affects 110 to 144 of every 1 million people in developed countries.

Secondary adrenal insufficiency occurs when the pituitary gland—a pea-sized gland at the base of the brain—fails to produce enough adrenocorticotropin (ACTH), a hormone that stimulates the adrenal glands to produce the hormone cortisol. If ACTH output is too low, cortisol production drops. Eventually, the adrenal glands can shrink due to lack of ACTH stimulation. Secondary adrenal insufficiency is much more common than Addison disease.

What Do Adrenal Hormones Do?

Adrenal hormones, such as cortisol and aldosterone, play key roles in the functioning of the human body, such as regulating blood pressure; metabolism, the way the body uses digested food for energy; and the body's response to stress. In addition, the body uses the adrenal hormone dehydroepiandrosterone (DHEA) to make androgens and estrogens, the male and female sex hormones.

What Are the Symptoms of Adrenal Insufficiency and Adrenal Crisis?

Adrenal Insufficiency

The most common symptoms of adrenal insufficiency are:

- chronic, or long lasting, fatigue
- muscle weakness
- loss of appetite
- weight loss
- abdominal pain

Other symptoms of adrenal insufficiency can include:

- nausea
- vomiting
- diarrhea
- low blood pressure that drops further when a person stands up, causing dizziness or fainting
- irritability and depression
- craving salty foods
- hypoglycemia, or low blood sugar
- headache
- sweating
- irregular or absent menstrual periods
- in women, loss of interest in sex

Hyperpigmentation, or darkening of the skin, can occur in Addison disease, although not in secondary adrenal insufficiency. This darkening is most visible on scars; skin folds; pressure points such as the elbows, knees, knuckles, and toes; lips; and mucous membranes such as the lining of the cheek.

The slowly progressing symptoms of adrenal insufficiency are often ignored until a stressful event, such as surgery, a severe injury, an illness, or pregnancy, causes them to worsen.

Adrenal Crisis

Symptoms of adrenal crisis include:

- sudden, severe pain in the lower back, abdomen, or legs
- severe vomiting and diarrhea
- dehydration
- low blood pressure
- loss of consciousness

What Causes Addison Disease?

Autoimmune disorders cause most cases of Addison disease. Infections and medications may also cause the disease.

Autoimmune Disorders

Up to 80 percent of Addison disease cases are caused by an autoimmune disorder, which is when the body's immune system attacks the body's own cells and organs. In autoimmune Addison, which mainly occurs in middle-aged females, the immune system gradually destroys the adrenal cortex—the outer layer of the adrenal glands.

Primary adrenal insufficiency occurs when at least 90 percent of the adrenal cortex has been destroyed. As a result, both cortisol and aldosterone are often lacking. Sometimes only the adrenal glands are affected. Sometimes other endocrine glands are affected as well, as in polyendocrine deficiency syndrome.

Polyendocrine deficiency syndrome is classified into type 1 and type 2. Type 1 is inherited and occurs in children. In addition to adrenal insufficiency, these children may have

- underactive parathyroid glands, which are four pea-sized glands located on or near the thyroid gland in the neck; they produce a hormone that helps maintain the correct balance of calcium in the body.
- slow sexual development.
- pernicious anemia, a severe type of anemia; anemia is a condition in which red blood cells are fewer than normal, which means less oxygen is carried to the body's cells. With most types of anemia, red blood cells are smaller than normal; however, in pernicious anemia, the cells are bigger than normal.

- chronic fungal infections.
- chronic hepatitis, a liver disease.

Researchers think type 2, which is sometimes called Schmidt's syndrome, is also inherited. Type 2 usually affects young adults and may include

- an underactive thyroid gland, which produces hormones that regulate metabolism
- slow sexual development
- diabetes, in which a person has high blood glucose, also called high blood sugar or hyperglycemia
- vitiligo, a loss of pigment on areas of the skin

Infections

Tuberculosis (TB), an infection that can destroy the adrenal glands, accounts for 10 to 15 percent of Addison disease cases in developed countries. When primary adrenal insufficiency was first identified by Dr. Thomas Addison in 1849, TB was the most common cause of the disease. As TB treatment improved, the incidence of Addison disease due to TB of the adrenal glands greatly decreased. However, recent reports show an increase in Addison disease from infections such as TB and cytomegalovirus. Cytomegalovirus is a common virus that does not cause symptoms in healthy people; however, it does affect babies in the womb and people who have a weakened immune system—mostly due to human immunodeficiency virus (HIV)/Acquired immune deficiency syndrome (AIDS). Other bacterial infections, such as *Neisseria meningitidis*, which is a cause of meningitis, and fungal infections can also lead to Addison disease.

Other Causes

Less common causes of Addison disease are

- cancer cells in the adrenal glands
- amyloidosis, a serious, though rare, group of diseases that occurs when abnormal proteins, called amyloids, build up in the blood and are deposited in tissues and organs
- surgical removal of the adrenal glands
- bleeding into the adrenal glands

- genetic defects including abnormal adrenal gland development, an inability of the adrenal glands to respond to ACTH, or a defect in adrenal hormone production
- medication-related causes, such as from anti-fungal medications and the anesthetic etomidate, which may be used when a person undergoes an emergency intubation—the placement of a flexible, plastic tube through the mouth and into the trachea, or windpipe, to assist with breathing

What Causes Secondary Adrenal Insufficiency?

A lack of corticotropin-releasing hormone (CRH) or adrenocorticotropin (ACTH) causes secondary adrenal insufficiency. The lack of these hormones in the body can be traced to several possible sources.

Stoppage of Corticosteroid Medication

A temporary form of secondary adrenal insufficiency may occur when a person who has been taking a synthetic glucocorticoid hormone, called a corticosteroid, for a long time stops taking the medication. Corticosteroids are often prescribed to treat inflammatory illnesses such as rheumatoid arthritis, asthma, and ulcerative colitis. In this case, the prescription doses often cause higher levels than those normally achieved by the glucocorticoid hormones created by the body. When a person takes corticosteroids for prolonged periods, the adrenal glands produce less of their natural hormones. Once the prescription doses of corticosteroid are stopped, the adrenal glands may be slow to restart their production of the body's glucocorticoids. To give the adrenal glands time to regain function and prevent adrenal insufficiency, prescription corticosteroid doses should be reduced gradually over a period of weeks or even months. Even with gradual reduction, the adrenal glands might not begin to function normally for some time, so a person who has recently stopped taking prescription corticosteroids should be watched carefully for symptoms of secondary adrenal insufficiency.

Surgical Removal of Pituitary Tumors

Another cause of secondary adrenal insufficiency is surgical removal of the usually non-cancerous, ACTH-producing tumors of the pituitary gland that cause Cushing syndrome. Cushing syndrome is a hormonal disorder caused by prolonged exposure of the body's tissues to high levels of the hormone cortisol. When the tumors are removed, the source of extra ACTH is suddenly gone and a replacement hormone must be taken until the body's adrenal glands are able to resume their normal production of cortisol. The adrenal glands might not begin to function normally for some time, so a person who has had an ACTH-producing tumor removed and is going off of his or her prescription corticosteroid replacement hormone should be watched carefully for symptoms of adrenal insufficiency.

Changes in the Pituitary Gland

Less commonly, secondary adrenal insufficiency occurs when the pituitary gland either decreases in size or stops producing ACTH. These events can result from

- tumors or an infection in the pituitary
- loss of blood flow to the pituitary
- radiation for the treatment of pituitary or nearby tumors
- surgical removal of parts of the hypothalamus
- surgical removal of the pituitary

How Is Adrenal Insufficiency Diagnosed?

In its early stages, adrenal insufficiency can be difficult to diagnose. A healthcare provider may suspect it after reviewing a person's medical history and symptoms.

A diagnosis of adrenal insufficiency is confirmed through hormonal blood and urine tests. A healthcare provider uses these tests first to determine whether cortisol levels are too low and then to establish the cause. Imaging studies of the adrenal and pituitary glands can be useful in helping to establish the cause.

A lab technician performs the following tests in a healthcare provider's office, a commercial facility, or a hospital.

How Is Adrenal Insufficiency Treated?

Adrenal insufficiency is treated by replacing, or substituting, the hormones that the adrenal glands are not making. The dose of each medication is adjusted to meet the needs of the patient.

Cortisol is replaced with a corticosteroid, such as hydrocortisone, prednisone, or dexamethasone, taken orally one to three times each day, depending on which medication is chosen.

If aldosterone is also deficient, it is replaced with oral doses of a mineralocorticoid hormone, called fludrocortisone acetate (Florinef), taken once or twice daily. People with secondary adrenal insufficiency normally maintain aldosterone production, so they do not require aldosterone replacement therapy.

What Problems Can Occur with Adrenal Insufficiency?

Problems can occur in people with adrenal insufficiency who are undergoing surgery, suffer a severe injury, have an illness, or are pregnant. These conditions place additional stress on the body, and people with adrenal insufficiency may need additional treatment to respond and recover.

Surgery

People with adrenal insufficiency who need any type of surgery requiring general anesthesia must be treated with intravenous (IV) corticosteroids and IV saline. IV treatment begins before surgery and continues until the patient is fully awake after surgery and is able to take medication by mouth. The "stress" dosage is adjusted as the patient recovers until the regular, presurgery dose is reached.

In addition, people who are not currently taking corticosteroids, yet have taken long-term corticosteroids in the past year, should tell their healthcare provider before surgery. These people may have sufficient ACTH for normal events; however, they may need IV treatment for the stress of surgery.

Severe Injury

Patients who suffer severe injury may need a higher, "stress" dosage of corticosteroids immediately following the injury and during recovery. Often, these stress doses must be given intravenously. Once the patient recovers from the injury, dosing is returned to regular, pre-injury levels.

Illness

During an illness, a person taking corticosteroids orally may take an adjusted dose to mimic the normal response of the adrenal glands to this stress on the body. Significant fever or injury may require a triple dose. Once the person recovers from the illness, dosing is then returned to regular, pre-illness levels. People with adrenal insufficiency should know how to increase medication during such periods of stress, as advised by their healthcare provider. Immediate medical attention is needed if severe infections, vomiting, or diarrhea occur. These conditions can lead to an adrenal crisis.

Pregnancy

Women with adrenal insufficiency who become pregnant are treated with the same hormone therapy taken prior to pregnancy. However, if nausea and vomiting in early pregnancy interfere with taking medication orally, injections of corticosteroids may be necessary. During delivery, treatment is similar to that of people needing surgery. Following delivery, the dose is gradually lessened, and the regular dose is reached about 10 days after childbirth.

How Is Adrenal Crisis Treated?

Adrenal crisis is treated with adrenal hormones. People with adrenal crisis need immediate treatment. Any delay can cause death. When people with adrenal crisis are vomiting or unconscious and cannot take their medication, the hormones can be given as an injection.

A person with adrenal insufficiency should carry a corticosteroid injection at all times and make sure that others know how and when to administer the injection, in case the person becomes unconscious.

The dose of corticosteroid needed may vary with a person's age or size. For example, a child younger than 2 years of age can receive 25 milligrams (mg), a child between 2 and 8 years of age can receive 50 mg, and a child older than 8 years should receive the adult dose of 100 mg.

Section 22.2

Constitutional Growth Delay

Constitutional growth delay is a relatively common condition in which physical development and maturation occurs at a much later age than average. Children with this condition are sometimes called "late bloomers" because they grow more slowly than their peers and reach puberty several years later. Although children with constitutional growth delay tend to be short in stature during their teen years, in most cases the condition is temporary. Once the growth spurt associated with puberty finally occurs, they continue growing after their peers have stopped and eventually reach an adult height similar to that of their parents. As a result, constitutional growth delay is not considered a disease. Rather, it is viewed as a variant of normal growth patterns in otherwise healthy teenagers.

Although constitutional growth delay can occur in either sex, it is more common among boys than girls. Children who are diagnosed with the condition tend to have a characteristic pattern of growth. After being born at a normal weight and length, they typically have a slow growth rate during the first two years of life. Their growth rate usually returns to normal around age three, however, so children with constitutional growth delay typically will be small for their age but keep pace with their peers. This situation changes when peers' growth rate accelerates upon reaching puberty. For children with congenital growth delay, the onset of puberty—and the associated growth spurt—may not occur for several more years. Consequently, their growth and physical maturation falls significantly behind at this time, sometimes resulting in social and psychological challenges.

Causes of Growth Delay

Experts believe that constitutional growth delay has a genetic component, since between 60 percent and 90 percent of children affected by the condition have a family member who was also affected. Heredity may account for delays in the release of hormones that are responsible for initiating the changes associated with puberty, such as the maturation of the ovaries and testicles.

In children with constitutional growth delay, the pattern of development of secondary sexual characteristics is normal, but the age at which it begins is much later than average. The absence or disruption of this normal pattern may indicate hormonal deficiencies that warrant further investigation. Growth that is delayed or slower than expected can also result from other medical conditions, such as chronic diseases or infections, endocrine disorders, autoimmune disorders, inflammatory bowel disease, or poor nutrition. Some of the syndromes that can mimic constitutional growth delay include Turner syndrome, Noonan syndrome, Kallmann syndrome, and Russell-Silver syndrome. These conditions must be ruled out in order to form a diagnosis of constitutional growth delay.

Diagnosis

In diagnosing constitutional growth delay, a doctor will begin by taking a complete medical history of the child. The doctor is likely to inquire about the child's growth pattern over time, eating habits or feeding schedule, and any medications or supplements they might take. The doctor is also likely to ask about any other symptoms that might be present, especially delays in social interactions or other skill development. Finally, the doctor will likely inquire about the child's biological parents, including their height, weight, and age upon reaching puberty.

Next, the doctor will perform a physical examination that includes measurements of the child's height, weight, and head circumference. The doctor may order additional laboratory tests as well, including blood tests, urine tests, and stool samples to rule out infections, diseases, and nutritional deficiencies. In addition, an X ray will typically be conducted on the child's left hand and wrist to determine the child's "bone age," or degree of skeletal maturation. The growth plates on long bones in the forearm remain open until the growth spurt that accompanies puberty. Afterward, the bones begin to fuse, meaning that further growth will be limited. The extent of skeletal maturation provides valuable clues about whether a child's growth is merely delayed or is being limited by some other biological factor.

Social and Psychological Effects

Once other causes of growth delay have been ruled out, the main priority is helping the child cope with the social and psychological challenges that often accompany the condition. Children with constitutional growth delay are likely to be quite short for their age and appear much younger than their friends. As their peers reach puberty and show signs of sexual maturation, they may feel self-conscious, left out, and anxious about their future sexual function and fertility.

Since adolescence is fraught with social changes, concerns surrounding delayed growth can create a serious emotional or psychological disturbance for some teenagers. Some may respond by behaving immaturely, or acting the age they appear rather than their chronological age. Others may respond to teasing or bullying with aggressive, antisocial behavior. Under most circumstances, constitutional growth delay does not require treatment. Doctors merely provide reassurance that children with the condition are developing normally, will experience the onset of puberty soon, and will eventually reach an appropriate adult height. But children who have trouble coping with the condition may need therapeutic help to accelerate the timing of puberty and growth.

Treatment

While medical treatment is not necessary for most cases of constitutional growth delay, it may be indicated for patients who experience psychological distress due to their slow patterns of growth and development. Short courses of therapy with growth hormones or sex hormones can accelerate growth and advance the onset of puberty. Although hormone therapy does not increase adult height, it does help speed up the process so that teenagers feel less different than their peers.

One potential benefit of medical treatment for constitutional growth delay is that it may help protect adult bone mass. Because of the activity of sex hormones and growth hormones, puberty is the peak period for bone mineralization. In fact, more than half of all bone calcium accumulates between the ages of 11 and 14 for girls, and 14 and 17 for boys. As a result, delays in the circulation of these hormones may increase the risk of osteopenia, or reduced bone mass, in adulthood. Hormone therapy thus has the potential to increase adult bone mass in children with constitutional growth delay.

References

1. Alter, Craig, and Sue Smith. "Constitutional Delay of Growth," MAGIC Foundation, n.d.
2. Clark, Pamela A. "Constitutional Growth Delay Clinical Presentation," Medscape, July 28, 2016.
3. "Delayed Growth," Agency for Health Care Administration, 2016.
4. Stanhope, Richard. "Constitutional Delay of Growth and Puberty," Child Growth Foundation, September 2000.

Section 22.3

Growth Hormone Deficiency

This section includes text excerpted from "Isolated Growth Hormone Deficiency," Genetics Home Reference (GHR), National Institutes of Health (NIH), September 20, 2016.

What Is Growth Hormone Deficiency?

Isolated growth hormone deficiency is a condition caused by a severe shortage or absence of growth hormone. Growth hormone is a protein that is necessary for the normal growth of the body's bones and tissues. Because they do not have enough of this hormone, people with isolated growth hormone deficiency commonly experience a failure to grow at the expected rate and have unusually short stature. This condition is usually apparent by early childhood.

What Are the Types of Growth Hormone Deficiency?

There are four types of isolated growth hormone deficiency differentiated by the severity of the condition, the gene involved, and the inheritance pattern.

Isolated growth hormone deficiency **type IA** is caused by an absence of growth hormone and is the most severe of all the types. In people with type IA, growth failure is evident in infancy as affected babies are shorter than normal at birth.

People with isolated growth hormone deficiency **type IB** produce very low levels of growth hormone. As a result, type IB is characterized by short stature, but this growth failure is typically not as severe as in type IA. Growth failure in people with type IB is usually apparent in early to mid-childhood.

Individuals with isolated growth hormone deficiency **type II** have very low levels of growth hormone and short stature that varies in severity. Growth failure in these individuals is usually evident in early to mid-childhood. It is estimated that nearly half of the individuals with type II have underdevelopment of the pituitary gland (pituitary hypoplasia). The pituitary gland is located at the base of the brain and produces many hormones, including growth hormone.

Isolated growth hormone deficiency **type III** is similar to type II in that affected individuals have very low levels of growth hormone and short stature that varies in severity. Growth failure in type III is usually evident in early to mid-childhood. People with type III may also have a weakened immune system and are prone to frequent infections. They produce very few B cells, which are specialized white blood cells that help protect the body against infection (agammaglobulinemia).

Frequency

The incidence of isolated growth hormone deficiency is estimated to be 1 in 4,000 to 10,000 individuals worldwide.

Section 22.4

Hypothyroidism and Hyperthyroidism (Graves' Disease)

This section contains text excerpted from the following sources: Text beginning with the heading "Hypothyroidism" is excerpted from "Hypothyroidism (Underactive Thyroid)," National Institute of Diabetes and Digestive and Kidney Diseases (NIDDK), July 2016; Text beginning with the heading "What Is Hyperthyroidism (Graves' Disease)?" is excerpted from "Graves' Disease," National Institute of Diabetes and Digestive and Kidney Diseases (NIDDK), August 2012. Reviewed October 2016.

Hypothyroidism

What Is Hypothyroidism?

Hypothyroidism, also called underactive thyroid, is when the thyroid gland doesn't make enough thyroid hormones to meet your body's needs. The thyroid is a small, butterfly-shaped gland in the front of your neck. Thyroid hormones control the way the body uses energy, so they affect nearly every organ in your body, even the way your heart beats. Without enough thyroid hormones, many of your body's functions slow down.

How Common Is Hypothyroidism?

About 4.6 percent of the U.S. population ages 12 and older has hypothyroidism, although most cases are mild. That's almost 5 people out of 100.

Who Is More Likely to Develop Hypothyroidism?

Women are much more likely than men to develop hypothyroidism. The disease is also more common among people older than age 60.

You are more likely to have hypothyroidism if you

- have had a thyroid problem before, such as a goiter
- have had surgery to correct a thyroid problem
- have received radiation treatment to the thyroid, neck, or chest
- have a family history of thyroid disease
- were pregnant in the past 6 months
- have Turner syndrome, a genetic disorder that affects females
- have other health problems, including
    - Sjögren syndrome, a disease that causes dry eyes and mouth
    - pernicious anemia, a condition caused by a vitamin B12 deficiency
    - type 1 diabetes
    - rheumatoid arthritis, an autoimmune disease that affects the joints
    - lupus, a chronic inflammatory condition

What Are the Symptoms of Hypothyroidism?

Hypothyroidism has many symptoms that can vary from person to person. Some common symptoms of hypothyroidism include

- fatigue
- weight gain
- a puffy face

- trouble tolerating cold
- joint and muscle pain
- constipation
- dry skin
- dry, thinning hair
- decreased sweating
- heavy or irregular menstrual periods
- fertility problems
- depression
- slowed heart rate
- goiter

Because hypothyroidism develops slowly, many people don't notice symptoms of the disease for months or even years.

Many of these symptoms, especially fatigue and weight gain, are common and don't always mean that someone has a thyroid problem.

What Causes Hypothyroidism?

Hypothyroidism has several causes, including

- Hashimoto disease
- thyroiditis, or inflammation of the thyroid
- congenital hypothyroidism, or hypothyroidism that is present at birth
- surgical removal of part or all of the thyroid
- radiation treatment of the thyroid
- some medicines

Less often, hypothyroidism is caused by too much or too little iodine in the diet or by pituitary disease.

How Do Doctors Diagnose Hypothyroidism?

Your doctor will take a medical history and do a physical exam, but also will need to do some tests to confirm a diagnosis of hypothyroidism.

Many symptoms of hypothyroidism are the same as those of other diseases, so doctors usually can't diagnose hyperthyroidism based on symptoms alone.

Because hypothyroidism can cause fertility problems, women who have trouble getting pregnant often get tested for thyroid problems.

Your doctor may use several blood tests to confirm a diagnosis of hypothyroidism and find its cause. Learn more about thyroid tests and what the results mean.

How Is Hypothyroidism Treated?

Hypothyroidism is treated by replacing the hormone that your own thyroid can no longer make. You will take levothyroxine, a thyroid hormone medicine that is identical to a hormone the thyroid normally makes. Your doctor may recommend taking the medicine in the morning before eating.

Your doctor will give you a blood test about 6 to 8 weeks after you begin taking thyroid hormone and adjust your dose if needed. Each time your dose is adjusted, you'll have another blood test. Once you've reached a dose that's working for you, your healthcare provider will probably repeat the blood test in 6 months and then once a year.

Your hypothyroidism most likely can be completely controlled with thyroid hormone medicine, as long as you take the recommended dose as instructed. Never stop taking your medicine without talking with your healthcare provider first.

What Is Hyperthyroidism (Graves' Disease)?

Graves' disease, also known as toxic diffuse goiter, is the most common cause of hyperthyroidism in the United States. Hyperthyroidism is a disorder that occurs when the thyroid gland makes more thyroid hormone than the body needs.

What Are the Symptoms of Hyperthyroidism (Graves' Disease)

People with Graves' disease may have common symptoms of hyperthyroidism such as:

- nervousness or irritability
- fatigue or muscle weakness
- heat intolerance

- trouble sleeping
- hand tremors
- rapid and irregular heartbeat
- frequent bowel movements or diarrhea
- weight loss
- goiter, which is an enlarged thyroid that may cause the neck to look swollen and can interfere with normal breathing and swallowing

Who Is Likely to Develop Hyperthyroidism (Graves' Disease)

Scientists cannot predict who will develop Graves' disease. However, factors such as age, sex, heredity, and emotional and environmental stress are likely involved.

Graves' disease usually occurs in people younger than age 40 and is seven to eight times more common in women than men. Women are most often affected between ages 30 and 60. And a person's chance of developing Graves' disease increases if other family members have the disease.

Researchers have not been able to find a specific gene that causes the disease to be passed from parent to child. While scientists know some people inherit an immune system that can make antibodies against healthy cells, predicting who will be affected is difficult.

People with other autoimmune diseases have an increased chance of developing Graves' disease. Conditions associated with Graves' disease include type 1 diabetes, rheumatoid arthritis, and vitiligo—a disorder in which some parts of the skin are not pigmented.

How Is Hyperthyroidism (Graves' Disease) Diagnosed?

Healthcare providers can sometimes diagnose Graves' disease based only on a physical examination and a medical history. Blood tests and other diagnostic tests, such as the following, then confirm the diagnosis.

- TSH test
- T_3 and T_4 test
- Radioactive iodine uptake test

- Thyroid scan
- TSI test

How Is Hyperthyroidism (Graves' Disease) Treated?

People with Graves' disease have three treatment options: radioiodine therapy, medications, and thyroid surgery. Radioiodine therapy is the most common treatment for Graves' disease in the United States. Graves' disease is often diagnosed and treated by an endocrinologist—a doctor who specializes in the body's hormone-secreting glands.

Section 22.5

Idiopathic Short Stature

Idiopathic short stature (ISS) is the term used to describe a child who is considerably shorter than others of the same age, sex, and genetic background when there is no known medical cause for the condition. ("Idiopathic" refers to a condition that arises spontaneously with no discernable origin.) Although ISS is not itself considered a disease, children who fit the definition need to be evaluated by a growth specialist in order to rule out the numerous diseases and disorders that can cause short stature before a diagnosis of ISS can be made.

When to See a Growth Specialist

Accurate height measurement is an ongoing process that should be charted by a pediatrician or family doctor throughout a child's growth years. The American Academy of Pediatrics recommends measuring height and weight at birth, at age 2-4 days, periodically from 1 to 24 months, and then yearly until age 21. In this way, growth can be monitored and compared to established standards, and if there is significant deviation further evaluation and testing can be initiated.

If parents suspect that their child is small for his or her age, or if the child appears to have stopped growing, the regular physician should be consulted first for an opinion. The doctor will compare the child's height and rate of growth to demographic standards, perform a physical examination, and perhaps order some preliminary tests, such as blood work. If appropriate, the physician may then refer the child to a specialist, such as a pediatric endocrinologist.

Diagnosis

One of the first things a specialist will do is confirm that the child is actually of short stature, beginning with measurements of height, weight, and arm and leg lengths. Technically, that would mean that he or she is 2 standard deviations (SD) or more below average for someone of the same age, race, ethnic background, and geographical origin. The doctor will also take a thorough family history, both to learn about the height of close relatives and to ask about genetic disorders that might affect growth.

If short stature is confirmed, the next step is to determine whether it is idiopathic (ISS) or the result of a medical condition. Beginning with a physical examination, the doctor would then likely order a series of tests that might include:

- complete blood count (CBC)
- other blood work to check kidney, liver, and immune system function
- thyroid function tests
- growth hormone stimulation
- insulin growth factor 1 test to identify growth hormone deficiency
- bone tests, including X-rays and scans, such as an MRI

Because short stature can be the result of such a wide variety of diseases or genetic disorders, diagnosing the underlying pathology, if any, can be a lengthy process. Eliminating possible causes can take weeks, or even months, depending on the condition and the individual child.

Causes of Short Stature

Since growth rate and height are the result of so many factors, ranging from genetic traits to nutrition to disease, the causes of short stature are numerous and varied. Some possible causes include:

- growth hormone deficiency
- thyroid disorders, such as Cushing disease and hypothyroidism
- juvenile rheumatoid arthritis
- celiac disease
- kidney disorders
- genetic conditions, like Turner syndrome and Down syndrome
- sickle cell anemia
- gastrointestinal disease
- rickets
- malnutrition

If no specific medical cause of short stature can be determined, then it may be diagnosed as ISS. In that case, assuming all relevant tests have been completed and the conditions is not judged to be dangerous, the physician may recommend regular follow-up examinations, testing, and measurement to monitor the child's condition and growth patterns.

Treatment

If testing reveals an underlying medical cause of short stature, then treatment will be based on that disease or disorder. For example, hypothyroidism is normally treated with thyroid hormone replacement pills; juvenile rheumatoid arthritis could be treated with nonsteroidal anti-inflammatory drugs, such as ibuprofen or naproxen; and celiac disease would be addressed with a gluten-free diet.

Children for whom testing reveals growth hormone deficiency are commonly treated with growth hormone (GH) injections. These can be given at home, usually once per day, and have proven effective, particularly when treatment is begun at least five years before the onset of puberty.

In 2003, the use of GH was approved by the U.S. Food and Drug Administration for the treatment of children with ISS, if a doctor predicts that they will attain a very short final height (under 4 feet 11 inches for a girl, and under 5 feet 4 inches for a boy). Again, the treatments, when started well before puberty, have been shown to aid growth and increase final height. But the use of GH to treat ISS is not without controversy.

For one thing, children with ISS, by definition, have normal GH levels, and some healthcare professionals are not comfortable administering medicine that tests indicate is not required. Others feel it unwise to administer hormone treatments—or any medication—when the condition is not physically harmful and the underlying cause is unknown. Another point of contention is that response to GH is highly variable, with some children experiencing only a moderate increase in height.

In addition, GH treatments can be very expensive and, if low hormone levels have not been supported by tests, some insurance plans won't cover the cost. And although GH is generally considered a safe treatment, its benefits must be weighed against the possible side effects, which can include allergic reactions, headaches, blurred vision, nervousness, and, in rare cases, chest pain, abdominal pain, rash, nausea, and vomiting.

References

1. "Childhood Growth and Height Issues," Children's Hospital of Philadelphia, n.d.
2. "Controversies in the Definition and Treatment of Idiopathic Short Stature (ISS)," National Center for Biotechnology Information, February 1, 2009.
3. Geffner, Mitchell, MD. "Idiopathic Short Stature," MAGIC Foundation, n.d.
4. Lee, Kimberly G., MD, MSc, IBCLC. "Short Stature," University of Maryland Medical Center, December 12, 2014.
5. Rogol, Alan D., MD, PhD. "Causes of Short Stature," UpToDate.com, August 16, 2016.
6. Rosenbloom, Arlan L., MD. " Idiopathic Short Stature: Conundrums of Definition and Treatment," National Center for Biotechnology Information, March 12, 2009.
7. Sinha, Sunil, MD. "Short Stature," Medscape, June 17, 2016.

Section 22.6

Klinefelter Syndrome

This section includes text excerpted from "Klinefelter Syndrome (KS)," *Eunice Kennedy Shriver* National Institute of Child Health and Human Development (NICHD), October 25, 2013.

What Is Klinefelter Syndrome (KS)?

The term "Klinefelter syndrome," or KS, describes a set of features that can occur in a male who is born with an extra X chromosome in his cells. It is named after Dr. Henry Klinefelter, who identified the condition in the 1940s.

Usually, every cell in a male's body, except sperm and red blood cells, contains 46 chromosomes. The 45th and 46th chromosomes—the X and Y chromosomes—are sometimes called "sex chromosomes" because they determine a person's sex. Normally, males have one X and one Y chromosome, making them XY. Males with KS have an extra X chromosome, making them XXY.

KS is sometimes called "47,XXY" (47 refers to total chromosomes) or the "XXY condition." Those with KS are sometimes called "XXY males."

Some males with KS may have both XY cells and XXY cells in their bodies. This is called "mosaic." Mosaic males may have fewer symptoms of KS depending on the number of XY cells they have in their bodies and where these cells are located. For example, males who have normal XY cells in their testes may be fertile.

In very rare cases, males might have two or more extra X chromosomes in their cells, for instance XXXY or XXXXY, or an extra Y, such as XXYY. This is called poly-X Klinefelter syndrome, and it causes more severe symptoms.

What Causes Klinefelter Syndrome (KS)?

The extra chromosome results from a random error that occurs when a sperm or egg is formed; this error causes an extra X cell to be included each time the cell divides to form new cells. In very rare cases, more than one extra X or an extra Y is included.

How Many People Are Affected by or at Risk for Klinefelter Syndrome (KS)?

Researchers estimate that 1 male in about 500 newborn males has an extra X chromosome, making KS among the most common chromosomal disorders seen in all newborns. The likelihood of a third or fourth X is much rarer:

Table 22.1. Prevalence of Klinefelter Syndrome Variants

Number of extra X chromosomes	One (XXY)	Two (XXXY)	Three (XXXXY)
Number of newborn males with the condition	1 in 500	1 in 50,000	1 in 85,000 to 100,000

Scientists are not sure what factors increase the risk of KS. The error that produces the extra chromosome occurs at random, meaning the error is not hereditary or passed down from parent to child. Research suggests that older mothers might be slightly more likely to have a son with KS. However, the extra X chromosome in KS comes from the father about one-half of the time.

What Are Common Symptoms of Klinefelter Syndrome (KS)?

Because XXY males do not really appear different from other males and because they may not have any or have mild symptoms, XXY males often don't know they have KS.

In other cases, males with KS may have mild or severe symptoms. Whether or not a male with KS has visible symptoms depends on many factors, including how much testosterone his body makes, if he is mosaic (with both XY and XXY cells), and his age when the condition is diagnosed and treated.

KS symptoms fall into these main categories:

Physical Symptoms

Many physical symptoms of KS result from low testosterone levels in the body. The degree of symptoms differs based on the amount of testosterone needed for a specific age or developmental stage and the amount of testosterone the body makes or has available.

During the first few years of life, when the need for testosterone is low, most XXY males do not show any obvious differences from typical male infants and young boys. Some may have slightly weaker muscles, meaning they might sit up, crawl, and walk slightly later than average. For example, on average, baby boys with KS do not start walking until age 18 months.

After age 5 years, when compared to typically developing boys, boys with KS may be slightly:

- Taller
- Fatter around the belly
- Clumsier
- Slower in developing motor skills, coordination, speed, and muscle strength

Puberty for boys with KS usually starts normally. But because their bodies make less testosterone than non-KS boys, their pubertal development may be disrupted or slow. In addition to being tall, KS boys may have:

- Smaller testes and penis
- Breast growth (about one-third of teens with KS have breast growth)
- Less facial and body hair
- Reduced muscle tone
- Narrower shoulders and wider hips
- Weaker bones, greater risk for bone fractures
- Decreased sexual interest
- Lower energy
- Reduced sperm production

An adult male with KS may have these features:

- Infertility: Nearly all men with KS are unable to father a biologically-related child without help from a fertility specialist.
- Small testes, with the possibility of testes shrinking slightly after the teen years
- Lower testosterone levels, which lead to less muscle, hair, and sexual interest and function

- Breasts or breast growth (called gynecomastia).

In some cases, breast growth can be permanent, and about 10% of XXY males need breast-reduction surgery.

Language and Learning Symptoms

Most males with KS have normal intelligence quotients (IQs) and successfully complete education at all levels. (IQ is a frequently used intelligence measure, but does not include emotional, creative, or other types of intelligence.) Between 25% and 85% of all males with KS have some kind of learning or language-related problem, which makes it more likely that they will need some extra help in school. Without this help or intervention, KS males might fall behind their classmates as schoolwork becomes harder.

KS males may experience some of the following learning and language-related challenges:

- A delay in learning to talk. Infants with KS tend to make only a few different vocal sounds. As they grow older, they may have difficulty saying words clearly. It might be hard for them to distinguish differences between similar sounds.
- **Trouble using language to express their thoughts and needs.** Boys with KS might have problems putting their thoughts, ideas, and emotions into words. Some may find it hard to learn and remember some words, such as the names of common objects.
- **Trouble processing what they hear.** Although most boys with KS can understand what is being said to them, they might take longer to process multiple or complex sentences. In some cases, they might fidget or "tune out" because they take longer to process the information. It might also be difficult for KS males to concentrate in noisy settings. They might also be less able to understand a speaker's feelings from just speech alone.
- **Reading difficulties.** Many boys with KS have difficulty understanding what they read (called poor reading comprehension). They might also read more slowly than other boys.

By adulthood, most males with KS learn to speak and converse normally, although they may have a harder time doing work that involves extensive reading and writing.

Social and Behavioral Symptoms

Many of the social and behavioral symptoms in KS may result from the language and learning difficulties. For instance, boys with KS who have language difficulties might hold back socially and could use help building social relationships.

Boys with KS, compared to typically developing boys, tend to be:

- Quieter
- Less assertive or self-confident
- More anxious or restless
- Less physically active
- More helpful and eager to please
- More obedient or more ready to follow directions

In the teenage years, boys with KS may feel their differences more strongly. As a result, these teen boys are at higher risk of depression, substance abuse, and behavioral disorders. Some teens might withdraw, feel sad, or act out their frustration and anger.

As adults, most men with KS have lives similar to those of men without KS. They successfully complete high school, college, and other levels of education. They have successful and meaningful careers and professions. They have friends and families.

Contrary to research findings published several decades ago, males with KS are no more likely to have serious psychiatric disorders or to get into trouble with the law.

Symptoms of Poly-X KS

Males with poly-X Klinefelter syndrome have more than one extra X chromosome, so their symptoms might be more pronounced than in males with KS. In childhood, they may also have seizures, crossed eyes, constipation, and recurrent ear infections. Poly-KS males might also show slight differences in other physical features.

Some common additional symptoms for several poly-X Klinefelter syndromes are listed below.

48,XXYY

- Long legs
- Little body hair

- Lower IQ, average of 60 to 80 (normal IQ is 90 to 110)
- Leg ulcers and other vascular disease symptoms
- Extreme shyness, but also sometimes aggression and impulsiveness

48,XXXY (or tetrasomy)

- Eyes set further apart
- Flat nose bridge
- Arm bones connected to each other in an unusual way
- Short
- Fifth (smallest) fingers curve inward (clinodactyly)
- Lower IQ, average 40 to 60
- Immature behavior

49,XXXXY (or pentasomy)

- Low IQ, usually between 20 and 60
- Small head
- Short
- Upward-slanted eyes
- Heart defects, such as when the chambers do not form properly
- High feet arches
- Shy, but friendly
- Difficulty with changing routines

What Are the Treatments for Symptoms in Klinefelter Syndrome (KS)?

It's important to remember that because symptoms can be mild, many males with KS are never diagnosed ore treated.

The earlier in life that KS symptoms are recognized and treated, the more likely it is that the symptoms can be reduced or eliminated. It is especially helpful to begin treatment by early puberty. Puberty is a time of rapid physical and psychological change, and treatment can successfully limit symptoms. However, treatment can bring benefits at any age.

The type of treatment needed depends on the type of symptoms being treated.

How Do Healthcare Providers Diagnose Klinefelter Syndrome (KS)?

The only way to confirm the presence of an extra chromosome is by a karyotype test. A healthcare provider will take a small blood or skin sample and send it to a laboratory, where a technician inspects the cells under a microscope to find the extra chromosome. A karyotype test shows the same results at any time in a person's life.

Tests for chromosome disorders, including KS, may be done before birth. To obtain tissue or liquid for this test, a pregnant woman undergoes chorionic villus sampling or amniocentesis. These types of prenatal testing carry a small risk for miscarriage and are not routinely conducted unless the woman has a family history of chromosomal disorders, has other medical problems, or is above 35 years of age.

Is There a Cure for Klinefelter Syndrome (KS)?

Currently, there is no way to remove chromosomes from cells to "cure" the XXY condition.

But many symptoms can be successfully treated, minimizing the impact the condition has on length and quality of life. Most adult XXY men have full independence and have friends, families, and normal social relationships. They live about as long as other men, on average.

Can KS Lead to Cancer?

Compared with the general male population, men with KS may have a higher chance over time of getting breast cancer, non-Hodgkin lymphoma, and lung cancer. There are ways to reduce this risk, such as removing the breasts and avoiding use of tobacco products. In general, XXY males are also at lower risk for prostate cancer.

If My Son, Family Member, Partner, Or Spouse Is Diagnosed with XXY Condition, How Can I Help Him and The Family?

If someone you know is diagnosed with KS:

- **Recognize your feelings.** It is natural for parents or family members to feel that they have done something to cause KS. But, remember it is a genetic disorder that occurs at random—there is nothing you could have done or not done to prevent it from happening. Allow yourself and your family time to deal with your feelings. Talk with your healthcare provider about your concerns.
- **Educate yourself about the disorder.** It is common to fear the unknown. Educate yourself about the XXY condition and its symptoms so you know how you can help your son, family member, or partner/spouse.
- **Support your son, family member, or partner/spouse.** Provide appropriate education about KS and give him the emotional support and encouragement he needs. Remember, most XXY males go through life with few problems, and many never find out they have the condition.
- **Be actively involved in your son's, family member's, or partner's/spouse's care.** Talk with your healthcare provider and his healthcare provider about his treatment. If counseling for behavioral problems is needed, or if special learning environments or methods are needed, get help from qualified professionals who have experience working with XXY males.
- **Encourage your son, family member, partner/spouse to do activities** to improve his physical motor skills, such as karate or swimming.
- **Work with your teachers/educators and supervisors/ co-workers.**
- Contact these people regularly to compare how he is doing at home and at school/work.
- When appropriate, encourage him to talk with his teachers, educators, supervisor, and co-workers. Suggest using brief notes, telephone calls, and meetings to identify problems and propose solutions.

- **Encourage your son's, family member's, partner's/ spouse's independence**. Although it is important to be supportive, realize that watching over too much can send the message that you think he is not able to do things on his own.
- **Share the following information with healthcare providers about XXY problems:**

Table 22.2. Recommendations

XXY males may have	Consider recommending
Delayed early expressive language and speech milestones	Early speech therapy and language evaluation
Difficulty during transition from elementary school to middle school or high school	Re-testing to identify learning areas that require extra attention at or before entrance to middle/high school
Difficulty with math at all ages	Testing to identify problem areas and remediation for math disabilities
Difficulty with complex language processing, specifically with understanding and creating spoken language	Language evaluation, increased opportunities to communicate through written language, possibly getting written notes from lectures/discussions
Decreased running speed, agility, and overall strength in childhood	Physical therapy, occupational therapy, activities that build strength

Section 22.7

Precocious Puberty and Delayed Puberty

This section includes text excerpted from "Puberty and Precocious Puberty: Condition Information," *Eunice Kennedy Shriver* National Institute of Child Health and Human Development (NICHD), December 16, 2013.

What Are Normal Puberty, Precocious Puberty, and Delayed Puberty?

Normal Puberty

The time in one's life when sexual maturity takes place is known as puberty. The physical changes that mark puberty typically begin in girls between ages 8 and 13 and in boys between ages 9 and 14.

Precocious Puberty

Precocious puberty is a condition that occurs when sexual maturity begins earlier than normal. Precocious (meaning prematurely developed) puberty begins before age 8 for girls and before age 9 for boys.

Children affected by precocious puberty may experience problems such as:

- Failure to reach their full height because their growth halts too soon
- Psychological and social problems, such as anxiety over being "different" from their peers. However, many children do not experience major psychological or social problems, particularly when the onset of puberty is only slightly early.

Delayed Puberty

Delayed puberty is the term for a condition in which the body's timing for sexual maturity is later than the normal range of ages.

Many children with delayed puberty will eventually go through an otherwise normal puberty, just at a late age. Other children have a long-lasting condition known as hypogonadism in which the sex glands (the testes in men and the ovaries in women) produce few or no hormones. For example, hypogonadism can occur in girls with Turner syndrome or in individuals with hypogonadotropic hypogonadism, which occurs when the hypothalamus produces little to no gonadotropin-releasing hormone (GnRH).

What Are the Symptoms of Puberty, Precocious Puberty, and Delayed Puberty?

Normal Puberty

In Girls

The signs of puberty include:

- Growth of pubic and other body hair
- Growth spurt
- Breast development
- Onset of menstruation (after puberty is well advanced)
- Acne

In Boys

The signs of puberty include:

- Growth of pubic hair, other body hair, and facial hair
- Enlargement of testicles and penis
- Muscle growth
- Growth spurt
- Acne
- Deepening of the voice

Precocious Puberty

The symptoms of precocious puberty are similar to the signs of normal puberty but they manifest earlier—before the age of 8 in girls and before age 9 in boys.

Delayed Puberty

Delayed puberty is characterized by the lack of onset of puberty within the normal range of ages.

How Many Children Are Affected by/at Risk of Precocious Puberty?

Precocious puberty affects about 1% of the U.S. population (roughly 3 million children). Many more girls are affected than boys. One study suggests that African American girls have some early breast development or some early pubic hair more often than white girls or Hispanic girls.

Who Is at Risk?

There is a greater chance of being affected by precocious puberty if a child is:

- Female
- African American
- Obese

What Causes Normal Puberty, Precocious Puberty, and Delayed Puberty?

Normal Puberty

Puberty is the body's natural process of sexual maturation. Puberty's trigger lies in a small part of the brain called the hypothalamus, a gland that secretes gonadotropin-releasing hormone (GnRH). GnRH stimulates the pituitary gland, a pea-sized organ connected to the bottom of the hypothalamus, to emit two hormones: luteinizing hormone (LH) and follicle-stimulating hormone (FSH). These two hormones signal the female and male sex organs (ovaries and testes, respectively) to begin releasing the appropriate sex hormones, including estrogens and testosterone, which launch the other signs of puberty in the body.

Precocious Puberty

In approximately 90% of girls who experience precocious puberty, no underlying cause can be identified—although heredity and being overweight may contribute in some cases. When a cause cannot be identified, the condition is called idiopathic precocious puberty. In boys with precocious puberty, approximately 50% of cases are idiopathic. In the remaining 10% of girls and 50% of boys with precocious puberty, an underlying cause can be identified.

Sometimes the cause is an abnormality involving the brain. In other children, the signs of puberty occur because of a problem such as a tumor or genetic abnormality in the ovaries, testes, or adrenal glands, causing overproduction of sex hormones.

Precocious puberty can be divided into two categories, depending on where in the body the abnormality occurs—central precocious puberty and peripheral precocious puberty.

Central Precocious Puberty

This type of early puberty, also known as gonadotropin-dependent precocious puberty, occurs when the abnormality is located in the brain. The brain signals the pituitary gland to begin puberty at an early age. Central precocious puberty is the most common form of precocious puberty and affects many more girls than boys. The causes of central precocious puberty include:

- Brain tumors
- Prior radiation to the brain
- Prior infection of the brain
- Other brain abnormalities

Often, however, there is no identifiable abnormality in the brain; this is called *idiopathic central precocious puberty*.

Peripheral Precocious Puberty

This form of early puberty is also called gonadotropin-independent precocious puberty. In peripheral precocious puberty, the abnormality is not in the brain but in the testicles, ovaries, or adrenal glands, causing overproduction of sex hormones, like testosterone and estrogens. Peripheral precocious puberty may be caused by:

- Tumors of the ovary, testis, or adrenal gland
- In boys, tumors that secrete a hormone called hCG, or human chorionic gonadotropin
- Certain rare genetic syndromes, such as McCune-Albright syndrome or familial male precocious puberty
- Severe hypothyroidism, in which the thyroid gland secretes abnormally low levels of hormones

- Disorders of the adrenal gland, such as congenital adrenal hyperplasia
- Exposure of the child to medicines or creams that contain estrogens or androgens

Delayed Puberty

Many children with delayed puberty will eventually go through an otherwise normal puberty, just at a late age. Sometimes, this delay occurs because the child is just maturing more slowly than average, a condition called *constitutional delay of puberty*. This condition often runs in families.

Puberty can be delayed in children who have not gotten proper nutrition due to long-term illnesses. Also, some young girls who undergo intense physical training for a sport, such as running or gymnastics, start puberty later than normal.

In other cases, the delay in puberty is not just due to slow maturation but occurs because the child has a long-term medical condition known as hypogonadism, in which the sex glands (the testes in men and the ovaries in women) produce few or no hormones. Hypogonadism can be divided into two categories: *secondary hypogonadism and primary hypogonadism*.

- *Secondary hypogonadism* (also known as central hypogonadism or hypogonadotropic hypogonadism), is caused by a problem with the pituitary gland or hypothalamus (part of the brain). In secondary hypogonadism, the hypothalamus and the pituitary gland fail to signal the gonads to properly release sex hormones. Causes of secondary hypogonadism include:
- Kallmann syndrome, a genetic problem that also diminishes the sense of smell
- Isolated hypogonadotropic hypogonadism, a genetic condition that only affects sexual development but not the sense of smell
- Prior radiation, trauma, surgery, or other injury to the brain or pituitary
- Tumors of the brain or pituitary
- In *primary hypogonadism*, the problem lies in the ovaries or testes, which fail to make sex hormones normally. Some causes include:
- Genetic disorders, especially Turner syndrome (in women) and Klinefelter syndrome (in men)

- Certain autoimmune disorders
- Developmental disorders
- Radiation or chemotherapy
- Infection
- Surgery

How Do Healthcare Providers Diagnose Precocious Puberty and Delayed Puberty?

To identify whether a child is entering puberty, a pediatrician (a physician specializing in the treatment of children) will carefully examine the following:

- In girls, the growth of pubic hair and breasts
- In boys, the increase in size of the testicles and penis and the growth of pubic hair

The pediatrician will compare what he or she finds against the Tanner scale, a 5-point scale that gauges the extent of puberty development in children.

Precocious Puberty

After giving a child a complete physical examination and analyzing his or her medical history, a healthcare provider may perform tests to diagnose precocious puberty, including:

- Blood test
- Gonadotropin-releasing hormone agonist (GnRHa) stimulation test
- Blood 17-hydroxyprogesterone test
- "bone age" X-ray

The healthcare provider may also use imaging techniques to rule out a tumor or other organ abnormality as a cause. These imaging methods may include:

- Ultrasound (sonography) to examine the gonads. An ultrasound painlessly creates an image on a computer screen of blood vessels and tissues, allowing a healthcare provider to monitor organs and blood flow in real time

- An MRI (magnetic resonance imaging) scan of the brain and pituitary gland using an instrument that produces detailed images of organs and bodily structures

Delayed Puberty

To diagnose hypogonadotropic hypogonadism, a healthcare provider may prescribe these tests:

- Blood tests to measure hormone levels
- Blood tests to measure if the pituitary gland can correctly respond to GnRH
- An MRI of the brain and pituitary gland

What Are Common Treatments for Problems of Puberty?

Precocious Puberty

There are a number of reasons to treat precocious puberty.

Treatment for precocious puberty can help stop puberty until the child is closer to the normal time for sexual development. One reason to consider treating precocious puberty is that rapid growth and bone maturation, caused by precocious puberty, can prevent a child from reaching his or her full height potential. Children grow rapidly in height during puberty and reach their final adult height after puberty. Children who go through puberty too early may not reach their full adult height potential because their growth stops too soon.

Another reason to consider treating precocious puberty is that a young child may not be psychologically ready for the physical and hormonal changes that occur in puberty.

However, not all children with precocious puberty require treatment, particularly if the onset of puberty is only slightly early. The goal of treatment is to prevent the production of sex hormones to prevent the early halt of growth, short stature in adulthood, emotional effects, social problems, and problems with libido (especially in boys).

If precocious puberty is caused by a specific medical problem, treating the underlying problem can often stop the progression of precocious puberty. In addition, precocious puberty can often be stopped by medical treatment to block the hormones that cause puberty. For example, medications called gonadotropin-releasing hormone agonists (GnRHa) are used to treat central precocious puberty. These medications, some of which are injected, suppress production of luteinizing hormone (LH) and follicle-stimulating hormone (FSH).

Delayed Puberty

With delayed puberty or hypogonadism, treatment varies with the origin of the problem but may involve:

- In males, testosterone injections, skin patches, or gel
- In females, estrogen and/or progesterone given as pills or skin patches

Section 22.8

Turner Syndrome

This section includes text excerpted from "Turner Syndrome," *Eunice Kennedy Shriver* National Institute of Child Health and Human Development (NICHD), August 23, 2013.

What Is Turner Syndrome?

Turner syndrome is a disorder caused by a partially or completely missing X chromosome. This condition affects only females.

Most people have 46 chromosomes in each cell—23 from their mother and 23 from their father. The 23rd pair of chromosomes are called the sex chromosomes—X and Y—because they determine whether a person is male or female. Females have two X chromosomes (XX) in most of their cells, and males have one X chromosome and one Y chromosome (XY) in most of their cells. A female with all of her chromosomes is referred to as 46,XX. A male is 46,XY.

Turner syndrome most often occurs when a female has one normal X chromosome, but the other X chromosome is missing (45,X). Other forms of Turner syndrome result when one of the two chromosomes is partially missing or altered in some way.

What Are the Symptoms of Turner Syndrome?

Turner syndrome causes a variety of symptoms in girls and women. For some people, symptoms are mild, but for others, Turner syndrome can cause serious health problems. In general, women with Turner syndrome have female sex characteristics, but these characteristics are underdeveloped compared to the typical female. Turner syndrome can affect:

- Appearance
- Stature
- Puberty
- Reproduction
- Cardiovascular
- Kidney
- Osteoporosis
- Diabetes
- Thyroid
- Cognitive

How Many People Are Affected or at Risk?

Turner syndrome affects about 1 of every 2,500 female live births worldwide.

This disorder affects all races and regions of the world equally. There are no known environmental risks for Turner syndrome. Parents who have had many unaffected children can still have a child with Turner syndrome later on.

Generally, Turner syndrome is not passed on from mother to child. In most cases, women with Turner syndrome are infertile.

What Causes Turner Syndrome?

Turner syndrome occurs when part or all of an X chromosome is missing from most or all of the cells in a girl's body. A girl normally receives one X chromosome from each parent. The error that leads to the missing chromosome appears to happen during the formation of the egg or sperm.

Most commonly, a girl with Turner syndrome has only one X chromosome. Occasionally, she may have a partial second X chromosome. Because she is missing part or all of a chromosome, certain genes are missing. The loss of these genes leads to the symptoms of Turner syndrome.

Sometimes, girls with Turner syndrome have some cells that are missing one X chromosome (45,X) and some that are normal. This is because not every cell in the body is exactly the same, so some cells might have the chromosome, while others might not. This condition is called mosaicism. If the second sex chromosome is lost from most of a girl's cells, then it's likely that she will have symptoms of Turner syndrome. If the chromosome is missing from only some of her cells, she may have no symptoms or only mild symptoms.

How Do Healthcare Providers Diagnose Turner Syndrome?

Healthcare providers use a combination of physical symptoms and the results of a genetic blood test, called a karyotype, to determine the chromosomal characteristics of the cells in a female's body. The test will show if one of the X chromosomes is partially or completely missing.

Turner syndrome also can be diagnosed during pregnancy by testing the cells in the amniotic fluid. Newborns may be diagnosed after heart problems are detected or after certain physical features, such as swollen hands and feet or webbed skin on the neck, are noticed. Other characteristics, like widely spaced nipples or low-set ears, also may lead to a suspicion of Turner syndrome. Some girls may be diagnosed as teenagers because of a slow growth rate or a lack of puberty-related changes. Still others may be diagnosed as adults when they have difficulty becoming pregnant.

What Are Common Treatments for Turner Syndrome?

Although there is no cure for Turner syndrome, some treatments can help minimize its symptoms. These include:

- **Human growth hormone.** If given in early childhood, hormone injections can often increase adult height by a few inches.
- **Estrogen replacement therapy (ERT).** ERT can help start the secondary sexual development that normally begins at puberty (around age 12). This includes breast development and

the development of wider hips. Healthcare providers may prescribe a combination of estrogen and progesterone to girls who haven't started menstruating by age 15. ERT also provides protection against bone loss.

Regular health checks and access to a wide variety of specialists are important to care for the various health problems that can result from Turner syndrome. These include ear infections, high blood pressure, and thyroid problems.

Is Turner Syndrome Inherited?

Turner syndrome is usually not inherited, but it is genetic. It is caused by a random error that leads to a missing X chromosome in the sperm or egg of a parent.

Only about 1% of pregnancies in which the fetus has Turner syndrome result in live births. The others end in miscarriage.

Most women with Turner syndrome cannot get pregnant naturally. In one study, as many as 40% of women with Turner syndrome got pregnant using donated eggs. However, pregnant women with Turner syndrome are at increased risk for high blood pressure during pregnancy, which can result in complications, including preterm birth and fetal growth restriction.

Women with Turner syndrome also are at risk for aortic dissection during pregnancy. This happens about 2% of the time. An aortic dissection is a tear in or damage to the inner wall of the aorta, the major artery carrying blood to the heart. Damage to the aorta's inner wall causes blood to flow rapidly into the lining of the aorta. This can restrict the main flow of blood through the aorta or cause the aorta to balloon—a condition called an aneurysm. An aneurysm can rupture, which can be life-threatening.

Can Turner Syndrome Be Prevented?

Turner syndrome cannot be prevented. It is a genetic problem that is caused by a random error that leads to a missing X chromosome in the sperm or egg of a parent. There is nothing the father or mother can do to prevent the error from occurring. However, there are many options for treatment.

Is Turner Syndrome Considered a Disability?

Turner syndrome is not considered a disability, although it can cause certain learning challenges, including problems learning mathematics and with memory. Most girls and women with Turner syndrome lead a normal, healthy, productive life with proper medical care.

My Daughter Has Been Diagnosed with Turner Syndrome. Now What?

If your daughter has been diagnosed with Turner syndrome, you may be wondering what to expect as she grows up. A few of these questions, with answers, are listed here.

- Will she mature normally?
- Most girls with Turner syndrome do not mature typically. They may not develop breasts or start getting a period. Estrogen treatment can replace hormones that the body doesn't naturally produce, spurring development and preventing osteoporosis.
- Will she have problems in school?
- Some girls with Turner syndrome have difficulty with arithmetic, visual memory, and visio-spatial skills (such as determining the relative positions of objects in space). They may also have some trouble understanding nonverbal communication (body language, facial expression) and interacting with peers.
- What care will she need as she grows up?
- Girls and women with Turner syndrome usually require care from a variety of specialists throughout their lives.
- Will she be able to have a normal sex life as an adult?
- Women with Turner syndrome can enjoy normal sex lives.
- Will she be able to have children?
- Most women with Turner syndrome cannot get pregnant naturally. Those who can are at risk for blood pressure-related complications, which can lead to premature birth or fetal growth restriction. Pregnancy also is associated with increased risk for maternal complications, including aortic dissection and rupture.

Chapter 23

Gastrointestinal Disorders in Children

Chapter Contents

Section 23.1

Abdominal Pain

"Abdominal Pain," © 2017 Omnigraphics.
Reviewed October 2016.

Functional abdominal pain (FAP) in children refers to chronic stomachaches that have no apparent underlying physical cause. The pain may be intermittent or constant and is usually experienced in the area surrounding the navel. According to the medical definition, functional abdominal pain occurs at least once per week over a period of two months or more. Even if the child undergoes extensive medical examination and testing, no abnormality, infection, or blockage will be found to explain the condition. FAP is relatively common, affecting between 10 and 15 percent of school-aged children—most of whom are otherwise healthy—and accounting for one-fourth of all visits to gastroenterologists by children and adolescents.

Although the exact mechanism is not well understood, doctors believe that FAP is caused by increased nerve sensitivity in the digestive organs. This sensitivity may be triggered by psychological stress, constipation, or some sort of infection in the digestive system. As a result, the nerves and muscles that help move food through the stomach and intestines overreact to normal functions, such as gas or bloating, that usually only cause mild discomfort. Instead, children with FAP experience recurrent episodes of significant pain that may interfere with their participation in school, sports, and family activities. While the pain is real, the lack of an identifiable cause can be frustrating or frightening for children and parents.

Causes and Risk Factors

Occasional, mild abdominal pain is common in children and does not usually require medical attention. It may be caused by such issues as constipation, gas, food allergy, lactose intolerance, food poisoning, colic, or a viral, bacterial, or parasitic infestation of the digestive tract. Chronic abdominal pain also has many possible causes, including appendicitis, acid reflux, ulcers, gallstones, hernia, intestinal obstruction, urinary tract infection, and cancer. These conditions warrant medical examination and treatment.

If a child experiences frequent, recurring abdominal pain—but medical examination and testing rules out other possible causes—then the likely cause is functional abdominal pain. The triggers for FAP vary depending on the individual and may be difficult to identify. In many cases the condition appears to be related to traumatic experiences or emotional disturbances. FAP also tends to affect children with underlying anxiety or depression, as these conditions are often associated with an increased or exaggerated pain response. Many children with FAP have previously contracted a gastrointestinal infection. The condition may also have a genetic component, as many children with FAP have a family member who also experienced recurrent abdominal pain in childhood.

Symptoms

The main symptom of FAP is recurrent pain that centers around the navel, although the characteristics of the pain may vary. FAP includes several different types or categories, each of which has its own distinct symptoms:

- functional dyspepsia (FD) includes upper abdominal pain along with nausea, vomiting, and loss of appetite;
- irritable bowel syndrome (IBS) includes abdominal pain along with changes in bowel movements, such as constipation or diarrhea, or abdominal pain that is relieved by bowel movements;
- abdominal migraine includes recurring attacks of stomach pain along with nausea, vomiting, and pallor that last between 2 and 72 hours.

Diagnosis

The first step in diagnosing involves taking a medical history. The doctor is likely to inquire about the location and severity of the child's abdominal pain, how often it occurs, and how long each episode lasts. The doctor may also ask the patient to keep a food log to identify any relationships between foods and beverages and abdominal pain. Finally, the doctor is likely to inquire about the patient's overall health, including sleep, exercise, and psychological stress.

The next step in diagnosis involves physical examination and testing to rule out underlying health conditions that could be contributing to the abdominal pain. The initial screening tests are likely to include blood, urine, and stool samples. If any concerning symptoms are present—such as weight loss, poor growth, fever, joint pains, unusual rashes, or blood in the vomit or stool—then further testing may be indicated. Additional tests that may be performed include an ultrasound or computerized tomography (CT) scan of the abdomen or an endoscopy of the digestive tract. If all of these tests fail to turn up evidence of abnormalities, infections, blockages, or other disorders, then the diagnosis for an otherwise healthy child is likely to be FAP.

Treatment

One of the challenges in treating FAP is that no specific cause of the symptoms can be found. It is important to note that FAP symptoms are nonetheless real and not simply a product of the child's imagination or an example of attention-seeking behavior. Although no single cure is available, many patients find relief from some combination of the following treatment options:

- identifying sources of emotional or psychological stress and assisting the child in developing coping skills and relaxation techniques
- undergoing psychological treatments, such as cognitive behavioral therapy
- implementing dietary changes, such as avoiding greasy and spicy foods, cabbage, beans, caffeine, fruit juices, carbonated beverages, and anything sweetened with sorbitol
- taking medications, such as tricyclic antidepressants, anti-spasmodic medications, laxatives, or acid reducers

Nearly half of all children with FAP experience improvement in symptoms within a few months, either on their own or with some form of treatment. Studies have shown that parental acceptance of the reality of the condition, along with family support for the emotional needs of the child, is key to recovery. The outlook is not as positive for children whose FAP is related to family dysfunction, sexual abuse, or stressful life events. Up to 30 percent of children with FAP may continue to experience chronic abdominal pain in adulthood, and evidence also suggests that FAP in childhood may increase the risk of emotional and psychiatric disorders later in life.

References

1. "Functional Abdominal Pain," GI Kids, 2016.
2. Khan, Seema. "Functional Abdominal Pain in Children," American College of Gastroenterology, December 2012.
3. Tidy, Colin. "Recurrent Abdominal Pain in Children," Patient, July 27, 2016.

Section 23.2

Appendicitis

This section includes text excerpted from "Definition and Facts for Appendicitis," National Institute of Diabetes and Digestive and Kidney Diseases (NIDDK), November 13, 2014.

What Is Appendicitis?

Appendicitis is inflammation of your appendix.

How Common Is Appendicitis

In the United States, appendicitis is the most common cause of acute abdominal pain requiring surgery. Over 5% of the population develops appendicitis at some point.

Who Is More Likely to Develop Appendicitis?

Appendicitis most commonly occurs in the teens and twenties but may occur at any age.

What Are the Complications of Appendicitis?

If appendicitis is not treated, it may lead to complications. The complications of a ruptured appendix are:

- peritonitis, which can be a dangerous condition. Peritonitis happens if your appendix bursts and infection spreads in your abdomen. If you have peritonitis, you may be very ill and have:

- fever
- nausea
- severe tenderness in your abdomen
- vomiting
- an abscess of the appendix called an appendiceal abscess.

What Are the Symptoms of Appendicitis?

The most common symptom of appendicitis is pain in your abdomen. If you have appendicitis, you'll most often have pain in your abdomen that:

- begins near your belly button and then moves lower and to your right
- gets worse in a matter of hours
- gets worse when you move around, take deep breaths, cough, or sneeze
- is severe and often described as different from any pain you've felt before
- occurs suddenly and may even wake you up if you're sleeping
- occurs before other symptoms

Other symptoms of appendicitis may include:

- loss of appetite
- nausea
- vomiting
- constipation or diarrhea
- an inability to pass gas
- a low-grade fever
- swelling in your abdomen
- the feeling that having a bowel movement will relieve discomfort

Symptoms can be different for each person and can seem like the following conditions that also cause pain in the abdomen:

- abdominal adhesions

- constipation
- inflammatory bowel disease, which includes Crohn's disease and ulcerative colitis, long-lasting disorders that cause irritation and ulcers in the GI tract
- intestinal obstruction
- pelvic inflammatory disease

What Causes Appendicitis?

Appendicitis can have more than one cause, and in many cases the cause is not clear. Possible causes include:

- Blockage of the opening inside the appendix
- enlarged tissue in the wall of your appendix, caused by infection in the gastrointestinal (GI) tract or elsewhere in your body
- inflammatory bowel disease
- stool, parasites, or growths that can clog your appendiceal lumen
- trauma to your abdomen

When Should I Seek a Doctor's Help?

Appendicitis is a medical emergency that requires immediate care. See a healthcare professional or go to the emergency room right away if you think you or a child has appendicitis. A doctor can help treat the appendicitis and reduce symptoms and the chance of complications.

How Do Doctors Diagnose Appendicitis?

Most often, healthcare professionals suspect the diagnosis of appendicitis based on your symptoms, your medical history, and a physical exam. A doctor can confirm the diagnosis with an ultrasound, X-ray, or Magnetic resonance imaging (MRI) exam.

How Do Doctors Treat Appendicitis?

Doctors typically treat appendicitis with surgery to remove the appendix. Surgeons perform the surgery in a hospital with general anesthesia. Your doctor will recommend surgery if you have continuous abdominal pain and fever, or signs of a burst appendix and infection. Prompt surgery decreases the chance that your appendix will burst.

Healthcare professionals call the surgery to remove the appendix an appendectomy. A surgeon performs the surgery using one of the following methods:

- **Laparoscopic surgery.** During laparoscopic surgery, surgeons use several smaller incisions and special surgical tools that they feed through the incisions to remove your appendix. Laparoscopic surgery leads to fewer complications, such as hospital-related infections, and has a shorter recovery time.
- **Laparotomy.** Surgeons use laparotomy to remove the appendix through a single incision in the lower right area of your abdomen.

After surgery, most patients completely recover from appendicitis and don't need to make changes to their diet, exercise, or lifestyle. Surgeons recommend that you limit physical activity for the first 10 to 14 days after a laparotomy and for the first 3 to 5 days after laparoscopic surgery.

How Do Doctors Treat Complications of a Burst Appendix?

Treating the complications of a burst appendix will depend on the type of complication. In most cases of peritonitis, a surgeon will remove your appendix immediately with surgery. The surgeon will use laparotomy to clean the inside of your abdomen to prevent infection and then remove your appendix. Without prompt treatment, peritonitis can cause death.

A surgeon may drain the pus from an appendiceal abscess during surgery or, more commonly, before surgery. To drain an abscess, the surgeon places a tube in the abscess through the abdominal wall. You leave the drainage tube in place for about 2 weeks while you take antibiotics to treat infection. When the infection and inflammation are under control, about 6 to 8 weeks later, surgeons operate to remove what remains of the burst appendix.

Section 23.3

Celiac Disease

This section includes text excerpted from "Celiac Disease," National Institute of Diabetes and Digestive and Kidney Diseases (NIDDK), June 2016.

What Is Celiac Disease?

Celiac disease is a digestive disorder that damages the small intestine. The disease is triggered by eating foods containing gluten. Gluten is a protein found naturally in wheat, barley, and rye, and is common in foods such as bread, pasta, cookies, and cakes. Many pre-packaged foods, lip balms and lipsticks, hair and skin products, toothpastes, vitamin and nutrient supplements, and, rarely, medicines, contain gluten.

Celiac disease can be very serious. The disease can cause long-lasting digestive problems and keep your body from getting all the nutrients it needs. Celiac disease can also affect the body outside the intestine.

Celiac disease is different from gluten sensitivity or wheat intolerance. If you have gluten sensitivity, you may have symptoms similar to those of celiac disease, such as abdominal pain and tiredness. Unlike celiac disease, gluten sensitivity does not damage the small intestine.

Celiac disease is also different from a wheat allergy. In both cases, your body's immune system reacts to wheat. However, some symptoms in wheat allergies, such as having itchy eyes or a hard time breathing, are different from celiac disease. Wheat allergies also do not cause long-term damage to the small intestine.

How Common Is Celiac Disease?

As many as one in 141 Americans has celiac disease, although most don't know it.

Who Is More Likely to Develop Celiac Disease?

Although celiac disease affects children and adults in all parts of the world, the disease is more common in Caucasians and more often diagnosed in females. You are more likely to develop celiac disease if someone in your family has the disease. Celiac disease also is more common among people with certain other diseases, such as Down syndrome, Turner syndrome, and type 1 diabetes.

What Other Health Problems Do People with Celiac Disease Have?

If you have celiac disease, you also may be at risk for:

- Addison disease
- Hashimoto disease
- primary biliary cirrhosis
- type 1 diabetes

What Are the Complications of Celiac Disease?

Long-term complications of celiac disease include:

- malnutrition, a condition in which you don't get enough vitamins, minerals, and other nutrients you need to be healthy
- accelerated osteoporosis or bone softening, known as osteomalacia
- nervous system problems
- problems related to reproduction

Rare complications can include:

- intestinal cancer
- liver diseases
- lymphoma, a cancer of part of the immune system called the lymph system that includes the gut

In rare cases, you may continue to have trouble absorbing nutrients even though you have been following a strict gluten-free diet. If you have this condition, called refractory celiac disease, your intestines are severely damaged and can't heal. You may need to receive nutrients through an intravenous (IV).

Symptoms of Celiac Disease

Most people with celiac disease have one or more symptoms. However, some people with the disease may not have symptoms or feel sick. Sometimes health issues such as surgery, a pregnancy, childbirth, bacterial gastroenteritis, a viral infection, or severe mental stress can trigger celiac disease symptoms.

If you have celiac disease, you may have digestive problems or other symptoms. Digestive symptoms are more common in children and can include:

- bloating, or a feeling of fullness or swelling in the abdomen
- chronic diarrhea
- constipation
- gas
- nausea
- pale, foul-smelling, or fatty stools that float
- stomach pain
- vomiting

For children with celiac disease, being unable to absorb nutrients when they are so important to normal growth and development can lead to:

- damage to the permanent teeth's enamel
- delayed puberty
- failure to thrive in infants
- mood changes or feeling annoyed or impatient
- slowed growth and short height
- weight loss

Celiac disease also can produce a reaction in which your immune system, or your body's natural defense system, attacks healthy cells in your body. This reaction can spread outside your digestive tract to other areas of your body, including your:

- bones
- joints
- nervous system
- skin
- spleen

Depending on how old you are when a doctor diagnoses your celiac disease, some symptoms, such as short height and tooth defects, will not improve.

What Causes Celiac Disease?

Research suggests that celiac disease only happens to individuals who have particular genes. These genes are common and are carried by about one-third of the population. Individuals also have to be eating food that contains gluten to get celiac disease. Researchers do not know exactly what triggers celiac disease in people at risk who eat gluten over a long period of time. Sometimes the disease runs in families. About 10 to 20 percent of close relatives of people with celiac disease also are affected.

Your chances of developing celiac disease increase when you have changes in your genes, or variants. Certain gene variants and other factors, such as things in your environment, can lead to celiac disease.

How Do Doctors Diagnose Celiac Disease?

Celiac disease can be hard to diagnose because some of the symptoms are like symptoms of other diseases, such as irritable bowel syndrome (IBS) and lactose intolerance. Your doctor may diagnose celiac disease with a medical and family history, physical exam, and tests. Tests may include blood tests, genetic tests, and biopsy.

What Tests Do Doctors Use to Diagnose Celiac Disease?

- Blood Tests
- Genetic Tests
- Intestinal Biopsy
- Skin Biopsy

Do Doctors Screen for Celiac Disease?

Screening is testing for diseases when you have no symptoms. Doctors in the United States do not routinely screen people for celiac disease. However, blood relatives of people with celiac disease and those with type 1 diabetes should talk with their doctor about their chances of getting the disease.

Many researchers recommend routine screening of all family members, such as parents and siblings, for celiac disease. However, routine genetic screening for celiac disease is not usually helpful when diagnosing the disease.

How Do Doctors Treat Celiac Disease?

A gluten-free diet.

Doctors treat celiac disease with a gluten-free diet. Gluten is a protein found naturally in wheat, barley, and rye that triggers a reaction if you have celiac disease. Symptoms greatly improve for most people with celiac disease who stick to a gluten-free diet. In recent years, grocery stores and restaurants have added many more gluten-free foods and products, making it easier to stay gluten free.

Your doctor may refer you to a dietitian who specializes in treating people with celiac disease. The dietitian will teach you how to avoid gluten while following a healthy diet. He or she will help you

- check food and product labels for gluten
- design everyday meal plans
- make healthy choices about the types of foods to eat

For most people, following a gluten-free diet will heal damage in the small intestine and prevent more damage. You may see symptoms improve within days to weeks of starting the diet. The small intestine usually heals in 3 to 6 months in children. Complete healing can take several years in adults. Once the intestine heals, the villi, which were damaged by the disease, regrow and will absorb nutrients from food into the bloodstream normally.

Gluten-free diet and dermatitis herpetiformis.

If you have dermatitis herpetiformis—an itchy, blistering skin rash—skin symptoms generally respond to a gluten-free diet. However, skin symptoms may return if you add gluten back into your diet. Medicines such as dapsone, taken by mouth, can control the skin symptoms. People who take dapsone need to have regular blood tests to check for side effects from the medicine.

Dapsone does not treat intestinal symptoms or damage, which is why you should stay on a gluten-free diet if you have the rash. Even when you follow a gluten-free diet, the rash may take months or even years to fully heal—and often comes back over the years.

What If Changing to a Gluten-Free Diet Isn't Working?

If you don't improve after starting a gluten-free diet, you may still be eating or using small amounts of gluten. You probably will start responding to the gluten-free diet once you find and cut out all hidden sources of gluten. Hidden sources of gluten include additives made with wheat, such as:

- modified food starch
- malt flavoring
- preservatives
- stabilizers

If you still have symptoms even after changing your diet, you may have other conditions or disorders that are more common with celiac disease, such as irritable bowel syndrome (IBS), lactose intolerance, microscopic colitis, dysfunction of the pancreas, and small intestinal bacterial overgrowth.

What Should I Avoid Eating If I Have Celiac Disease?

Avoiding foods with gluten, a protein found naturally in wheat, rye, and barley, is critical in treating celiac disease. Removing gluten from your diet will improve symptoms, heal damage to your small intestine, and prevent further damage over time. While you may need to avoid certain foods, the good news is that many healthy, gluten-free foods and products are available.

You should avoid all products that contain gluten, such as most cereal, grains, and pasta, and many processed foods. Be sure to always read food ingredient lists carefully to make sure the food you want to eat doesn't have gluten. In addition, discuss gluten-free food choices with a dietitian or healthcare professional who specializes in celiac disease.

Is a Gluten-Free Diet Safe If I Don't Have Celiac Disease?

In recent years, more people without celiac disease have adopted a gluten-free diet, believing that avoiding gluten is healthier or could help them lose weight. No current data suggests that the general public should maintain a gluten-free diet for weight loss or better health.

A gluten-free diet isn't always a healthy diet. For instance, a gluten-free diet may not provide enough of the nutrients, vitamins, and minerals the body needs, such as fiber, iron, and calcium. Some gluten-free products can be high in calories and sugar.

If you think you might have celiac disease, don't start avoiding gluten without first speaking with your doctor. If your doctor diagnoses you with celiac disease, he or she will put you on a gluten-free diet.

Section 23.4

Crohn's Disease

This section includes text excerpted from "Definition and Facts for Crohn's Disease," National Institute of Diabetes and Digestive and Kidney Diseases (NIDDK), July 2016.

What Is Crohn's Disease?

Crohn's disease is a chronic disease that causes inflammation and irritation in your digestive tract. Most commonly, Crohn's disease affects your small intestine and the beginning of your large intestine. However, the disease can affect any part of your digestive tract, from your mouth to your anus.

Crohn's disease is an inflammatory bowel disease (IBD). Ulcerative colitis and microscopic colitis are other common types of IBD.

Crohn's disease most often begins gradually and can become worse over time. You may have periods of remission that can last for weeks or years.

How Common Is Crohn's Disease?

Researchers estimate that more than half a million people in the United States have Crohn's disease. Studies show that, over time, Crohn's disease has become more common in the United States and other parts of the world. Experts do not know the reason for this increase.

Who Is More Likely to Develop Crohn's Disease?

Crohn's disease can develop in people of any age and is more likely to develop in people:

- between the ages of 20 and 29
- who have a family member, most often a sibling or parent, with IBD
- who smoke cigarettes

What Are the Complications of Crohn's Disease?

Complications of Crohn's disease can include the following:

- **Intestinal obstruction.** Crohn's disease can thicken the wall of your intestines. Over time, the thickened areas of your intestines can narrow, which can block your intestines. A partial or complete intestinal obstruction, also called a bowel blockage, can block the movement of food or stool through your intestines.
- **Fistulas.** In Crohn's disease, inflammation can go through the wall of your intestines and create tunnels, or fistulas. Fistulas are abnormal passages between two organs, or between an organ and the outside of your body. Fistulas may become infected.
- **Abscesses.** Inflammation that goes through the wall of your intestines can also lead to abscesses. Abscesses are painful, swollen, pus-filled pockets of infection.
- **Anal fissures.** Anal fissures are small tears in your anus that may cause itching, pain, or bleeding.
- **Ulcers.** Inflammation anywhere along your digestive tract can lead to ulcers or open sores in your mouth, intestines, anus, or perineum.
- **Malnutrition.** Malnutrition develops when your body does not get the right amount of vitamins, minerals, and nutrients it needs to maintain healthy tissues and organ function.
- **Inflammation in other areas of your body.** You may have inflammation in your joints, eyes, and skin.

What Are the Symptoms of Crohn's Disease?

The most common symptoms of Crohn's disease are:

- diarrhea
- cramping and pain in your abdomen
- weight loss

Other symptoms include:

- anemia
- eye redness or pain
- feeling tired
- fever
- joint pain or soreness
- nausea or loss of appetite
- skin changes that involve red, tender bumps under the skin

Your symptoms may vary depending on the location and severity of your inflammation.

Some research suggests that stress, including the stress of living with Crohn's disease, can make symptoms worse. Also, some people may find that certain foods can trigger or worsen their symptoms.

What Causes Crohn's Disease?

Doctors aren't sure what causes Crohn's disease. Experts think the following factors may play a role in causing Crohn's disease.

Autoimmune Reaction

One cause of Crohn's disease may be an autoimmune reaction—when your immune system attacks healthy cells in your body. Experts think bacteria in your digestive tract can mistakenly trigger your immune system. This immune system response causes inflammation, leading to symptoms of Crohn's disease.

Genes

Crohn's disease sometimes runs in families. Research has shown that if you have a parent or sibling with Crohn's disease, you may be more likely to develop the disease. Experts continue to study the link between genes and Crohn's disease.

Other factors

Some studies suggest that other factors may increase your chance of developing Crohn's disease:

- Smoking may double your chance of developing Crohn's disease.
- Nonsteroidal anti-inflammatory drugs (NSAIDs) such as aspirin or ibuprofen, antibiotics, and birth-control pills may slightly increase the chance of developing Crohn's disease.
- A high-fat diet may also slightly increase your chance of getting Crohn's disease.
- Stress and eating certain foods do not cause Crohn's disease.

How Do Doctors Diagnose Crohn's Disease?

Doctors typically use a combination of tests to diagnose Crohn's disease. Your doctor will also ask you about your medical history—including medicines you are taking—and your family history and will perform a physical exam.

What Tests Do Doctors Use to Diagnose Crohn's Disease?

Your doctor may perform the following tests to help diagnose Crohn's disease.

Lab Tests

Lab tests to help diagnose Crohn's disease include:

Blood tests. A healthcare professional may take a blood sample from you and send the sample to a lab to test for changes in

- red blood cells. If your red blood cells are fewer or smaller than normal, you may have anemia.
- white blood cells. When your white blood cell count is higher than normal, you may have inflammation or infection somewhere in your body.

Stool tests. A stool test is the analysis of a sample of stool. Your doctor will give you a container for catching and storing the stool. You will receive instructions on where to send or take the kit for analysis. Doctors use stool tests to rule out other causes of digestive diseases.

Intestinal Endoscopy

Intestinal endoscopies are the most accurate methods for diagnosing Crohn's disease and ruling out other possible conditions, such as ulcerative colitis, diverticular disease, or cancer. Intestinal endoscopies include the following:

- Colonoscopy
- Upper GI endoscopy and enteroscopy
- Capsule endoscopy

Upper GI Series

- An upper GI series is a procedure in which a doctor uses X-rays, fluoroscopy, and a chalky liquid called barium to view your upper GI tract.
- CT Scan
    - A CT scan uses a combination of X-rays and computer technology to create images of your digestive tract.

How Do Doctors Treat Crohn's Disease?

Doctors treat Crohn's disease with medicines, bowel rest, and surgery. No single treatment works for everyone with Crohn's disease. The goals of treatment are to decrease the inflammation in your intestines, to prevent flare-ups of your symptoms, and to keep you in remission.

Eating, Diet, and Nutrition for Crohn's Disease

How Can My Diet Help the Symptoms of Crohn's Disease?

Changing your diet can help reduce symptoms. Your doctor may recommend that you make changes to your diet such as

- avoiding carbonated, or "fizzy," drinks
- avoiding popcorn, vegetable skins, nuts, and other high-fiber foods
- drinking more liquids
- eating smaller meals more often
- keeping a food diary to help identify foods that cause problems

Depending on your symptoms or medicines, your doctor may recommend a specific diet, such as a diet that is

- high calorie
- lactose free
- low fat
- low fiber
- low salt

Talk with your doctor about specific dietary recommendations and changes.

Your doctor may recommend nutritional supplements and vitamins if you do not absorb enough nutrients. For safety reasons, talk with your doctor before using dietary supplements, such as vitamins, or any complementary or alternative medicines or medical practices.

Section 23.5

Constipation

This section includes text excerpted from "Definition and Facts for Constipation in Children," National Institute of Diabetes and Digestive and Kidney Diseases (NIDDK), November 13, 2014.

What Is Constipation in Children?

Constipation in children is a condition in which a child may have

- fewer than two bowel movements a week
- bowel movements with stools that are hard, dry, and small, making them painful or difficult to pass

In most cases, constipation in children lasts a short time and is not dangerous.

How Common Is Constipation in Children?

Almost 5 percent of visits to pediatricians are for constipation. About 25 percent of the children who visit gastroenterologists are constipated.

What Are the Complications of Constipation in Children?

Constipation can lead to health problems such as fecal impaction, anal fissures, or rectal prolapse.

Fecal Impaction

Fecal impaction happens when hard stool packs a child's intestine and rectum so tightly that the normal pushing action of the colon is not enough to push the stool out.

Anal Fissures

Anal fissures are small tears in the anus that may cause itching, pain, or bleeding.

Rectal Prolapse

Rectal prolapse happens when a child's rectum slips so that it sticks out from his or her anus. Rectal prolapse in children is not common in developed countries. Rectal prolapse can happen if a child strains during bowel movements, among other reasons. Rectal prolapse may cause mucus to leak from the child's anus.

What Are the Symptoms of Constipation in Children?

If a child is constipated, he or she may have the following symptoms:

Posturing or Changing Positions

Posturing or changing positions can show that a child is trying to hold in stool or is constipated. When a child postures or changes position, he or she may

- stand on tiptoes and then rock back on his or her heels
- clench his or her buttocks muscles
- do unusual, dance like movements

Parents or caretakers often mistake these postures as ways to try and have a bowel movement.

Abdominal Pain and Bloating

A child may feel pain or bloating in his or her abdomen.

Stool in a Child's Underwear

If a child delays having a bowel movement, he or she may develop a large amount of stool in the rectum—something healthcare professionals call a fecal impaction. Some of this stool may leak and soil a child's underwear. Parents or caretakers often mistake this soiling as a sign of diarrhea.

Urinary Incontinence

Stool in a child's colon can press against his or her bladder. This pressure may cause daytime or nighttime wetting called urinary incontinence.

When Should a Child with Constipation See a Doctor?

A child should see a doctor if his or her symptoms of constipation last for more than 2 weeks. You should take a child to see a doctor right away if he or she has one or more of the following symptoms:

- fever
- vomiting
- blood in his or her stool
- a swollen abdomen
- weight loss

What Causes Constipation in Children?

Constipation happens when stool stays too long in a child's colon. Causes of constipation in children may include the following:

Ignoring the Urge to Have a Bowel Movement

Children most often get constipated from holding in stool. When a child holds in stool, the colon absorbs too much fluid and his or her stool becomes hard, dry, and difficult to pass.

Children may hold in stool because they

- are feeling stressed about potty training

- are embarrassed to use a public bathroom
- do not want to interrupt playtime
- are worried about having a painful or an unpleasant bowel movement

Functional GI Disorders

Functional GI disorders happen when something changes the way a child's GI tract works, yet doesn't cause damage. Functional constipation happens when the muscles in a child's colon or anus move stool more slowly, and it often happens during one of three times:

- when infants transition from breastmilk to formula or when they start eating solid foods
- when parents or caretakers are potty training toddlers, and toddlers are learning how to control bowel movements
- when children start school and avoid using the bathroom at school for bowel movements

Irritable bowel syndrome (IBS) is also a functional GI disorder. Children with IBS can be constipated.

How Do Doctors Diagnose Constipation in Children?

To find out why a child is constipated, the child's doctor will take a medical history and perform a physical exam, and may order tests.

Medical History

The medical history will include questions about the child's constipation, such as

- what are the child's bowel movement patterns, including how often the child has bowel movements
- when the first bowel movement after birth happened
- what are the child's eating habits, including when and what the child most often eats and drinks
- what are the child's social situations like, including
- his or her day care attendance
- his or her potty training

- whether the child has any health problems
- whether the child is taking medicine that can cause constipation
- what is the family's history of constipation

Doctors primarily use a child's medical history to diagnose functional constipation. The child's history and symptoms may be different depending on his or her age.

Physical Exam

During a physical exam, a doctor will listen for bowel sounds and feel the child's abdomen for

- swelling
- tenderness
- masses, or lumps

The physical exam may include a rectal exam. After putting on a glove, a doctor will slide a lubricated finger into a child's anus to check for tenderness, blockage, or blood.

Diagnostic Tests

Since functional constipation is so common in children, doctors do not normally use diagnostic tests for children with constipation unless they do not respond to treatment or the doctor suspects a specific cause.

What Test Do Doctors Use to Diagnose Constipation in Children?

A doctor may use one or more of the following tests to diagnose constipation:

Blood Test

A blood test might show an abnormality, such as anemia, indicating that a disease might be the cause of a child's constipation.

X-Ray

A doctor may order an X-ray of the child's abdomen to look for problems causing the constipation. The child will lie on a table or stand during the X-ray. A healthcare professional positions the X-ray machine over the child's abdomen. The child will hold his or her breath while the healthcare professional takes the X-ray so that the picture will not be blurry. The healthcare professional may ask the child to change position for more X-rays.

How Do Doctors Treat Constipation in Children?

Parents or caretakers can most often treat a child at home. However, if a child does not respond to treatment, call the child's doctor. Treatment for constipation in children may include changes in eating, diet, and nutrition; behavioral changes; and enemas and laxatives:

Changes in Eating, Diet, and Nutrition

Changes in a child's eating, diet, and nutrition can treat constipation. These changes include

- drinking liquids throughout the day. A healthcare professional can recommend how much and what kind of liquids a child should drink.
- eating more fruits and vegetables.
- eating more fiber.

Read what a child should eat to help prevent and relieve constipation and foods to avoid if a child is constipated.

Behavioral Changes

Changing a child's patterns and behaviors about having bowel movements can help treat constipation. You can help the child by

- encouraging older children to use the toilet shortly after meals to build a routine
- using a reward system when children use the bathroom regularly
- taking a break from potty training until the constipation stops

Enemas and Laxatives

Some children need to have an enema or take medicines to treat constipation. Most often, a doctor will first recommend using an enema. Cleansing a child's bowel with an enema flushes water or a laxative into his or her anus using a special squirt bottle, which helps the child pass stool.

A doctor may prescribe a laxative for a child to take by mouth until his or her bowel movements are normal. Laxatives clean out the bowel and help a child have a bowel movement. Once a child has better eating and bowel habits, the doctor will recommend stopping the laxative. If you stop giving a child the laxative too soon then the child could become constipated again. You should not give a child laxatives unless told to do so by a doctor.

How Can a Child's Diet Help Prevent or Relieve Constipation?

A child should drink water and other fluids, such as fruit and vegetable juices and clear soups, to help the fiber in his or her diet work better. This change should make the child's stools more normal and regular. A doctor can help you plan a diet with the appropriate amount of fiber to help treat a child with constipation. A list of high-fiber foods appears below. Use this table as a tool to help replace less healthy foods with foods that have fiber.

Children ages 1 to 18, depending on their age and sex, should get 14 to 31 grams of fiber a day. Fiber guidelines are not available for infants less than 1 year old, who normally eat little to no solid food yet. Talk with the infant's doctor about possibly breastfeeding the infant or what kind of foods he or she should eat.

Table 23.1. Examples of Food That Have Fiber

Examples of Food That Have Fiber 1	
Beans, cereals, and breads	**Fiber**
½ cup of beans (navy, pinto, kidney, etc.), cooked	6.2–9.6 grams
½ cup of shredded wheat, ready-to-eat cereal	2.7–3.8 grams
? cup of 100% bran, ready-to-eat cereal	9.1 grams
1 small oat bran muffin	3.0 grams
1 whole-wheat English muffin	4.4 grams
Fruits	
1 small apple, with skin	3.6 grams
1 medium pear, with skin	5.5 grams
½ cup of raspberries	4.0 grams
½ cup of stewed prunes	3.8 grams

Table 23.1. Continued

Examples of Food That Have Fiber 1	
Beans, cereals, and breads	**Fiber**
Vegetables	
½ cup of winter squash, cooked	2.9 grams
1 medium sweet potato, baked in skin	3.8 grams
½ cup of green peas, cooked	3.5–4.4 grams
1 small potato, baked, with skin	3.0 grams
½ cup of mixed vegetables, cooked	4.0 grams
½ cup of broccoli, cooked	2.6–2.8 grams
½ cup of greens (spinach, collards, turnip greens), cooked	2.5–3.5 grams

If a child is constipated, try not to give him or her too many foods with little or no fiber, such as:

- cheese
- chips
- fast food
- ice cream
- meat
- prepared foods, such as some frozen meals and snack foods, such as saltine or animal crackers, angel food cake, and vanilla wafers
- processed foods, such as hot dogs or some microwavable dinners, such as pizza, Salisbury steak, and pot pie

Section 23.6

Chronic Diarrhea

This section includes text excerpted from "Chronic Diarrhea in Children," National Institute of Diabetes and Digestive and Kidney Diseases (NIDDK), March 2014.

What Is Chronic Diarrhea?

Diarrhea is loose, watery stools. Chronic, or long lasting, diarrhea typically lasts for more than 4 weeks. Children with chronic diarrhea may have loose, watery stools continually, or diarrhea may come and go. Chronic diarrhea may go away without treatment, or it may be a symptom of a chronic disease or disorder. Treating the disease or disorder can relieve chronic diarrhea.

Chronic diarrhea can affect children of any age:

- infants—ages 0 to 12 months
- toddlers—ages 1 to 3 years
- preschool-age children—ages 3 to 5 years
- grade school-age children—ages 5 to 12 years
- adolescents—ages 12 to 18 years

Diarrhea that lasts only a short time is called acute diarrhea. Acute diarrhea, a common problem, usually lasts a few days and goes away on its own.

What Causes Chronic Diarrhea in Children?

Many diseases and disorders can cause chronic diarrhea in children. Common causes include:

- infections
- functional gastrointestinal (GI) disorders
- food allergies and intolerances
- inflammatory bowel disease (IBD)

What Other Symptoms May Accompany Chronic Diarrhea in Children?

Symptoms that accompany chronic diarrhea in children depend on the cause of the diarrhea. Symptoms can include:

- cramping
- abdominal pain
- nausea or vomiting
- fever
- chills
- bloody stools

Children with chronic diarrhea who have malabsorption can experience:

- bloating and swelling, also called distention, of the abdomen
- changes in appetite
- weight loss or poor weight gain

How Do HealthCare Providers Determine the Cause of Chronic Diarrhea in Children?

To determine the cause of chronic diarrhea in children, the healthcare provider will take a complete medical and family history and conduct a physical exam, and may perform tests.

How Is Chronic Diarrhea in Children Treated?

The treatment for chronic diarrhea will depend on the cause. Some common causes of chronic diarrhea are treated as follows:

- **Infections.** If a child has prolonged problems digesting certain carbohydrates or proteins after an acute infection, a healthcare provider may recommend changes in diet. A child may need antibiotics or medications that target parasites to treat infections that do not go away on their own. A healthcare provider may also prescribe antibiotics to treat small intestinal bacterial overgrowth.
- **Functional GI disorders.** For toddler's diarrhea, treatment is usually not needed. Most children outgrow toddler's diarrhea by the time they start school. In many children, limiting fruit juice

intake and increasing the amount of fiber and fat in the diet may improve symptoms of toddler's diarrhea.

A healthcare provider may treat IBS with:

- changes in diet.
- medication.
- probiotics—live microorganisms, usually bacteria, that are similar to microorganisms normally found in the GI tract. Studies have found that probiotics, specifically Bifidobacteria and certain probiotic combinations, improve symptoms of IBS when taken in large enough amounts. However, researchers are still studying the use of probiotics to treat IBS.
- psychological therapy.
- Food allergies and intolerances. A healthcare provider will recommend changes in diet to manage symptoms of food allergies and intolerances. To treat food allergies, the child's parent or caretaker should remove the food that triggers the allergy from the child's diet.

For children with celiac disease, following a gluten-free diet will stop symptoms, heal existing intestinal damage, and prevent further damage.

The child's parent or caretaker can manage the symptoms of lactose intolerance with changes in the child's diet and by using products that contain the lactase enzyme. Most children with lactose intolerance can tolerate some amount of lactose in their diet. The amount of change needed in the diet depends on how much lactose a child can consume without symptoms.

For children with dietary fructose intolerance, reducing the amount of fructose in the diet can relieve symptoms.

- **Inflammatory Bowel Disease (IBD).** A healthcare provider may use medications, surgery, and changes in diet to treat IBD.

Section 23.7

Cyclic Vomiting Syndrome

This section includes text excerpted from "Cyclic Vomiting Syndrome," National Institute of Diabetes and Digestive and Kidney Diseases (NIDDK), March 2014.

What Is Cyclic Vomiting Syndrome?

Cyclic vomiting syndrome, sometimes referred to as CVS, is an increasingly recognized disorder with sudden, repeated attacks—also called episodes—of severe nausea, vomiting, and physical exhaustion that occur with no apparent cause. The episodes can last from a few hours to several days. Episodes can be so severe that a person has to stay in bed for days, unable to go to school or work. A person may need treatment at an emergency room or a hospital during episodes. After an episode, a person usually experiences symptom-free periods lasting a few weeks to several months. To people who have the disorder, as well as their family members and friends, cyclic vomiting syndrome can be disruptive and frightening.

The disorder can affect a person for months, years, or decades. Each episode of cyclic vomiting syndrome is usually similar to previous ones, meaning that episodes tend to start at the same time of day, last the same length of time, and occur with the same symptoms and level of intensity.

What Is the Gastrointestinal (GI) Tract?

The GI tract is a series of hollow organs joined in a long, twisting tube from the mouth to the anus—the opening through which stool leaves the body. The body digests food using the movement of muscles in the GI tract, along with the release of hormones and enzymes. Cyclic vomiting syndrome affects the upper GI tract, which includes the mouth, esophagus, stomach, small intestine, and duodenum, the first part of the small intestine. The esophagus is the muscular tube that carries food and liquids from the mouth to the stomach. The stomach slowly pumps the food and liquids through the duodenum and into the rest of the small intestine, which absorbs nutrients from food particles. This process is automatic and people are usually not aware of it, though people sometimes feel food in their esophagus when they swallow something too large, try to eat too quickly, or drink hot or cold liquids.

What Causes Cyclic Vomiting Syndrome?

The cause of cyclic vomiting syndrome is unknown. However, some experts believe that some possible problems with bodily functions may contribute to the cause, such as the following:

- gastrointestinal motility—the way food moves through the digestive system
- central nervous system function—includes the brain, spinal cord, and nerves that control bodily responses
- autonomic nervous system function—nerves that control internal organs such as the heart
- hormone imbalances—hormones are a chemical produced in one part of the body and released into the blood to trigger or regulate particular bodily functions
- in children, an abnormal inherited gene may also contribute to the condition

Specific conditions or events may trigger an episode of cyclic vomiting:

- emotional stress, anxiety, or panic attacks—for example, in children, common triggers of anticipatory anxiety are school exams or events, birthday parties, holidays, family conflicts, or travel
- infections, such as a sinus infection, a respiratory infection, or the flu
- eating certain foods, such as chocolate or cheese, or additives such as caffeine, nitrites—commonly found in cured meats such as hot dogs—and monosodium glutamate, also called MSG
- hot weather
- menstrual periods
- motion sickness
- overeating, fasting, or eating right before bedtime
- physical exhaustion or too much exercise

How Common Is Cyclic Vomiting Syndrome?

Cyclic vomiting syndrome is more common in children than adults, although reports of the syndrome in adults have increased in recent years. Usually, children are about 5 years old when diagnosed with cyclic vomiting syndrome, which occurs in every three out of 100,000 children.

Who Is More Likely to Develop Cyclic Vomiting Syndrome?

Children who suffer from migraines—severe, throbbing headaches with nausea, vomiting, and sensitivity to light and sound—are more likely to develop cyclic vomiting syndrome. Up to 80 percent of children and 25 percent of adults who develop cyclic vomiting syndrome also get migraine headaches. People with a family history of migraines may be more likely to develop the syndrome.

People with a history of chronic marijuana use may also be more likely to develop cyclic vomiting syndrome.

What Are the Symptoms of Cyclic Vomiting Syndrome?

The main symptoms of cyclic vomiting syndrome are severe nausea and sudden vomiting lasting hours to days. A person may also experience one or more of the following symptoms:

- retching, or making an attempt to vomit
- heaving or gagging
- lack of appetite
- abdominal pain
- diarrhea
- fever
- dizziness
- headache
- sensitivity to light

Intensity of symptoms will vary as a person cycles through four distinct phases of an episode:

- **Prodrome phase.** During the prodrome phase, the person feels that an episode of nausea and vomiting is about to start.

Often marked by intense sweating and nausea—with or without abdominal pain—this phase can last from a few minutes to several hours. The person may appear unusually pale.

- **Vomiting phase.** This phase consists of intense nausea, vomiting, and retching. Periods of vomiting and retching can last 20 to 30 minutes at a time. The person may be subdued and responsive, immobile and unresponsive, or writhing and moaning with intense abdominal pain. An episode can last from hours to days.
- **Recovery phase.** This phase begins when the vomiting and retching stop and the nausea subsides. Improvement of symptoms during the recovery phase can vary. Healthy color, appetite, and energy return gradually or right away.
- **Well phase.** This phase occurs between episodes when no symptoms are present.

How Is Cyclic Vomiting Syndrome Diagnosed?

A specific test to diagnose cyclic vomiting syndrome does not exist; instead, a healthcare provider will rule out other conditions and diagnose the syndrome based upon

- a medical and family history
- a physical exam
- a pattern or cycle of symptoms
- blood tests
- urine tests
- imaging tests
- upper GI endoscopy
- a gastric emptying test

Often, it is suspected that one of the following is causing their symptoms:

- gastroparesis—a disorder that slows or stops the movement of food from the stomach to the small intestine
- gastroenteritis—inflammation of the lining of the stomach, small intestine, and large intestine

A diagnosis of cyclic vomiting syndrome may be difficult to make until the person sees a healthcare provider. A healthcare provider will suspect cyclic vomiting syndrome if the person suffers from repeat episodes of vomiting.

How Is Cyclic Vomiting Syndrome Treated?

A healthcare provider may refer patients to a gastroenterologist for treatment.

People with cyclic vomiting syndrome should get plenty of rest and take medications to prevent a vomiting episode, stop an episode in progress, speed up recovery, or relieve associated symptoms.

The healthcare team tailors treatment to the symptoms experienced during each of the four cyclic vomiting syndrome phases:

Prodrome phase treatment. The goal during the prodrome phase is to stop an episode before it progresses. Taking medication early in the phase can help stop an episode from moving to the vomiting phase or becoming severe; however, people do not always realize an episode is coming. For example, a person may wake up in the morning and begin vomiting. A healthcare provider may recommend the following medications for both children and adults:

- ondansetron (Zofran) or lorazepam (Ativan) for nausea
- ibuprofen for abdominal pain
- ranitidine (Zantac), lansoprazole (Prevacid), or omeprazole (Prilosec, Zegerid) to control stomach acid production
- sumatriptan (Imitrex)—prescribed as a nasal spray, an injection, or a pill that dissolves under the tongue—for migraines

Vomiting phase treatment. Once vomiting begins, people should call or see a healthcare provider as soon as possible. Treatment usually requires the person to stay in bed and sleep in a dark, quiet room. A healthcare provider may recommend the following for both children and adults:

- medication for pain, nausea, and reducing stomach acid and anxiety
- anti-migraine medications such as sumatriptan to stop symptoms of a migraine or possibly stop an episode in progress
- hospitalization for severe nausea and vomiting
- IV fluids and medications to prevent dehydration and treat symptoms

- IV nutrition if an episode continues for several days

Recovery phase treatment. During the recovery phase, drinking and eating will replace lost electrolytes. A person may need IV fluids for a period of time. Some people find their appetite returns to normal right away, while others start by drinking clear liquids and then moving slowly to other liquids and solid food. A healthcare provider may prescribe medications during the recovery phase and well phase to prevent future episodes.

Well phase treatment. During the well phase, a healthcare provider may use medications to treat people whose episodes are frequent and long lasting in an effort to prevent or ease future episodes. A person may need to take a medication daily for 1 to 2 months before evaluating whether it helps prevent episodes. A healthcare provider may prescribe the following medications for both children and adults during the well phase to prevent cyclic vomiting syndrome episodes, lessen their severity, and reduce their frequency:

- amitriptyline (Elavil)
- propranolol (Inderal)
- cyproheptadine (Periactin)

How Can a Person Prevent Cyclic Vomiting Syndrome?

A person should stay away from known triggers, especially during the well phase, as well as

- get adequate sleep to prevent exhaustion
- treat sinus problems or allergies
- seek help on reducing stress and anxiety
- avoid foods that trigger episodes or foods with additives

A healthcare provider may refer people with cyclic vomiting syndrome and anxiety to a stress management specialist for relaxation therapy or other treatments.

A healthcare provider may prescribe medications to prevent migraines for people with cyclic vomiting syndrome.

Eating, Diet, And Nutrition

During the prodrome and vomiting phases of cyclic vomiting syndrome, a person will generally take in little or no nutrition by mouth. During the recovery phase, the person may be quite hungry as soon as the vomiting stops. As eating resumes, a person or his or her family should watch for the return of nausea. In some cases, a person can start with clear liquids and proceed slowly to a regular diet.

During the well phase, a balanced diet and regular meals are important. People should avoid any trigger foods and foods with additives. Eating small, carbohydrate-containing snacks between meals, before exercise, and at bedtime may help prevent future attacks. A healthcare provider will assist with planning a return to a regular diet.

Section 23.8

Dysphagia (Difficulty Swallowing)

Dysphagia, which literally means "difficulty swallowing," is a condition in which people have trouble passing foods or liquids from their mouth to their digestive system. The process of swallowing involves four stages. The brain controls this process through nerves that connect to the mouth, throat, esophagus, and stomach. Dysphagia can result from problems occurring in any of the four stages.

In the oral stage, food is placed in the mouth, where it is moistened by saliva, broken down by chewing, and pushed back toward the throat by the tongue. In the pharyngeal phase, food enters the throat (pharynx). The voice box (larynx) closes briefly to prevent food from entering the airway and lungs, and then the food passes down the throat and into the esophagus. In the esophageal stage, food is pushed downward through the esophagus by wave-like muscle contractions known as peristalsis. Finally, the food passes into the stomach through the lower esophageal sphincter, a band of muscle that relaxes to allow food to enter and tightens to prevent stomach contents from moving back upward into the esophagus.

Causes of Dysphagia

Swallowing difficulties have many possible causes, including the following:

- cleft lip, cleft palate, or other problems with craniofacial development
- dental problems
- large tongue
- large tonsils
- tumors, masses, or congenital abnormalities in the throat
- foreign objects in the esophagus
- gastrointestinal problems that irritate or damage the esophagus, such as acid reflux
- malformations of the digestive tract, such as esophageal atresia or tracheoesophageal fistula
- compression of the esophagus by enlarged thyroid gland, lymph nodes, or blood vessels
- premature birth or low birth weight
- autism or other developmental delays
- nervous system disorders, such as cerebral palsy
- diseases or injuries that affect the nerves and muscles of the face and neck, such as stroke, brain injury, or muscular dystrophy
- respiratory problems
- tracheostomy
- oral sensitivity or irritation of the airway from prolonged use of a ventilator
- vocal cord paralysis
- certain medications that decrease appetite
- dysfunctional parent-child interaction at mealtimes

Symptoms of Dysphagia

Swallowing difficulties manifest themselves in many ways, some of which may not be obvious or may mimic other medical conditions.

Some of the more common symptoms of dysphagia include the following:

- eating very slowly
- chewing with difficulty
- attempting to swallow a mouthful of food several times
- feeling as if food becomes stuck in the throat
- trouble coordinating breathing and swallowing
- frequent coughing, gagging, or choking during meals
- frequent spitting up or vomiting
- drooling
- stuffy nose at mealtime, or food or liquid coming out of the nose
- hoarse, raspy, or gurgling voice during or after meals
- chest congestion after eating, or recurring respiratory infections
- weight loss, or less than normal weight gain and growth
- aversion to certain textures of food
- arching the back or stiffening while feeding
- irritability or lack of alertness while feeding

Diagnosis of Dysphagia

The medical professional that is most often involved in diagnosing swallowing difficulties is a speech-language pathologist (SLP). The SLP may consult with a team that also includes a physician or pediatrician, a dietician or nutritionist, and a physical or occupational therapist. The team will ask about the patient's medical history, including the development of the condition, symptoms experienced, and overall health. They may also evaluate the patient's posture and behavior while eating, as well as their oral movements and the strength of muscles involved in chewing and swallowing. As needed, various tests and imaging studies may be performed to further analyze the actions of the mouth, throat, and esophagus. Some of the possible tests used to diagnose dysphagia include the following:

Modified Barium Swallow Study (MBSS)

The patient consumes a small amount of a liquid containing barium, a metallic chemical that shows up well on X-rays. A series of X-rays are taken as the barium moves through the throat and esophagus, providing the SLP with valuable information about the source of swallowing difficulties.

Fiberoptic Endoscopic Evaluation of Swallowing (FEES)

A small, flexible tube with a tiny camera on the end is inserted through the patient's nose to provide an internal view of the throat. The patient then consumes several varieties of solid and liquid foods while the SLP observes the function of the throat, vocal cords, and larynx.

Laryngoscopy

With the patient under anesthesia, the doctor uses a small tube with a light on the end to examine the patient's throat and larynx for abnormalities or narrow areas.

Gastroesophageal endoscopy

With the patient under anesthesia, the doctor inserts a small tube with a camera on the end into the patient's mouth. The tube is gently threaded through the throat and esophagus into the stomach, and the camera captures images of the internal structures. If the doctor notices any abnormalities, the endoscope can be used to take a tissue sample.

Esophageal manometry

A small tube containing a pressure gauge is inserted through the mouth into the esophagus, where it measures the pressure. This test is used to evaluate the effectiveness of the esophagus in moving food downward to the stomach.

Gastrointestinal reflux testing

Tiny probes are inserted into the patient's esophagus or stomach to measure the amount of acid present. The pH probes are used to analyze whether acid reflux may contribute to throat irritation and swallowing problems.

Treatment of Dysphagia

Based on the results of the physical examination and special tests, the medical team will recommend a course of treatment for the patient's swallowing difficulties. The treatment depends on the extent and underlying cause of the dysphagia, as well as the patient's overall health. Some of the possible forms of treatment include the following:

- nutritional changes, including different types, tastes, textures, and temperatures of foods

- thickening liquids to make them easier to swallow
- medications to treat acid reflux
- behavioral interventions
- posture or positioning changes
- exercises recommended by an SLP to improve chewing or sucking, strengthen muscles in the mouth, and increase tongue movement
- referral to a dentist or craniofacial surgeon
- surgical procedures to widen the esophagus or keep food and acid in the stomach

Prognosis

Dysphagia in children can result in dehydration, poor nutrition, and a failure to gain weight or grow properly. In addition, they may develop aversion to certain foods or liquids, embarrassment in social situations involving eating, or behavioral resistance to eating. Dysphagia can also result in aspiration of food into the windpipe (trachea) and lungs. Aspiration can create a choking hazard, and it also increases the risk of respiratory infections, pneumonia, and chronic lung disease. Medical treatment can help many children with dysphagia learn to swallow more effectively so that they can eat and drink with minimal difficulty. Some patients may not experience much improvement, however, especially those with health issues that affect the nerves and muscles.

References

1. "Difficulty Swallowing (Dysphagia)—Overview," WebMD, 2016.
2. "Dysphagia," Ann and Robert H. Lurie Children's Hospital of Chicago, 2016.
3. "Feeding and Swallowing Disorders (Dysphagia) in Children," American Speech-Language-Hearing Association, 2016.
4. "Swallowing Problems (Dysphagia)," Stanford Children's Health, 2016.

Section 23.9

Gastroenteritis

This section includes text excerpted from "Viral Gastroenteritis," National Institute of Diabetes and Digestive and Kidney Diseases (NIDDK), April 2012. Reviewed October 2016.

What Is Viral Gastroenteritis?

Viral gastroenteritis is inflammation of the lining of the stomach, small intestine, and large intestine. Several different viruses can cause viral gastroenteritis, which is highly contagious and extremely common. Viral gastroenteritis causes millions of cases of diarrhea each year.

Anyone can get viral gastroenteritis and most people recover without any complications, unless they become dehydrated.

What Are the Symptoms of Viral Gastroenteritis?

The main symptoms of viral gastroenteritis are

- watery diarrhea
- vomiting

Other symptoms include

- headache
- fever
- chills
- abdominal pain

Symptoms usually appear within 12 to 48 hours after exposure to a gastroenteritis-causing virus and last for 1 to 3 days. Some viruses cause symptoms that last longer.

What Causes Viral Gastroenteritis?

Four types of viruses cause most cases of viral gastroenteritis.

Rotavirus

Rotavirus is the leading cause of gastroenteritis among infants and young children. Rotavirus infections are most common in infants 3 to 15 months old. Symptoms usually appear 1 to 3 days after exposure. Rotavirus typically causes vomiting and watery diarrhea for 3 to 7 days, along with fever and abdominal pain. Rotavirus can also infect adults who are in close contact with infected children, but the symptoms in adults are milder.

Caliciviruses

Caliciviruses cause infection in people of all ages. Norovirus is the most common calicivirus and the most common cause of viral gastroenteritis in adults. Norovirus is usually responsible for epidemics of viral gastroenteritis. Norovirus outbreaks occur all year but are more frequent from October to April. People infected with norovirus typically experience nausea, vomiting, diarrhea, abdominal cramps, fatigue, headache, and muscle aches. The symptoms usually appear 1 to 2 days after exposure to the virus and last for 1 to 3 days.

Adenovirus

Adenovirus mainly infects children younger than 2 years old. Of the 49 types of adenoviruses, one strain affects the gastrointestinal tract, causing vomiting and diarrhea. Symptoms typically appear 8 to 10 days after exposure and last 5 to 12 days. Adenovirus infections occur year-round.

Astrovirus

Astrovirus primarily infects infants and young children, but adults may also be infected. This virus causes vomiting and watery diarrhea. Symptoms usually appear 3 to 4 days after exposure and last 2 to 7 days. The symptoms are milder than the symptoms of norovirus or rotavirus infections. Infections occur year-round, but the virus is most active during the winter months.

Viral gastroenteritis is often mistakenly called "stomach flu," but it is not caused by the influenza virus. Some forms of gastroenteritis are caused by bacteria or parasites rather than viruses.

How Is Viral Gastroenteritis Transmitted?

Viral gastroenteritis is transmitted from person to person. Viruses are present in the stool and vomit of people who are infected.

Infected people may contaminate surfaces, objects, food, and drinks with viruses, especially if they do not wash their hands thoroughly after using the bathroom. When an infected person with unwashed hands shakes hands with or touches another person, the virus can spread. When an infected person vomits, the virus can become airborne.

People may be infected with viruses by:

- touching contaminated surfaces or objects and then touching their mouths
- sharing food, drink, or eating utensils with infected people
- eating foods that are contaminated with the virus, such as oysters from contaminated waters
- swallowing airborne particles that contain viruses

How Is Viral Gastroenteritis Diagnosed?

Viral gastroenteritis is usually diagnosed based on symptoms alone. People who have symptoms that are severe or last for more than a few days may want to see a healthcare provider for additional tests. A healthcare provider may ask for a stool sample to test for rotavirus or norovirus or to rule out bacteria or parasites as the cause of the gastroenteritis.

During an epidemic of viral gastroenteritis, healthcare providers or public health officials may test stool samples to find out which virus is responsible for the outbreak.

How Is Viral Gastroenteritis Treated?

Most cases of viral gastroenteritis resolve over time without specific treatment. Antibiotics are not effective against viral infections. The primary goal of treatment is to reduce symptoms and prevent complications.

Over-the-counter medicines such as loperamide (Imodium) and bismuth subsalicylate (Pepto-Bismol) can help relieve symptoms in adults. These medicines are not recommended for children.

How Can Viral Gastroenteritis Be Prevented?

People can reduce their chances of getting or spreading viral gastroenteritis if they:

- wash their hands thoroughly with soap and warm water for 20 seconds after using the bathroom or changing diapers and before eating or handling food
- disinfect contaminated surfaces such as countertops and baby changing tables with a mixture of 2 cups of household bleach and 1 gallon of water
- avoid foods and drinks that might be contaminated

Section 23.10

Gastroesophageal Reflux

This section includes text excerpted from "Definition and Facts for GER and GERD in Children and Teens," National Institute of Diabetes and Digestive and Kidney Diseases (NIDDK), April 8, 2015.

What Is Gastroesophageal Reflux (GER)?

Gastroesophageal reflux (GER) happens when stomach contents come back up into the esophagus. Stomach acid that touches the lining of the esophagus can cause heartburn, also called acid indigestion.

Does GER Have Another Name?

Doctors also refer to GER as:

- acid indigestion
- acid reflux
- acid regurgitation
- heartburn
- reflux

How Common Is GER in Children and Teens?

Occasional GER is common in children and teens—ages 2 to 19—and doesn't always mean that they have gastroesophageal reflux disease (GERD).

What Is Gastroesophageal Reflux Disease (GERD)?

GERD is a more serious and long-lasting form of GER in which acid reflux irritates the esophagus.

How Common Is GERD in Children and Teens?

Up to 25 percent of children and teens have symptoms of GERD, although GERD is more common in adults.

What Are the Complications of GERD in Children and Teens?

Without treatment, GERD can sometimes cause serious complications over time, such as:

Esophagitis

Esophagitis may lead to ulcerations, a sore in the lining of the esophagus.

Esophageal Stricture

An esophageal stricture happens when a person's esophagus becomes too narrow. Esophageal strictures can lead to problems with swallowing.

Respiratory Problems

A child or teen with GERD might breathe stomach acid into his or her lungs. The stomach acid can then irritate his or her throat and lungs, causing respiratory problems or symptoms, such as

- asthma—a long-lasting lung disease that makes a child or teen extra sensitive to things that he or she is allergic to
- chest congestion, or extra fluid in the lungs
- a dry, long-lasting cough or a sore throat
- hoarseness—the partial loss of a child or teen's voice
- laryngitis—the swelling of a child or teen's voice box that can lead to a short-term loss of his or her voice
- pneumonia—an infection in one or both lungs—that keeps coming back

- wheezing—a high-pitched whistling sound that happens while breathing

A pediatrician should monitor children and teens with GERD to prevent or treat long-term problems.

What Is the Difference between GER and GERD?

GER that occurs more than twice a week for a few weeks could be GERD. GERD can lead to more serious health problems over time. If you think your child or teen has GERD, you should take him or her to see a doctor or a pediatrician.

What Are the Symptoms of GER and GERD in Children and Teens?

If a child or teen has gastroesophageal reflux (GER), he or she may taste food or stomach acid in the back of the mouth.

Symptoms of gastroesophageal reflux disease (GERD) in children and teens can vary depending on their age. The most common symptom of GERD in children 12 years and older is regular heartburn, a painful, burning feeling in the middle of the chest, behind the breastbone, and in the middle of the abdomen. In many cases, children with GERD who are younger than 12 don't have heartburn.

Other common GERD symptoms include

- bad breath
- nausea
- pain in the chest or the upper part of the abdomen
- problems swallowing or painful swallowing
- respiratory problems
- vomiting
- the wearing away of teeth

What Causes GER and GERD in Children and Teens?

GER and GERD happen when a child or teen's lower esophageal sphincter becomes weak or relaxes when it shouldn't, causing stomach contents to rise up into the esophagus. The lower esophageal sphincter becomes weak or relaxes due to certain things, such as

- increased pressure on the abdomen from being overweight, obese, or pregnant
- certain medicines, including
- those used to treat asthma—a long-lasting disease in the lungs that makes a child or teen extra sensitive to things that he or she is allergic to
- antihistamines—medicines that treat allergy symptoms
- painkillers
- sedatives—medicines that help put someone to sleep
- antidepressants—medicines that treat depression
- smoking, which is more likely with teens than younger children, or inhaling secondhand smoke

Other reasons a child or teen develops GERD include

- previous esophageal surgery
- having a severe developmental delay or neurological condition, such as cerebral palsy

When Should I Seek a Doctor's Help?

Call a doctor right away if your child or teen

- vomits large amounts
- has regular projectile, or forceful, vomiting
- vomits fluid that is
- green or yellow
- looks like coffee grounds
- contains blood
- has problems breathing after vomiting
- has mouth of throat pain when he or she eats
- has problems swallowing or pain when swallowing
- refuses food repeatedly, causing weight loss or poor growth
- shows signs of dehydration, such as no tears when he or she cries

How Do Doctors Diagnose GER in Children and Teens?

In most cases, a doctor diagnoses gastroesophageal reflux (GER) by reviewing a child or teen's symptoms and medical history. If symptoms of GER do not improve with lifestyle changes and anti-reflux medicines, he or she may need testing.

How Do Doctors Diagnose GERD in Children and Teens?

If a child or teen's GER symptoms do not improve, if they come back frequently, or he or she has trouble swallowing, the doctor may recommend testing for gastroesophageal reflux disease (GERD).

The doctor may refer the child or teen to a pediatric gastroenterologist to diagnose and treat GERD.

What Tests Do Doctors Use to Diagnose GERD?

Several tests can help a doctor diagnose GERD. A doctor may order more than one test to make a diagnosis.

Upper GI Series

An upper GI series looks at the shape of the child or teen's upper GI tract.

An x-ray technician performs this procedure at a hospital or an outpatient center. A radiologist reads and reports on the x-ray images. The child or teen doesn't need anesthesia. If possible, the child or teen shouldn't eat or drink before the procedure. Check with the doctor about what to do to prepare the child or teen for an upper GI series.

During the procedure, the child or teen will drink liquid contrast (barium or gastrograffin) to coat the lining of the upper GI tract. The x-ray technician takes several x-rays as the contrast moves through the GI tract. The technician or radiologist will often change the position of the child or teen to get the best view of the GI tract. They may press on the child's abdomen during the x-ray procedure.

The upper GI series can't show mild irritation in the esophagus. It can find problems related to GERD, such as esophageal strictures, or problems with the anatomy that may cause symptoms of GERD.

Children or teens may have bloating and nausea for a short time after the procedure. For several days afterward, they may have white or light-colored stools from the barium. A healthcare professional will give you specific instructions about the child or teen's eating and drinking after the procedure.

Esophageal pH and Impedance Monitoring

The most accurate procedure to detect acid reflux is esophageal pH and impedance monitoring. Esophageal pH and impedance monitoring measures the amount of acid or liquid in a child or teen's esophagus while he or she does normal things, such as eating and sleeping.

This procedure takes place at a hospital or outpatient center. A nurse or physician places a thin flexible tube through the child or teen's nose into the stomach. The tube is then pulled back into the esophagus and taped to the child or teen's cheek. The end of the tube in the esophagus measures when and how much acid comes up into the esophagus. The other end of the tube attaches to a monitor outside his or her body that records the measurements. The placement of the tube is sometimes done while a child is sedated after an upper endoscopy, but can be done while a child is fully awake.

The child or teen will wear a monitor for the next 24 hours. He or she will return to the hospital or outpatient center to have the tube removed. Children may need to stay in the hospital for the esophageal pH and impedancemonitoring.

This procedure is most useful to the doctor if you keep a diary of when, what, and how much food the child or teen eats and his or her GERD symptoms after eating. The gastroenterologist can see how the symptoms, certain foods, and certain times of day relate to one another. The procedure can also help show whether acid reflux triggers any respiratory symptoms the child or teen might have.

Upper Gastro Intestinal (GI) Endoscopy and Biopsy

In an upper GI endoscopy, a gastroenterologist, surgeon, or other trained healthcare professional uses an endoscope to see inside a child or teen's upper GI tract. This procedure takes place at a hospital or an outpatient center.

An intravenous (IV) needle will be placed in the child or teen's arm to give him or her medicines that keep him or her relaxed and comfortable during the procedure. They may be given a liquid anesthetic to gargle or spray anesthetic on the back of his or her throat. The doctor carefully feeds the endoscope down the child or teen's esophagus then into the stomach and duodenum. A small camera mounted on the endoscope sends a video image to a monitor, allowing close examination of the lining of the upper GI tract. The endoscope pumps air into the child or teen's stomach and duodenum, making them easier to see.

The doctor may perform a biopsy with the endoscope by taking small pieces of tissue from the lining of the child or teen's esophagus, stomach, or duodenum. He or she won't feel the biopsy. A pathologist examines the tissue in a lab.

In most cases, the procedure only diagnoses GERD if the child or teen has moderate to severe symptoms.

How Do Doctors Treat GER and GERD in Children and Teens?

You can help control a child or teen's gastroesophageal reflux (GER) or gastroesophageal reflux disease (GERD) by having him or her

- not eat or drink items that may cause GER, such as greasy or spicy foods
- not overeat
- avoid smoking and secondhand smoke
- lose weight if he or she is overweight or obese
- avoid eating 2 to 3 hours before bedtime
- take over-the-counter medicines, such as Alka-Seltzer, Maalox, or Rolaids

How Do Doctors Treat GERD in Children and Teens?

Depending on the severity of the child's symptoms, a doctor may recommend lifestyle changes, medicines, or surgery.

Lifestyle changes

Helping a child or teen make lifestyle changes can reduce his or her GERD symptoms.

Over-the-Counter and Prescription Medicines

If a child or teen has symptoms that won't go away, you should take him or her to see a doctor. The doctor can prescribe medicine to relieve his or her symptoms. Some medicines are available over the counter.

Antacids

Doctors often first recommend antacids to relieve GER and other mild GERD symptoms. A doctor will tell you which over-the-counter antacids to give a child or teen.

H2 blockers

H2 blockers decrease acid production. They provide short-term or on-demand relief for many people with GERD symptoms. They can also help heal the esophagus, although not as well as other medicines. If a doctor recommends an H2 blocker for the child or teen, you can buy them over the counter or a doctor can prescribe one.

Proton pump inhibitors (PPIs)

PPIs lower the amount of acid the stomach makes. PPIs are better at treating GERD symptoms than H2 blockers. They can heal the esophageal lining in most people with GERD. Doctors often prescribe PPIs for long-term GERD treatment.

Prokinetics

Prokinetics help the stomach empty faster

Antibiotics

Antibiotics, including erythromycin, can help the stomach empty faster. Erythromycin has fewer side effects than prokinetics; however, it can cause diarrhea.

Surgery

A pediatric gastroenterologist may recommend surgery if a child or teen's GERD symptoms don't improve with lifestyle changes or medicines. A child or teen is more likely to develop complications from surgery than from medicines.

How Can Diet Help Prevent or Relieve GER or GERD in Children?

You can help a child or teen prevent or relieve their symptoms from gastroesophageal reflux (GER) or gastroesophageal reflux disease (GERD) by changing their diet. He or she may need to avoid certain foods and drinks that make his or her symptoms worse. Other dietary changes that can help reduce the child or teen's symptoms include

- decreasing fatty foods
- eating small, frequent meals instead of three large meals

Section 23.11

Irritable Bowel Syndrome

This section includes text excerpted from "Irritable Bowel Syndrome (IBS) in Children," National Institute of Diabetes and Digestive and Kidney Diseases (NIDDK), June 2014.

What Is Irritable Bowel Syndrome (IBS)?

Irritable bowel syndrome is a functional gastrointestinal (GI) disorder, meaning it is a problem caused by changes in how the GI tract works. Children with a functional GI disorder have frequent symptoms, but the GI tract does not become damaged. IBS is not a disease; it is a group of symptoms that occur together. The most common symptoms of IBS are abdominal pain or discomfort, often reported as cramping, along with diarrhea, constipation, or both. In the past, IBS was called colitis, mucous colitis, spastic colon, nervous colon, and spastic bowel. The name was changed to reflect the understanding that the disorder has both physical and mental causes and is not a product of a person's imagination.

IBS is diagnosed when a child who is growing as expected has abdominal pain or discomfort once per week for at least 2 months without other disease or injury that could explain the pain. The pain or discomfort of IBS may occur with a change in stool frequency or consistency or may be relieved by a bowel movement.

How Common Is IBS in Children?

Limited information is available about the number of children with IBS. Older studies have reported prevalence rates for recurrent abdominal pain in children of 10 to 20 percent. However, these studies did not differentiate IBS from functional abdominal pain, indigestion, and abdominal migraine. One study of children in North America found that 14 percent of high school students and 6 percent of middle school students have IBS. The study also found that IBS affects boys and girls equally.

What Are the Symptoms of IBS in Children?

The symptoms of IBS include abdominal pain or discomfort and changes in bowel habits. To meet the definition of IBS, the pain or discomfort should be associated with two of the following three symptoms:

- start with bowel movements that occur more or less often than usual
- start with stool that appears looser and more watery or harder and more lumpy than usual
- improve with a bowel movement

Other symptoms of IBS may include

- diarrhea—having loose, watery stools three or more times a day and feeling urgency to have a bowel movement
- constipation—having hard, dry stools; two or fewer bowel movements in a week; or straining to have a bowel movement
- feeling that a bowel movement is incomplete
- passing mucus, a clear liquid made by the intestines that coats and protects tissues in the GI tract
- abdominal bloating

Symptoms may often occur after eating a meal. To meet the definition of IBS, symptoms must occur at least once per week for at least 2 months.

What Causes IBS in Children?

The causes of IBS are not well understood. Researchers believe a combination of physical and mental health problems can lead to IBS. The possible causes of IBS in children include the following:

- Brain-gut signal problems
- GI motor problems

- Hypersensitivity
- Mental health problems
- Bacterial gastroenteritis
- Small intestinal bacterial overgrowth (SIBO)
- Genetics

How Is IBS in Children Diagnosed?

To diagnose IBS, a healthcare provider will conduct a physical exam and take a complete medical history. The medical history will include questions about the child's symptoms, family members with GI disorders, recent infections, medications, and stressful events related to the onset of symptoms. IBS is diagnosed when the physical exam does not show any cause for the child's symptoms and the child meets all of the following criteria:

- has had symptoms at least once per week for at least 2 months
- is growing as expected
- is not showing any signs that suggest another cause for the symptoms

How Is IBS in Children Treated?

Though there is no cure for IBS, the symptoms can be treated with a combination of the following:

- changes in eating, diet, and nutrition
- medications
- probiotics
- therapies for mental health problems

Section 23.12

Lactose Intolerance

This section includes text excerpted from "Lactose Intolerance," National Institute of Diabetes and Digestive and Kidney Diseases (NIDDK), June 2014.

What Is Lactose?

Lactose is a sugar found in milk and milk products. The small intestine—the organ where most food digestion and nutrient absorption take place—produces an enzyme called lactase. Lactase breaks down lactose into two simpler forms of sugar: glucose and galactose. The body then absorbs these simpler sugars into the bloodstream.

What Is Lactose Intolerance?

Lactose intolerance is a condition in which people have digestive symptoms—such as bloating, diarrhea, and gas—after eating or drinking milk or milk products.

Lactase deficiency and lactose malabsorption may lead to lactose intolerance:

- **Lactase deficiency.** In people who have a lactase deficiency, the small intestine produces low levels of lactase and cannot digest much lactose.
- **Lactose malabsorption.** Lactase deficiency may cause lactose malabsorption. In lactose malabsorption, undigested lactose passes to the colon. The colon, part of the large intestine, absorbs water from stool and changes it from a liquid to a solid form. In the colon, bacteria break down undigested lactose and create fluid and gas. Not all people with lactase deficiency and lactose malabsorption have digestive symptoms.

People have lactose intolerance when lactase deficiency and lactose malabsorption cause digestive symptoms. Most people with lactose intolerance can eat or drink some amount of lactose without having digestive symptoms. Individuals vary in the amount of lactose they can tolerate.

People sometimes confuse lactose intolerance with a milk allergy. While lactose intolerance is a digestive system disorder, a milk allergy is a reaction by the body's immune system to one or more milk proteins. An allergic reaction to milk can be life threatening even if the person eats or drinks only a small amount of milk or milk product. A milk allergy most commonly occurs in the first year of life, while lactose intolerance occurs more often during adolescence or adulthood.

Four Types of Lactase Deficiency

Four types of lactase deficiency may lead to lactose intolerance:

- **Primary lactase deficiency**, also called lactase non persistence, is the most common type of lactase deficiency. In people with this condition, lactase production declines over time. This decline often begins at about age 2; however, the decline may begin later. Children who have lactase deficiency may not experience symptoms of lactose intolerance until late adolescence or adulthood. Researchers have discovered that some people inherit genes from their parents that may cause a primary lactase deficiency.
- **Secondary lactase deficiency** results from injury to the small intestine. Infection, diseases, or other problems may injure the small intestine. Treating the underlying cause usually improves the lactose tolerance.
- **Developmental lactase deficiency** may occur in infants born prematurely. This condition usually lasts for only a short time after they are born.
- **Congenital lactase deficiency** is an extremely rare disorder in which the small intestine produces little or no lactase enzyme from birth. Genes inherited from parents cause this disorder.

Who Is More Likely to Have Lactose Intolerance?

In the United States, some ethnic and racial populations are more likely to have lactose intolerance than others, including African Americans, Hispanics/Latinos, American Indians, and Asian Americans. The condition is least common among Americans of European descent.

What Are the Symptoms of Lactose Intolerance?

Common symptoms of lactose intolerance include

- abdominal bloating, a feeling of fullness or swelling in the abdomen
- abdominal pain
- diarrhea
- gas
- nausea

Symptoms occur 30 minutes to 2 hours after consuming milk or milk products. Symptoms range from mild to severe based on the amount of lactose the person ate or drank and the amount a person can tolerate.

How Does Lactose Intolerance Affect Health?

In addition to causing unpleasant symptoms, lactose intolerance may affect people's health if it keeps them from consuming enough essential nutrients, such as calcium and vitamin D. People with lactose intolerance may not get enough calcium if they do not eat calcium-rich foods or do not take a dietary supplement that contains calcium. Milk and milk products are major sources of calcium and other nutrients in the diet. Calcium is essential at all ages for the growth and maintenance of bones. A shortage of calcium intake in children and adults may lead to bones that are less dense and can easily fracture later in life, a condition called osteoporosis.

How Is Lactose Intolerance Diagnosed?

A healthcare provider makes a diagnosis of lactose intolerance based on:

- medical, family, and diet history, including a review of symptoms
- a physical exam
- medical tests

How Much Lactose Can a Person with Lactose Intolerance Have?

Most people with lactose intolerance can tolerate some amount of lactose in their diet and do not need to avoid milk or milk products completely. Avoiding milk and milk products altogether may cause people to take in less calcium and vitamin D than they need. See the "Calcium and Vitamin D" section.

Individuals vary in the amount of lactose they can tolerate. A variety of factors—including how much lactase the small intestine produces—can affect how much lactose an individual can tolerate. For example, one person may have severe symptoms after drinking a small amount of milk, while another person can drink a large amount without having symptoms. Other people can easily eat yogurt and hard cheeses such as cheddar and Swiss, while they are not able to eat or drink other milk products without having digestive symptoms.

Research suggests that adults and adolescents with lactose malabsorption could eat or drink at least 12 grams of lactose in one sitting without symptoms or with only minor symptoms. This amount is the amount of lactose in 1 cup of milk. People with lactose malabsorption may be able to eat or drink more lactose if they eat it or drink it with meals or in small amounts throughout the day.

How Is Lactose Intolerance Managed?

Many people can manage the symptoms of lactose intolerance by changing their diet. Some people may only need to limit the amount of lactose they eat or drink. Others may need to avoid lactose altogether. Using lactase products can help some people manage their symptoms.

For people with secondary lactase deficiency, treating the underlying cause improves lactose tolerance. In infants with developmental lactase deficiency, the ability to digest lactose improves as the infants mature. People with primary and congenital lactase deficiency cannot change their body's ability to produce lactase.

Calcium and Vitamin D

Ensuring that children and adults with lactose intolerance get enough calcium is important, especially if their intake of milk and milk products is limited. The amount of calcium a person needs to maintain good health varies by age. Table 1 illustrates recommendations for calcium intake.

Table 23.2. Recommended Dietary Allowance of Calcium by Age Group

Age Group	Recommended Dietary Allowance (mg/day)
1–3 years	700 mg
4–8 years	1,000 mg
9–18 years	1,300 mg
19–50 years	1,000 mg
51–70 years, males	1,000 mg
51–70 years, females	1,200 mg
70+ years	1,200 mg
14–18 years, pregnant/breastfeeding	1,300 mg
19–50 years, pregnant/breastfeeding	1,000 mg

A U.S. Recommended Dietary Allowance for calcium has not been determined for infants. However, researchers suggest 200 mg of calcium per day for infants age 0 to 6 months and 260 mg for infants age 6 to 12 months.

Many foods can provide calcium and other nutrients the body needs. Non-milk products high in calcium include fish with soft bones, such as canned salmon and sardines, and dark green vegetables, such as spinach. Manufacturers may also add calcium to fortified breakfast cereals, fruit juices, and soy beverage—also called soy milk. Many fortified foods are also excellent sources of vitamin D and other essential nutrients, in addition to calcium.

Table 23.3. Calcium Content in Common Foods

Nonmilk Products	Calcium Content
sardines, with bone, 3.75 oz.	351 mg
rhubarb, frozen, cooked, 1 cup	348 mg
soy milk, original and vanilla, with added calcium and vitamins A and D	299 mg
spinach, frozen, cooked, 1 cup	291 mg
salmon, canned, with bone, 3 oz.	181 mg
pinto beans, cooked, 1 cup	79 mg
broccoli, cooked, 1 cup	62 mg
soy milk, original and vanilla, unfortified, 1 cup	61 mg

Table 23.3. Continued

Nonmilk Products	Calcium Content
orange, 1 medium	52 mg
lettuce, green leaf, 1 cup	13 mg
tuna, white, canned, 3 oz.	12 mg
Milk and Milk Products	
yogurt, plain, skim milk, 8 oz.	452 mg
milk, reduced fat, with added vitamins A and D, 1 cup	293 mg
Swiss cheese, 1 oz.	224 mg
cottage cheese, low fat, 1 cup	206 mg
ice cream, vanilla, 1/2 cup	84 mg

Vitamin D helps the body absorb and use calcium. Some people with lactose intolerance may not get enough vitamin D. Foods such as salmon, tuna, eggs, and liver naturally contain vitamin D. Most milk sold in the United States is fortified with vitamin D, and vitamin D is added to some non milk beverages, yogurts, and breakfast cereals. People's bodies also make vitamin D when the skin is exposed to sunlight.

People may find it helpful to talk with a healthcare provider or a registered dietitian to determine if their diet provides adequate nutrients—including calcium and vitamin D. To help ensure coordinated and safe care, people should discuss their use of complementary and alternative medical practices, including their use of dietary supplements, with their healthcare provider.

What Products Contain Lactose?

Lactose is present in many food products and in some medications.

Food Products

Lactose is in all milk and milk products. Manufacturers also often add milk and milk products to boxed, canned, frozen, packaged, and prepared foods. People who have digestive symptoms after consuming a small quantity of lactose should be aware of the many food products that may contain even small amounts of lactose, such as

- bread and other baked goods
- waffles, pancakes, biscuits, cookies, and the mixes to make them

- processed breakfast foods such as doughnuts, frozen waffles and pancakes, toaster pastries, and sweet rolls
- processed breakfast cereals
- instant potatoes, soups, and breakfast drinks
- potato chips, corn chips, and other processed snacks
- processed meats such as bacon, sausage, hot dogs, and lunch meats
- margarine
- salad dressings
- liquid and powdered milk-based meal replacements
- protein powders and bars
- candies
- nondairy liquid and powdered coffee creamers
- nondairy whipped toppings

People can check the ingredients on food labels to find possible sources of lactose in food products. If a food label includes any of the following words, the product contains lactose:

- milk
- lactose
- whey
- curds
- milk by-products
- dry milk solids
- nonfat dry milk powder

Medications

Some medications also contain lactose, including prescription medications such as birth control pills and over-the-counter medications such as products to treat stomach acid and gas. These medications most often cause symptoms in people with severe lactose intolerance. People with lactose intolerance who take medications that contain lactose should speak with their healthcare provider about other options.

Section 23.13

Motion Sickness

This section includes text excerpted from "Motion Sickness," Centers for Disease Control and Prevention (CDC), July 10, 2015.

Risk for Travelers

Motion sickness is the term attributed to physiologic responses of the body to motion by sea, car, train or air. Given sufficient stimulus all people with functional vestibular systems can develop motion sickness. However, people vary in their susceptibility. Risk factors include the following:

- Age—children aged 2–12 years are especially susceptible, but infants and toddlers are generally immune.
- Migraines—people who get migraine headaches are more prone to motion sickness, especially during a migraine.
- Medication—some prescriptions can worsen the nausea of motion sickness

Table 23.4. Medications That May Increase Nausea

Medication Class	Examples
Antibiotics	Azithromycin, metronidazole, erythromycin, trimethoprim-sulfamethoxazole
Antiparasitics	Albendazole, thiabendazole, iodoquinol, chloroquine, mefloquine
Estrogens	Oral contraceptives, estradiol
Cardiovascular	Digoxin, levodopa
Narcotic analgesics	Codeine, morphine, meperidine
Nonsteroidal analgesics	Ibuprophen, naproxen, indomethacin
Antidepressants	Fluoxetine, paroxitene, sertraline
Asthma medication	Aminophylline
Bisphosphonates	Alendronate sodium, ibandronate sodium, risedronate sodium

Treatment

Nonpharmacologic treatments for preventing and treating motion sickness can be effective with few adverse side effects (see Prevention below). However, these measures can be time-consuming and unpleasant for travelers. Many patients will prefer medication. A primary side effect of most efficacious medications used for motion sickness is drowsiness, along with other drug-specific side effects. Some medications may interfere with or delay acclimation to the offending movement. Because gastric stasis can occur with motion sickness, parenteral delivery may be advantageous.

Antihistamines are the most frequently used and widely available medications for motion sickness; non-sedating ones appear to be less effective. Antihistamines commonly used for motion sickness include cinnarizine (not currently available in the United States), cyclizine, dimenhydrinate, meclizine, and promethazine (oral and suppository). Other common medications used to treat motion sickness are scopolamine (hyoscine, oral and transdermal), antidopaminergic drugs (such as prochlorperazine), metoclopramide, sympathomimetics, and benzodiazepines. Clinical trials have not shown that ondansetron, a drug commonly used as an antiemetic in cancer patients, is effective in the prevention of nausea associated with motion sickness.

When recommending any of these medications to travelers, providers should make sure that patients understand the risks and benefits, possible undesirable side effects, and potential drug interactions. Travelers may consider trying the medication before travel to see what effect it has on them.

Medications in Children

For children aged 2–12 years, dimenhydrinate (Dramamine), 1–1.5 mg/kg per dose, or diphenhydramine (Benadryl), 0.5–1 mg/kg per dose up to 25 mg, can be given 1 hour before travel and every 6 hours during the trip. Because some children have paradoxical agitation with these medicines, a test dose should be given at home before departure.

Antihistamines are not approved by the Food and Drug Administration to treat motion sickness in children. Caregivers should be reminded to always ask a physician, pharmacist, or other clinician if they have any questions about how to use or dose antihistamines in children before they administer the medication. Oversedation of young children with antihistamines can be life-threatening.

Scopolamine can cause dangerous adverse effects in children and should not be used; prochlorperazine and metoclopramide should be used with caution in children.

Prevention

Nonpharmacologic interventions to prevent or treat motion sickness include the following:

- Being aware of and avoiding situations that tend to trigger symptoms.
- Optimizing position to reduce motion or motion perception—for example, driving a vehicle instead of riding in it, sitting in the front seat of a car or bus, or sitting over the wing of an aircraft.
- Reducing sensory input—lying prone, shutting eyes, or looking at the horizon.
- Maintaining hydration by drinking water, eating small meals frequently, and limiting alcoholic and caffeinated beverages.
- Adding distractions—listening to music or using aromatherapy scents such as mint or lavender. Flavored lozenges may also help, in particular ginger-flavored. Lozenges may also function as distractions or, in the case of ginger, may hasten gastric emptying.
- Using acupressure or magnets is advocated by some to prevent or treat nausea, although scientific data on efficacy of these interventions for preventing motion sickness are equivocal.

Chapter 24

Kidney and Urologic Disorders in Children

Chapter Contents

Section 24.1

Bedwetting and Urinary Incontinence

This section includes text excerpted from "Urinary Incontinence in Children," National Institute of Diabetes and Digestive and Kidney Diseases (NIDDK), June 2012. Reviewed October 2016.

What Is Urinary Incontinence (UI) In Children?

Urinary incontinence is the loss of bladder control, which results in the accidental loss of urine. A child with UI may not stay dry during the day or night. Some UI is caused by a health problem such as

- a urinary tract infection (UTI)
- diabetes, a condition where blood glucose, also called blood sugar, is too high
- kidney problems
- nerve problems
- constipation, a condition in which a child has fewer than two bowel movements a week and stools can be hard, dry, small, and difficult to pass
- obstructive sleep apnea (OSA), a condition in which breathing is interrupted during sleep, often because of inflamed or enlarged tonsils
- a structural problem in the urinary tract

How Common Is UI in Children?

By 5 years of age, more than 90 percent of children can control urination during the day. Nighttime wetting is more common than daytime wetting in children, affecting 30 percent of 4-year-olds. The condition resolves itself in about 15 percent of children each year; about 10 percent of 7-year-olds, 3 percent of 12-year-olds, and 1 percent of 18-year-olds continue to experience nighttime wetting.

What Causes Nighttime UI?

The exact cause of most cases of nighttime UI is not known. Though a few cases are caused by structural problems in the urinary tract, most cases probably result from a mix of factors including slower physical development, an overproduction of urine at night, and the inability to recognize bladder filling when asleep. Nighttime UI has also been associated with attention deficit hyperactivity disorder (ADHD), OSA, and anxiety. Children also may inherit genes from one or both parents that make them more likely to have nighttime UI.

Slower Physical Development

Between the ages of 5 and 10, bedwetting may be the result of a small bladder capacity, long sleeping periods, and underdevelopment of the body's alarms that signal a full or emptying bladder. This form of UI fades away as the bladder grows and the natural alarms become operational.

Overproduction of Urine at Night

The body produces antidiuretic hormone (ADH), a natural chemical that slows down the production of urine. More ADH is produced at night so the need to urinate lessens. If the body does not produce enough ADH at night, the production of urine may not slow down, leading to bladder overfilling. If a child does not sense the bladder filling and awaken to urinate, wetting will occur.

Structural Problems

A small number of UI cases are caused by physical problems in the urinary tract. Rarely, a blocked bladder or urethra may cause the bladder to overfill and leak. Nerve damage associated with the birth defect spina bifida can cause UI. In these cases, UI can appear as a constant dribbling of urine.

Attention Deficit Hyperactivity Disorder (ADHD)

Children with ADHD are three times more likely to have nighttime UI than children without ADHD. The connection between ADHD and bedwetting has not been explained, but some experts theorize that both conditions are related to delays in central nervous system development.

Obstructive Sleep Apnea (OSA)

Nighttime UI may be one sign of OSA. Other symptoms of OSA include snoring, mouth breathing, frequent ear and sinus infections, sore throat, choking, and daytime drowsiness. Experts believe that when the airway in people with OSA closes, a chemical may be released in the body that increases water production and inhibits the systems that regulate fluid volume. Successful treatment of OSA often resolves the associated nighttime UI.

Anxiety

Anxiety-causing events that occur between 2 and 4 years of age—before total bladder control is achieved—might lead to primary enuresis. Anxiety experienced after age 4 might lead to secondary enuresis in children who have been dry for at least 6 months. Events that cause anxiety in children include physical or sexual abuse; unfamiliar social situations, such as moving or starting at a new school; and major family events such as the birth of a sibling, a death, or divorce.

UI itself is an anxiety-causing event. Strong bladder contractions resulting in daytime leakage can cause embarrassment and anxiety that lead to nighttime wetting.

Genetics

Certain genes have been found to contribute to UI. Children have a 30 percent chance of having nighttime UI if one parent was affected as a child. If both parents were affected, there is a 70 percent chance of bedwetting.

What Causes Daytime UI?

Daytime UI can be caused by a UTI or structural problems in the urinary tract. Daytime UI that is not associated with UTI or structural problems is less common and tends to disappear much earlier than nighttime UI. Overactive bladder and infrequent or incomplete voiding, or urination, are common causes of daytime UI.

Overactive Bladder

Overactive bladder is a condition in which a child experiences at least two of the following conditions:

- urinary urgency—inability to delay urination

- urge urinary incontinence—urinary leakage when the bladder contracts unexpectedly
- urinary frequency—urination eight or more times a day or more than twice at night

Infrequent or Incomplete Voiding

Infrequent voiding is when children voluntarily hold urine for prolonged periods of time. For example, children may not want to use the toilets at school or may not want to interrupt enjoyable activities, so they ignore the body's signal of a full bladder. In these cases, the bladder can overfill and leak urine. In addition, these children often develop UTIs, leading to an irritated or overactive bladder.

Factors that may combine with infrequent voiding to produce daytime UI include

- small bladder capacity
- structural problems
- anxiety-causing events
- pressure from constipation
- drinks or foods that contain caffeine

Sometimes, overly demanding toilet training may make children unable to relax the sphincters enough to completely empty the bladder. Incomplete voiding may also lead to UTIs.

How Is UI in Children Treated?

Most UI fades away naturally as a child grows and develops and does not require treatment. When treatment is needed, options include bladder training and related strategies, moisture alarms, and medications.

Growth and Development

As children mature

- bladder capacity increases
- natural body alarms become activated
- an overactive bladder settles down

- production of ADH becomes normal
- response to the body's signal that it is time to void improves

Bladder Training and Related Strategies

Bladder training consists of exercises to strengthen the bladder muscles to better control urination. Gradually lengthening the time between trips to the bathroom can also help by stretching the bladder so it can hold more urine. Additional techniques that may help control daytime UI include

- urinating on a schedule—timed voiding—such as every 2 hours
- avoiding food or drinks with caffeine
- following suggestions for healthy urination, such as relaxing muscles and taking enough time to allow the bladder to empty completely

Waking children up to urinate can help decrease nighttime UI. Ensuring children drink enough fluids throughout the day so they do not drink a lot of fluids close to bedtime may also help. A healthcare provider can give guidance about how much a child needs to drink each day, as the amount depends on a child's age, physical activity, and other factors.

Moisture Alarms

At night, moisture alarms can wake children when they begin to urinate. These devices use a water-sensitive pad connected to an alarm that sounds when moisture is first detected. A small pad can clip to the pajamas, or a larger pad can be placed on the bed. For the alarm to be effective, children must awaken as soon as the alarm goes off, stop the urine stream, and go to the bathroom. Children using moisture alarms may need to have someone sleep in the same room to help wake them up.

Medications

Nighttime UI may be treated by increasing ADH levels. The hormone can be boosted by a synthetic version known as desmopressin (DDAVP), which is available in pill form, nasal spray, and nose drops. DDAVP is approved for use in children. Another medication, called imipramine (Tofranil), is also used to treat nighttime UI, though the way this medication prevents bedwetting is not known. Although both of these medications may help children achieve short-term success, relapse is common once the medication is withdrawn.

UI resulting from an overactive bladder may be treated with oxybutynin (Ditropan), a medication that helps calm the bladder muscle and control muscle spasms.

Section 24.2

Childhood Nephrotic Syndrome

This section includes text excerpted from "Childhood Nephrotic Syndrome," National Institute of Diabetes and Digestive and Kidney Diseases (NIDDK), September 2014.

What Is Childhood Nephrotic Syndrome?

Childhood nephrotic syndrome is not a disease in itself; rather, it is a group of symptoms that

- indicate kidney damage—particularly damage to the glomeruli, the tiny units within the kidney where blood is filtered
- result in the release of too much protein from the body into the urine

When the kidneys are damaged, the protein albumin, normally found in the blood, will leak into the urine. Proteins are large, complex molecules that perform a number of important functions in the body.

The two types of childhood nephrotic syndrome are

- primary—the most common type of childhood nephrotic syndrome, which begins in the kidneys and affects only the kidneys
- secondary—the syndrome is caused by other diseases

A healthcare provider may refer a child with nephrotic syndrome to a nephrologist—a doctor who specializes in treating kidney disease. A child should see a pediatric nephrologist, who has special training to take care of kidney problems in children, if possible. However, in many parts of the country, pediatric nephrologists are in short supply, so the child may need to travel. If traveling is not possible, some nephrologists who treat adults can also treat children.

What Causes Childhood Nephrotic Syndrome?

While idiopathic, or unknown, diseases are the most common cause of primary childhood nephrotic syndrome, researchers have linked certain diseases and some specific genetic changes that damage the kidneys with primary childhood nephrotic syndrome.

The cause of secondary childhood nephrotic syndrome is an underlying disease or infection. Called a primary illness, it's this underlying disease or infection that causes changes in the kidney function that can result in secondary childhood nephrotic syndrome.

Congenital diseases—diseases that are present at birth—can also cause childhood nephrotic syndrome.

Which Children Are More Likely to Develop Childhood Nephrotic Syndrome?

In cases of primary childhood nephrotic syndrome for which the cause is idiopathic, researchers are unable to pinpoint which children are more likely to develop the syndrome. However, as researchers continue to study the link between genetics and childhood nephrotic syndrome, it may be possible to predict the syndrome for some children.

Children are more likely to develop secondary childhood nephrotic syndrome if they

- have diseases that can damage their kidneys
- take certain medications
- develop certain types of infections

What Are the Signs and Symptoms of Childhood Nephrotic Syndrome?

The signs and symptoms of childhood nephrotic syndrome may include

- edema—swelling, most often in the legs, feet, or ankles and less often in the hands or face
- albuminuria—when a child's urine has high levels of albumin

- hypoalbuminemia—when a child's blood has low levels of albumin
- hyperlipidemia—when a child's blood cholesterol and fat levels are higher than normal

In addition, some children with nephrotic syndrome may have

- blood in their urine
- symptoms of infection, such as fever, lethargy, irritability, or abdominal pain
- loss of appetite
- diarrhea
- high blood pressure

What Are the Complications of Childhood Nephrotic Syndrome?

The complications of childhood nephrotic syndrome may include

- **Infection.** When the kidneys are damaged, a child is more likely to develop infections because the body loses proteins that normally protect against infection. Healthcare providers will prescribe medications to treat infections. Children with childhood nephrotic syndrome should receive the pneumococcal vaccine and yearly flu shots to prevent those infections. Children should also receive age-appropriate vaccinations, although a healthcare provider may delay certain live vaccines while a child is taking certain medications.
- **Blood clots.** Blood clots can block the flow of blood and oxygen through a blood vessel anywhere in the body. A child is more likely to develop clots when he or she loses proteins through the urine. The healthcare provider will treat blood clots with blood-thinning medications.
- **High blood cholesterol.** When albumin leaks into the urine, the albumin levels in the blood drop. The liver makes more albumin to make up for the low levels in the blood. At the same time, the liver makes more cholesterol. Sometimes children may need treatment with medications to lower blood cholesterol levels.

How Is Childhood Nephrotic Syndrome Diagnosed?

A healthcare provider diagnoses childhood nephrotic syndrome with

- a medical and family history
- a physical exam
- urine tests
- a blood test
- ultrasound of the kidney
- kidney biopsy

How Is Childhood Nephrotic Syndrome Treated?

Healthcare providers will decide how to treat childhood nephrotic syndrome based on the type:

- primary childhood nephrotic syndrome: medications
- secondary childhood nephrotic syndrome: treat the underlying illness or disease
- congenital nephrotic syndrome: medications, surgery to remove one or both kidneys, and transplantation

How Can Childhood Nephrotic Syndrome Be Prevented?

Researchers have not found a way to prevent childhood nephrotic syndrome when the cause is idiopathic or congenital.

Section 24.3

Hemolytic Uremic Syndrome

This section includes text excerpted from "Hemolytic Uremic Syndrome in Children (HUS)," National Institute of Diabetes and Digestive and Kidney Diseases (NIDDK), June 2015.

What Is Hemolytic Uremic Syndrome?

Hemolytic uremic syndrome, or HUS, is a kidney condition that happens when red blood cells are destroyed and block the kidneys' filtering system. Red blood cells contain hemoglobin—an iron-rich protein that gives blood its red color and carries oxygen from the lungs to all parts of the body.

When the kidneys and glomeruli—the tiny units within the kidneys where blood is filtered—become clogged with the damaged red blood cells, they are unable to do their jobs. If the kidneys stop functioning, a child can develop acute kidney injury—the sudden and temporary loss of kidney function. Hemolytic uremic syndrome is the most common cause of acute kidney injury in children.

What Causes Hemolytic Uremic Syndrome in Children?

The most common cause of hemolytic uremic syndrome in children is an *Escherichia coli (E. coli)* infection of the digestive system. The digestive system is made up of the gastrointestinal (GI), tract—a series of hollow organs joined in a long, twisting tube from the mouth to the anus—and other organs that help the body break down and absorb food.

Normally, harmless strains, or types, of *E. coli* are found in the intestines and are an important part of digestion. However, if a child becomes infected with the *O157:H7* strain of *E. coli*, the bacteria will lodge in the digestive tract and produce toxins that can enter the bloodstream. The toxins travel through the bloodstream and can destroy the red blood cells. *E.coli O157:H7* can be found in

- undercooked meat, most often ground beef
- unpasteurized, or raw, milk

- unwashed, contaminated raw fruits and vegetables
- contaminated juice
- contaminated swimming pools or lakes

Which Children Are More Likely to Develop Hemolytic Uremic Syndrome?

Children who are more likely to develop hemolytic uremic syndrome include those who

- are younger than age 5 and have been diagnosed with an *E. coli O157:H7* infection
- have a weakened immune system
- have a family history of inherited hemolytic uremic syndrome

Hemolytic uremic syndrome occurs in about two out of every 100,000 children.

What Are the Signs and Symptoms of Hemolytic Uremic Syndrome in Children?

A child with hemolytic uremic syndrome may develop signs and symptoms similar to those seen with gastroenteritis—an inflammation of the lining of the stomach, small intestine, and large intestine— such as

- vomiting
- bloody diarrhea
- abdominal pain
- fever and chills
- headache

Seek Immediate Care

Parents or caretakers should seek immediate care for a child experiencing any urgent symptoms, such as

- unusual bleeding
- swelling
- extreme fatigue

- decreased urine output
- unexplained bruises

How Is Hemolytic Uremic Syndrome in Children Diagnosed

A healthcare provider diagnoses hemolytic uremic syndrome with

- a medical and family history
- a physical exam
- urine tests
- a blood test
- a stool test
- kidney biopsy

How Is Hemolytic Uremic Syndrome in Children Treated?

A healthcare provider will treat a child with hemolytic uremic syndrome by addressing

- urgent symptoms and preventing complications
- acute kidney injury
- chronic kidney disease (CKD)

How Can Hemolytic Uremic Syndrome in Children Be Prevented?

Parents and caregivers can help prevent childhood hemolytic uremic syndrome due to *E. coli O157:H7* by

- avoiding unclean swimming areas
- avoiding unpasteurized milk, juice, and cider
- cleaning utensils and food surfaces often
- cooking meat to an internal temperature of at least 160° F
- defrosting meat in the microwave or refrigerator
- keeping children out of pools if they have had diarrhea

- keeping raw foods separate
- washing hands before eating
- washing hands well after using the restroom and after changing diapers

When a child is taking medications that may cause hemolytic uremic syndrome, it is important that the parent or caretaker watch for symptoms and report any changes in the child's condition to the healthcare provider as soon as possible.

Section 24.4

Urinary Tract Infections

This section includes text excerpted from "What I Need to Know about My Child's Urinary Tract Infection," National Institute of Diabetes and Digestive and Kidney Diseases (NIDDK), June 2012. Reviewed October 2016.

What Is a Urinary Tract Infection (UTI)?

A UTI is an infection in the urinary tract. Infections are caused by microbes—organisms too small to be seen without a microscope. Bacteria are the most common cause of UTIs. Normally, bacteria that enter the urinary tract are quickly removed by the body before they cause symptoms. But sometimes bacteria overcome the body's natural defenses and cause infection.

What Is the Urinary Tract?

The urinary tract is the body's drainage system for removing wastes and extra water. The urinary tract includes two kidneys, two ureters, bladder, and a urethra. The kidneys are a pair of bean-shaped organs, each about the size of a fist. They are located below the ribs, one on each side of the spine, toward the middle of the back. Every minute, the two kidneys process about 3 ounces of blood, removing wastes and extra water. The wastes and extra water make up the 1 to 2 quarts of urine produced each day. Children produce less urine each day; the amount produced depends on their age. The urine travels from the kidneys down two narrow tubes called the ureters. The urine is then stored in a balloon like organ called the bladder and emptied through the urethra, a tube at the bottom of the bladder. The opening of the urethra is at the end of the penis in boys and in front of the vagina in girls.

What Causes UTIs?

Most UTIs are caused by bacteria that live in the bowel, the part of the digestive tract where stool is changed from liquid to solid. The bacterium Escherichia coli (E. coli) causes most UTIs. The urinary tract has several systems to prevent infection. The points where the ureters attach to the bladder act like one-way valves to prevent urine from backing up, or refluxing, toward the kidneys, and urination washes microbes out of the body. The body's natural defenses also prevent infection. But despite these safeguards, infections still occur.

Who Gets UTIs?

Any child can get a UTI, though girls get UTIs more often than boys.

Children with a condition called vesicoureteral reflux (VUR) are at higher risk for UTIs. VUR causes urine to reflux at the point where one or both ureters attach to the bladder. When urine stays in the urinary tract, bacteria have a chance to grow and spread. Infants and young children who get a UTI often have VUR.

Boys younger than 6 months who are not circumcised are at greater risk for a UTI than circumcised boys the same age. Boys who are circumcised have had the foreskin, which is the skin that covers the tip of the penis, removed.

Are UTIs Serious?

Most UTIs are not serious, but some infections can lead to serious problems. Chronic kidney infections—infections that recur or last a long time—can cause permanent damage. This damage can include kidney scars, poor kidney function, high blood pressure, and other problems. Some acute kidney infections—infections that develop suddenly—can be life threatening, especially if the bacteria enter the bloodstream.

What Are the Symptoms of A UTI?

A child with a UTI may not have any symptoms. When symptoms are present, they can range from mild to severe. UTI symptoms can include

- fever
- pain or burning during urination with only a few drops of urine at a time
- irritability
- not eating
- nausea
- diarrhea
- vomiting
- cloudy, dark, bloody, or foul-smelling urine
- urinating often
- pain in the back or side below the ribs
- leaking urine into clothes or bedding in older children

When Should I Call a Healthcare Provider?

Call a healthcare provider right away if your child has any of these symptoms:

- a fever of 100.4 degrees or higher in an infant or 101 degrees or higher in an older child
- a burning feeling during urination
- frequent or intense urges to urinate, even when there is little urine to pass
- pain in the back or side below the ribs
- cloudy, dark, bloody, or foul-smelling urine

How Are UTIs Diagnosed?

A UTI is diagnosed by testing a sample of your child's urine. The way the urine is collected depends on your child's age:

- If your child is still in diapers, the healthcare provider may place a plastic collection bag over your child's genital area after the area around the urethra has been washed with soap and warm water or a sterile wipe. The bag will be sealed to your child's skin with an adhesive strip. The bag should be removed as soon as your child urinates into it, and the urine sample should be processed right away.

For infants, urine may need to be collected using a thin tube called a catheter. When using a catheter, the healthcare provider first cleans the area around the opening of the urethra with a germ-killing solution. The catheter is inserted gently into the urethra until it reaches the bladder. The bladder is then drained into a clean container. Using a catheter prevents bacteria on the skin from getting into the urine sample.

- Another method for collecting a urine sample from infants is to insert a needle directly into the bladder through the skin of the lower stomach. Using a needle also prevents bacteria on the skin from getting into the urine sample.
- Older children are given a cup to urinate into.

How Are UTIs Treated?

Bacteria-fighting medicines called antibiotics are used to treat a UTI. While the lab is doing the urine culture, the healthcare provider may begin treatment with an antibiotic that treats the bacteria most likely to be causing the infection. Once culture results are known, the healthcare provider may switch your child to a different antibiotic that targets the specific type of bacteria.

Your child will need to take antibiotics for at least 3 to 5 days and maybe as long as several weeks. Be sure your child takes every pill or every dose of liquid. Your child should feel better after a couple of days, but the infection might come back if your child stops taking the antibiotic too early.

You should let your child drink as much as your child wants. But don't force your child to drink large amounts of fluid. Call your child's healthcare provider if your child doesn't want to or isn't able to drink. Also, talk with your child's healthcare provider if your child needs medicine for the pain of a UTI. The healthcare provider can recommend an over-the-counter pain medicine. A heating pad on the back or abdomen may also help.

Will My Child Need More Tests After The UTI Is Gone?

Talk with your child's healthcare provider after your child's UTI is gone. The healthcare provider may want to do more tests to check for VUR or a blockage in the urinary tract. Repeated infections in an abnormal urinary tract may cause kidney damage. The kinds of tests ordered will depend on the child and the type of infection. VUR and blockages in the urinary tract often go away as a child grows. In some cases, surgery may be needed to correct any defects in the urinary tract.

How Can UTIs Be Prevented?

You can take the following steps to help prevent your child from getting a UTI:

- Teach your child not to hold in urine and to go to the bathroom whenever your child feels the urge.
- Teach your child how to properly clean himself or herself after using the bathroom to keep bacteria from entering the urinary tract.
- Have your child wear loose-fitting clothes. Tight clothes can trap moisture, which allows bacteria to grow.
- Buy your child cotton underwear. Cotton lets in air to dry the area.
- If your child has constipation, talk with a healthcare provider about the best treatment options.

Chapter 25

Liver Disorders in Children

Chapter Contents

Section 25.1

Alpha-1 Antitrypsin Deficiency

This section includes text excerpted from "Alpha-1 Antitrypsin Deficiency," National Heart, Lung, and Blood Institute (NHLBI), October 11, 2011. Reviewed October 2016.

What Is Alpha-1 Antitrypsin Deficiency (AAT)?

Alpha-1 antitrypsin deficiency, or AAT deficiency, is a condition that raises your risk for lung disease (especially if you smoke) and other diseases.

Some people who have severe AAT deficiency develop emphysema—often when they're only in their forties or fifties. Emphysema is a serious lung disease in which damage to the airways makes it hard to breathe.

A small number of people who have AAT deficiency develop cirrhosis and other serious liver diseases.

Cirrhosis is a disease in which the liver becomes scarred. The scarring prevents the organ from working well. In people who have AAT deficiency, cirrhosis and other liver diseases usually occur in infancy and early childhood.

A very small number of people who have AAT deficiency have a rare skin disease called necrotizing panniculitis. This disease can cause painful lumps under or on the surface of the skin.

What Causes Alpha-1 Antitrypsin Deficiency?

Alpha-1 antitrypsin (AAT) deficiency is an inherited disease. "Inherited" means it's passed from parents to children through genes.

Children who have AAT deficiency inherit two faulty AAT genes, one from each parent. These genes tell cells in the body how to make AAT proteins.

In AAT deficiency, the AAT proteins made in the liver aren't the right shape. Thus, they get stuck in the liver cells. The proteins can't get to the organs in the body that they protect, such as the lungs. Without the AAT proteins protecting the organs, diseases can develop.

The most common faulty gene that can cause AAT deficiency is called PiZ. If you inherit two PiZ genes (one from each parent), you'll have AAT deficiency.

If you inherit a PiZ gene from one parent and a normal AAT gene from the other parent, you won't have AAT deficiency. However, you might pass the PiZ gene to your children.

Even if you inherit two faulty AAT genes, you may not have any related complications. You may never even realize that you have AAT deficiency.

Who Is at Risk for Alpha-1 Antitrypsin Deficiency?

Alpha-1 antitrypsin (AAT) deficiency occurs in all ethnic groups. However, the condition occurs most often in White people of European descent.

AAT deficiency is an inherited condition. "Inherited" means the condition is passed from parents to children through genes.

If you have bloodline relatives with known AAT deficiency, you're at increased risk for the condition. Even so, it doesn't mean that you'll develop one of the diseases related to the condition.

Some risk factors make it more likely that you'll develop lung disease if you have AAT deficiency. Smoking is the leading risk factor for serious lung disease if you have AAT deficiency. Your risk for lung disease also may go up if you're exposed to dust, fumes, or other toxic substances.

What Are the Signs and Symptoms of Alpha-1 Antitrypsin Deficiency?

The first lung-related symptoms of alpha-1 antitrypsin (AAT) deficiency may include shortness of breath, less ability to be physically active, and wheezing. These signs and symptoms most often begin between the ages of 20 and 40.

Other signs and symptoms may include repeated lung infections, tiredness, a rapid heartbeat upon standing, vision problems, and weight loss.

Some people who have severe AAT deficiency develop emphysema—often when they're only in their forties or fifties. Signs and symptoms of emphysema include problems breathing, wheezing, and a chronic (ongoing) cough.

At first, many people who have AAT deficiency are diagnosed with asthma. This is because wheezing also is a symptom of asthma. Also, people who have AAT deficiency respond well to asthma medicines.

How Is Alpha-1 Antitrypsin Deficiency Diagnosed?

Alpha-1 antitrypsin (AAT) deficiency usually is diagnosed after you develop a lung or liver disease that's related to the condition.

Your doctor may suspect AAT deficiency if you have signs or symptoms of a serious lung condition, especially emphysema, without any obvious cause. He or she also may suspect AAT deficiency if you develop emphysema when you're 45 years old or younger.

How Is Alpha-1 Antitrypsin Deficiency Treated?

Alpha-1 antitrypsin (AAT) deficiency has no cure, but its related lung diseases have many treatments. Most of these treatments are the same as the ones used for a lung disease called COPD (chronic obstructive pulmonary disease).

If you have symptoms related to AAT deficiency, your doctor may recommend:

- Medicines called inhaled bronchodilators and inhaled steroids. These medicines help open your airways and make breathing easier. They also are used to treat asthma and COPD.
- Flu and pneumococcal vaccines to protect you from illnesses that could make your condition worse. Prompt treatment of lung infections also can help protect your lungs.
- Pulmonary rehabilitation (rehab). Rehab involves treatment by a team of experts at a special clinic. In rehab, you'll learn how to manage your condition and function at your best.
- Extra oxygen, if needed.
- A lung transplant. A lung transplant may be an option if you have severe breathing problems. If you have a good chance of surviving the transplant surgery, you may be a candidate for it.

How Can Alpha-1 Antitrypsin Deficiency Be Prevented?

You can't prevent alpha-1 antitrypsin (AAT) deficiency because the condition is inherited (passed from parents to children through genes).

If you inherit two faulty AAT genes, you'll have AAT deficiency. Even so, you may never develop one of the diseases related to the condition.

You can take steps to prevent or delay lung diseases related to AAT deficiency. One important step is to quit smoking. If you don't smoke, don't start.

Talk with your doctor about programs and products that can help you quit smoking. If you have trouble quitting smoking on your own, consider joining a support group. Many hospitals, workplaces, and community groups offer classes to help people quit smoking.

Also, try to avoid secondhand smoke and places with dust, fumes, or other toxic substances that you may inhale.

Check your living and working spaces for things that may irritate your lungs. Examples include flower and tree pollen, ash, allergens, air pollution, wood burning stoves, paint fumes, and fumes from cleaning products and other household items.

If you have a lung disease related to AAT deficiency, ask your doctor whether you might benefit from augmentation therapy. This is a treatment in which you receive infusions of AAT protein.

Augmentation therapy raises the level of AAT protein in your blood and lungs.

Section 25.2

Hepatitis in Children

This section contains text excerpted from the following sources: Text beginning with the heading "Hepatitis A" is excerpted from "Hepatitis A," National Institute of Diabetes and Digestive and Kidney Diseases (NIDDK), December 2012. Reviewed October 2016; Text beginning with the heading "Hepatitis B" is excerpted from "Hepatitis B," National Institute of Diabetes and Digestive and Kidney Diseases (NIDDK), December 2012. Reviewed October 2016; Text beginning with the heading "Hepatitis C" is excerpted from "Hepatitis C," National Institute of Diabetes and Digestive and Kidney Diseases (NIDDK), December 2012. Reviewed October 2016.

Hepatitis A

What Is Hepatitis A?

Hepatitis A is a virus, or infection, that causes liver disease and inflammation of the liver. Viruses can cause sickness. For example, the flu is caused by a virus. People can pass viruses to each other.

Inflammation is swelling that occurs when tissues of the body become injured or infected. Inflammation can cause organs to not work properly.

Who Gets Hepatitis A?

Anyone can get hepatitis A, but those more likely to are people who

- travel to developing countries
- live with someone who currently has an active hepatitis A infection
- use illegal drugs, including noninjection drugs
- have unprotected sex with an infected person
- provide child care

Also, men who have sex with men are more likely to get hepatitis A.

How Could I Get Hepatitis A?

You could get hepatitis A through contact with an infected person's stool. This contact could occur by

- eating food made by an infected person who didn't wash his or her hands after using the bathroom
- drinking untreated water or eating food washed in untreated water
- placing a finger or object in your mouth that came into contact with an infected person's stool
- having close personal contact with an infected person, such as through sex or caring for someone who is ill

You cannot get hepatitis A from

- being coughed or sneezed on by an infected person
- sitting next to an infected person
- hugging an infected person
- A baby cannot get hepatitis A from breast milk.

What Are the Symptoms of Hepatitis A?

Most people do not have any symptoms of hepatitis A. If symptoms of hepatitis A occur, they include

- feeling tired
- muscle soreness
- upset stomach
- fever
- loss of appetite
- stomach pain
- diarrhea
- dark-yellow urine
- light-colored stools
- yellowish eyes and skin, called jaundice

Symptoms of hepatitis A can occur 2 to 7 weeks after coming into contact with the virus. Children younger than age 6 may have no symptoms. Older children and adults often get mild, flulike symptoms. See a doctor right away if you or a child in your care has symptoms of hepatitis A.

How Is Hepatitis A Diagnosed?

A blood test will show if you have hepatitis A. Blood tests are done at a doctor's office or outpatient facility. A blood sample is taken using a needle inserted into a vein in your arm or hand. The blood sample is sent to a lab to test for hepatitis A.

How Is Hepatitis A Treated?

Hepatitis A usually gets better in a few weeks without treatment. However, some people can have symptoms for up to 6 months. Your doctor may suggest medicines to help relieve your symptoms. Talk with your doctor before taking prescription and over-the-counter medicines.

See your doctor regularly to make sure your body has fully recovered. If symptoms persist after 6 months, then you should see your doctor again.

When you recover, your body will have learned to fight off a future hepatitis A infection. However, you can still get other kinds of hepatitis.

How Can I Avoid Getting Hepatitis A?

You can avoid getting hepatitis A by receiving the hepatitis A vaccine.

Vaccines are medicines that keep you from getting sick. Vaccines teach the body to attack specific viruses and infections. The hepatitis A vaccine teaches your body to attack the hepatitis A virus.

The hepatitis A vaccine is given in two shots. The second shot is given 6 to 12 months after the first shot. You should get both hepatitis A vaccine shots to be fully protected.

All children should be vaccinated between 12 and 23 months of age. Discuss the hepatitis A vaccine with your child's doctor.

Adults at higher risk of getting hepatitis A and people with chronic liver disease should also be vaccinated.

If you are traveling to countries where hepatitis A is common, including Mexico, try to get both shots before you go. If you don't have time to get both shots before you travel, get the first shot as soon as possible. Most people gain some protection within 2 weeks after the first shot.

You can also protect yourself and others from hepatitis A if you

- always wash your hands with warm, soapy water after using the toilet or changing diapers and before fixing food or eating
- use bottled water for drinking, making ice cubes, and washing fruits and vegetables when you are in a developing country
- tell your doctor and your dentist if you have hepatitis A

What Should I Do If I Think I Have Been in Contact with the Hepatitis a Virus?

See your doctor right away if you think you have been in contact with the hepatitis A virus. A dose of the hepatitis A vaccine or a medicine called hepatitis A immune globulin may protect you from getting sick if taken shortly after coming into contact with the hepatitis A virus.

What Is Hepatitis B?

Hepatitis B is a contagious liver disease caused by the hepatitis B virus. When a person is first infected with the virus, he or she can develop an "acute" (short-term) infection. Acute hepatitis B refers to the first 6 months after someone is infected with the hepatitis B virus. This infection can range from a very mild illness with few or no symptoms to a serious condition requiring hospitalization. Some people are able to fight the infection and clear the virus.

For others, the infection remains and is "chronic," or lifelong. Chronic hepatitis B refers to the infection when it remains active instead of getting better after 6 months. Over time, the infection can cause serious health problems, and even liver cancer.

What Are the Symptoms of Hepatitis B?

Infants and young children usually show no symptoms. But, in about 7 out of 10 older children and adults, recent hepatitis B infection causes the following:

- Loss of appetite (not wanting to eat)
- Fever
- Tiredness
- Pain in muscles, joints, and stomach
- Nausea, diarrhea, and vomiting
- Dark urine
- Yellow skin and eyes

These symptoms usually appear 3 or 4 months after being exposed to the virus.

Is It Serious?

Hepatitis B can be very serious. Most people with recent hepatitis B may feel sick for a few weeks to several months. In some people, the infection goes away on its own (i.e., resolves without treatment). For other people, the virus infection remains active in their bodies for the rest of their life.

Although people with lifelong hepatitis B usually don't have symptoms, the virus causes liver damage over time and could lead to liver cancer. For these people, there is no cure, but treatment can help prevent serious problems.

How Does Hepatitis B Spread?

Hepatitis B virus spreads through blood or other body fluids that contain small amounts of blood from an infected person. People can spread the virus even when they have no symptoms.

Babies and children can get hepatitis B in the following ways:

- At birth from their infected mother
- Being bitten by an infected person
- By touching open cuts or sores of an infected person

- Through sharing toothbrushes or other personal items used by an infected person
- From food that was chewed (for a baby) by an infected person

The virus can live on objects for 7 days or more. Even if you don't see any blood, there could be virus on an object.

The Hepatitis B Vaccine Dose at Birth

All babies should get the first shot of hepatitis B vaccine before they leave the hospital. This shot acts as a safety net, reducing the risk of getting the disease from mom's or family members who may not know they are infected with hepatitis B.

When a mom has hepatitis B, there's an additional medicine that can help protect the baby against hepatitis B, called the hepatitis B immune globulin (HBIG). HBIG gives a baby's body a "boost" or extra help to fight the virus as soon as he is born. This shot works best when the baby gets it within the first 12 hours of his life. The baby will also need to complete the full hepatitis B vaccination series for best protection.

Why Should My Child Get the Hepatitis B Shot?

The hepatitis B shot:

- Protects your child against hepatitis B, a potentially serious disease
- Protects other people from the disease because children with hepatitis B usually don't have symptoms, but they often pass the disease to others without anyone knowing they were infected
- Prevents your child from developing liver disease and cancer from hepatitis B
- Keeps your child from missing school or childcare (and keeps you from missing work to care for your sick child)

Is the Hepatitis B Shot Safe?

The hepatitis B vaccine is very safe, and it is effective at preventing hepatitis B. Vaccines, like any medicine, can have side effects. No serious side effects are known to be caused by the hepatitis B vaccine.

Most people who get the hepatitis B vaccine will have no side effects at all. When side effects do occur, they are very mild, such as a low fever (less than 101 degrees) or a sore arm from the shot.

Hepatitis C

What Is Hepatitis C?

Hepatitis C is a virus, or infection, that causes liver disease and inflammation of the liver. Viruses can cause sickness. For example, the flu is caused by a virus. People can pass viruses to each other.

Inflammation is swelling that occurs when tissues of the body become injured or infected. Inflammation can cause organs to not work properly.

Who Gets Hepatitis C?

Anyone can get hepatitis C, but those more likely to are people who

- were born to a mother with hepatitis C
- are in contact with blood or infected needles at work
- have had more than one sex partner in the last 6 months or have a history of sexually transmitted disease
- are on kidney dialysis—the process of filtering wastes and extra water from the body by means other than the kidneys
- are infected with HIV
- have injected illegal drugs
- have had tattoos or body piercings
- work or live in a prison
- had a blood transfusion or organ transplant before July 1992
- have hemophilia and received clotting factor before 1987

Also, men who have sex with men are more likely to get hepatitis C.

How Could I Get Hepatitis C?

You could get hepatitis C through contact with an infected person's blood. This contact could occur by

- being born to a mother with hepatitis C

- getting an accidental stick with a needle that was used on an infected person
- having unprotected sex with an infected person
- having contact with blood or open sores of an infected person
- sharing drug needles or other drug materials with an infected person
- being tattooed or pierced with unsterilized tools that were used on an infected person
- using an infected person's razor, toothbrush, or nail clippers

You cannot get hepatitis C from

- shaking hands or holding hands with an infected person
- being coughed or sneezed on by an infected person
- hugging an infected person
- sitting next to an infected person
- sharing spoons, forks, and other eating utensils
- drinking water or eating food

A baby cannot get hepatitis C from breast milk.

What Are the Symptoms of Hepatitis C?

Most people do not have any symptoms until the hepatitis C virus causes liver damage, which can take 10 or more years to happen. Others may have one or more of the following symptoms:

- feeling tired
- muscle soreness
- upset stomach
- stomach pain
- fever
- loss of appetite
- diarrhea
- dark-yellow urine
- light-colored stools
- yellowish eyes and skin, called jaundice

When symptoms of hepatitis C occur, they can begin 1 to 3 months after coming into contact with the virus. See a doctor right away if you or a child in your care has symptoms of hepatitis C.

What Is Acute Hepatitis C?

Acute hepatitis C is a short-term infection with the hepatitis C virus. Symptoms can last up to 6 months. The infection sometimes clears up because your body is able to fight off the infection and get rid of the virus.

What Is Chronic Hepatitis C?

Chronic hepatitis C is a long-lasting infection with the hepatitis C virus. Chronic hepatitis C occurs when the body can't get rid of the hepatitis C virus. Most hepatitis C infections become chronic.

Without treatment, chronic hepatitis C can cause liver cancer or severe liver damage that leads to liver failure. Liver failure occurs when the liver stops working properly.

How Is Hepatitis C Diagnosed?

A blood test will show if you have hepatitis C. Blood tests are done at a doctor's office or outpatient facility. A blood sample is taken using a needle inserted into a vein in your arm or hand. The blood sample is sent to a lab to test for hepatitis C.

If you are at higher risk of getting hepatitis C, get tested. Many people with hepatitis C do not know they are infected.

Your doctor may suggest getting a liver biopsy if chronic hepatitis C is suspected. A liver biopsy is a test to take a small piece of your liver to look for liver damage. The doctor may ask you to stop taking certain medicines before the test. You may be asked to fast for 8 hours before the test.

During the test, you lie on a table with your right hand resting above your head. Medicine is applied to numb the area where the biopsy needle will be inserted. If needed, sedatives and pain medicine are also given. The doctor uses a needle to take a small piece of liver tissue. After the test, you must lie on your right side for up to 2 hours. You will stay 2 to 4 hours after the test before being sent home.

A liver biopsy is performed at a hospital or outpatient center by a doctor. The liver sample is sent to a special lab where a doctor looks at the tissue with a microscope and sends a report to your doctor.

How Is Hepatitis C Treated?

Hepatitis C is usually not treated unless it becomes chronic. Chronic hepatitis C is treated with medicines that slow or stop the virus from damaging the liver. Your doctor will closely watch your symptoms and schedule regular blood tests to make sure the treatment is working.

Medicines for Chronic Hepatitis C

Chronic hepatitis C is most often treated with a medicine combination that attacks the hepatitis C virus. Treatment may last from 24 to 48 weeks.

Today, newer treatments with medicine for chronic hepatitis C are appearing quickly. Talk with your doctor if you have questions about treatment.

Talk with your doctor before taking other prescription medicines and over-the-counter medicines.

Liver Transplant

A liver transplant may be necessary if chronic hepatitis C causes severe liver damage that leads to liver failure. Symptoms of severe liver damage include the symptoms of hepatitis C and

- generalized itching
- a longer than usual amount of time for bleeding to stop
- easy bruising
- swollen stomach or ankles
- spider like blood vessels, called spider angiomas, that develop on the skin

Liver transplant is surgery to remove a diseased or injured liver and replace it with a healthy one from another person, called a donor. If your doctors tell you that you need a transplant, you should talk with them about the long-term demands of living with a liver transplant.

A team of surgeons—doctors who specialize in surgery—performs a liver transplant in a hospital. You will learn how to take care of yourself after you go home and about the medicines you'll need to take to protect your new liver. You will continue to take medicines because hepatitis C may come back after surgery.

Testing for Liver Cancer

Having hepatitis C increases your risk for liver cancer, so your doctor may suggest an ultrasound test of the liver every 6 to 12 months. Finding cancer early makes it more treatable. Ultrasound is a machine that uses sound waves to create a picture of your liver. Ultrasound is performed at a hospital or radiology center by a specially trained technician. The image, called a sonogram, can show the liver's size and the presence of cancerous tumors.

How Can I Avoid Getting Hepatitis C?

- You can protect yourself and others from getting hepatitis C if you
- do not share drug needles and other drug materials
- do not donate blood or blood products
- wear gloves if you have to touch another person's blood or open sores
- do not share or borrow a toothbrush, razor, or nail clippers
- make sure any tattoos or body piercings you get are done with sterile tools
- tell your doctor and your dentist if you have hepatitis C
- A vaccine for hepatitis C does not yet exist.

What Should I Do If I Think I Have Been in Contact with the Hepatitis C Virus?

See your doctor right away if you think you have been in contact with the hepatitis C virus. Early diagnosis and treatment of chronic hepatitis C can help prevent liver damage.

Chapter 26

Musculoskeletal Disorders in Children

Chapter Contents

Section 26.1

Knock Knees

"Knock Knees," © 2017 Omnigraphics.
Reviewed October 2016.

Knock knees, also known as genu valgum, is a condition in which an inward-turning alignment of the leg bones creates a large gap between a person's feet when they stand with their knees together. In young children, knock knees is generally considered to be a normal stage in the development of the lower extremities. Children are typically born with an outward-turning alignment of the leg bones due to their position in the womb, and they remain bow-legged until the age of about 18 months. Leg alignment gradually straightens by the age of 2, as children learn to walk. Knock knees usually appear between the ages of 2 and 4, as the alignment of the leg bones continues bending inward. As a result, about 20 percent of 3-year-olds have at least a 2-inch (5 cm) gap between their ankles while standing with their knees together. In about 99 percent of cases, however, the condition corrects itself by the time a child reaches the age of 7 or 8.

Although knock knees affect both genders, the condition is more common among girls. The inward bend is usually symmetrical in both legs, but it is not uncommon for one leg to remain straight. Knock knees are not usually associated with other health problems, although severe cases can cause pain in the knee or hip joints or an altered gait. If the condition persists into adulthood, it may increase the risk of arthritis in the knee joints. In very rare cases—especially when knock knees develop after the age of 6—the condition can be symptomatic of a health condition that requires medical attention.

Causes and Symptoms

Most cases of knock knees occur as part of the normal development of the leg bones. Cases that appear outside of the usual window of growth may have other causes, including bone diseases related to vitamin deficiencies, such as osteomalacia or rickets. Other possible contributing factors include obesity, injury to the growth plate of the tibia (shin bone), infection in the leg bones (osteomyelitis), and genetic conditions affecting development of the leg bones or joints.

The main symptom of knock knees is a gap between the ankles when the child is standing with the feet pointed straight ahead and the knees together. Since most children outgrow the condition, it is not necessary to seek medical attention except if the following symptoms appear:

- knock knees develop before age 2 or after age 6
- the child has knee pain or difficulty walking
- the gap between the ankles is greater than 3 inches (8 cm)
- the gap seems to be increasing
- only one leg seems to be affected

Diagnosis

Observation and measurement of the inward-turning alignment of the child's knees and ankles is the first step in diagnosing knock knees. The doctor is likely to conduct a physical examination that includes measurements of the child's height, weight, body mass index (BMI), leg length, leg symmetry, knee extension, and knee rotation. The doctor will also assess the child's gait and inquire about any knee pain or difficulty walking.

When knock knees appear in a child older than 6, or when the condition affects only one leg, the child may be referred to an orthopedic surgeon for further testing. Blood tests may be conducted to check for vitamin deficiencies or other underlying problems. In some cases, standing X-rays may be performed.

Treatment

Knock knees that occur as part of the normal development of the lower extremities do not require medical treatment. Instead, doctors will usually observe the child's growth to ensure that the condition corrects itself over time. For cases of knock knees that are related to an underlying health condition, such as a vitamin deficiency, the treatment would focus on addressing that condition.

For severe cases of knock knees, or those that do not improve as the child grows, the treatment options include leg braces and surgery. Children whose condition does not resolve itself by the age of 8 may need to wear a leg brace at night while they sleep. The brace gradually pulls the knee into a straighter position. Another nonsurgical option is an orthopedic shoe that helps adjust the alignment of the leg.

Surgery is only required in very rare cases where natural growth and leg braces fail to correct severe knock knees. The most common surgical procedure for children is called guided growth. It involves attaching metal plates to the growth centers on the inside of the knees. These plates usually remain in place for about one year. During this time, they prevent the inner part of the knee from growing, which gives the outer part of the knee a chance to catch up. Guided growth surgery is usually performed when a child is approaching puberty, or around age 11 for girls and 13 for boys. Although it requires general anesthesia, it is a minimally invasive procedure that allows children to get back on their feet within a few days.

Osteotomy, on the other hand, is major surgery that entails several months of recovery time. It involves cutting through the bone of the shin or thigh, removing a thin wedge of bone, realigning the legs in a straight position, and inserting metal screws or plates to hold the bones together. Osteotomies are usually performed only to correct severe deformities in adults and children who have stopped growing.

Prognosis

Most children with knock knees outgrow the condition and have a positive prognosis. Even those who require leg braces or surgery usually heal quickly with good results. When severe knock knees are left untreated, some children may experience difficulty walking or running that interferes with their enjoyment of sports and activities. If the condition continues into adolescence, some teens may experience embarrassment or low self-esteem related to their appearance or gait. Finally, knock knees that persist into adulthood can contribute to knee problems, such as pain, ligament tears, dislocation, or early arthritis.

References

1. Kaneshiro, Neil K. "Knock Knees," MedlinePlus, 2016.
2. "Knock Knees," NHS Choices, 2016.
3. "Knock Knees: Symptoms and Causes," Boston Children's Hospital, 2016.

Section 26.2

Flat Feet

What Is Pediatric Flat Feet?

Pediatric flatfoot is a medical condition in which the arch of the child's foot partially or totally collapses when the child is standing. Pediatric flatfoot can be present in one or both of the child's feet. The condition is most often an inherited disorder, although certain injuries and diseases may also cause pediatric flatfoot. There are two main types of pediatric flatfoot: flexible and rigid.

In cases of flexible pediatric flatfoot, the foot arch collapses when the child stands but reappears when the child is standing on tiptoe or sitting. Flexible pediatric flatfoot occurs most often in very young children and generally resolves without treatment by the time the child reaches age five.

Rigid pediatric flatfoot occurs when the foot arch does not appear when the child sits or stands on tiptoe. Rigid flatfoot can occur in children as young as newborn, or the condition may not develop until preadolescence. Tarsal coalition is a type of rigid pediatric flatfoot that is present from birth. In these cases, two or more bones in the child's foot are fused together abnormally. Children with tarsal coalition may not experience any pain or other symptoms, or symptoms may emerge during preadolescence years. Another type of rigid pediatric flatfoot is known as congenital vertical talus. This type of flatfoot is present at birth and is identified by the rigid "rocker bottom" appearance of the child's feet. Most children with this type of flatfoot will begin to experience symptoms at walking age, because the condition makes it painful for the child to walk or wear shoes.

Symptoms

The majority of children with pediatric flatfoot never experience symptoms. Pediatric flatfoot is generally identified by parents or other caregivers through visual observation of the appearance of the child's feet. Among children who do have symptoms of pediatric flatfoot, the most common indications include:

- Discomfort in the legs or bottom of the feet
- Discomfort while walking or a change in the way the child walks
- Discomfort during other physical activities such as sports or games, or voluntary withdrawal from physical activities
- Outward-tilting heels
- Discomfort while wearing shoes

Assessment and Testing

Pediatricians generally diagnose flatfoot in children through visual examination of the child's legs, knees, feet, and the wear patterns on the soles of the child's shoes, along with observation of the child sitting, standing, and walking. X-rays can help the pediatrician classify the type of pediatric flatfoot disorder as well as the severity of the condition. Magnetic resonance imaging (MRI) or other medical imaging tests may also be used in diagnosis of pediatric flatfoot.

Treatment

The majority of cases of pediatric flatfoot resolve untreated. In cases where the affected child complains of pain in their feet, recommendations often include the use of special shoe inserts to provide arch support, stretching exercises, and physical therapy. In severe cases of rigid pediatric flatfoot, surgery may be required. A pediatrician may refer the child to a foot and ankle surgeon for evaluation. Various surgical techniques can be used to correct pediatric flatfoot depending upon a range of factors including the child's age, the severity of the child's condition, the extent of the child's symptoms, and the type of flatfoot disorder.

References

1. "Flatfoot," St. Louis Children's Hospital. 2016.
2. "Flatfoot in Children," Cleveland Clinic. November 27, 2013.
3. "Pediatric Flatfoot," American College of Foot and Ankle Surgeons. 2005.

Section 26.3

Growing Pains

Text in this section is excerpted from "Growing Pains," © 1995–2016. The Nemours Foundation/KidsHealth®. Reprinted with permission.

Your 8-year-old son wakes up crying in the night complaining that his legs are throbbing. You rub them and soothe him as much as you can, but you're uncertain about whether to give him any medicine or take him to the doctor.

Sound familiar? Your son is probably having growing pains, which about 25% to 40% of kids do. They usually strike during two periods: in early childhood among 3- to 5-year-olds and, later, in 8- to 12-year-olds.

Signs and Symptoms

Growing pains always concentrate in the muscles, rather than the joints. Most kids report pains in the front of their thighs, in the calves, or behind the knees. Joints affected by more serious diseases are swollen, red, tender, or warm—the joints of kids having growing pains look normal.

Although growing pains often strike in late afternoon or early evening before bed, pain can sometimes wake a sleeping child. The intensity of the pain varies from child to child, and most kids don't have the pains every day.

What Causes Them?

Bone growth hasn't been proved to cause pain. So "growing" pains might just be aches and discomfort from the jumping, climbing, and running that active kids do during the day. The pains can happen after a child has had a particularly athletic day.

Diagnosing Growing Pains

One symptom that doctors find most helpful in making a diagnosis of growing pains is how a child responds to touch while in pain. Kids who have pain from a serious medical cause don't like to be handled because movement can make the pain worse. But those with growing pains respond differently—they feel better when they're held, massaged, and cuddled.

Growing pains are what doctors call a diagnosis of exclusion. This means that other conditions will be ruled out before a diagnosis of growing pains is made. This usually is done by taking a medical history and doing a physical exam. In rare cases, blood tests and X-rays might be done before a doctor diagnoses growing pains.

Helping Your Child

Things that may help ease growing pains include:

- massaging the area
- stretching
- placing a heating pad on the area
- giving ibuprofen or acetaminophen

Do not give aspirin to a child or teen, as it has been linked to a rare but serious illness called Reye syndrome.

When to Call the Doctor

Call your doctor if any of these symptoms happen with your child's pain:

- long-lasting pain, pain in the morning, or swelling or redness in one particular area or joint
- pain associated with an injury
- fever
- limping
- unusual rashes
- loss of appetite
- weakness
- tiredness
- unusual behavior

These signs are not related to growing pains and should be checked out by the doctor.

While growing pains aren't usually related to illness, they can upset kids—and parents. Because the aches are usually gone in the morning, parents sometimes think that a child faked the pains. But this usually isn't true. Instead, offer support and reassurance that growing pains will pass as kids grow up.

Section 26.4

Intoeing

Text in this section is excerpted from "In-Toeing and Out-Toeing in Toddlers," © 1995–2016. The Nemours Foundation/KidsHealth®. Reprinted with permission.

Whether your baby rises from a crawl with a shaky first step or a full-on sprint across the living room, chances are you'll be on the edge of your seat. But remember—a child's first steps usually aren't picture perfect.

Learning to walk takes time and practice, and it's common for kids to start walking with their toes and feet turned at an angle. When feet turn inward—a tendency referred to as walking "pigeon-toed"—doctors call it in-toeing. When feet point outward, it's called out-toeing.

It can be upsetting to see your child develop an abnormal gait, but for most toddlers with in-toeing or out-toeing, it's usually nothing to worry about. The conditions do not cause pain and usually improve as kids grow older.

Almost all healthy kids who toe-in or -out as toddlers learn to run, jump, and play sports as they grow up, just the same as kids without gait problems.

In-Toeing and Out-Toeing

Most toddlers toe-in or -out because of a slight rotation, or twist, of the upper or lower leg bones.

Tibial torsion, the most common cause of intoeing, occurs when the lower leg bone (tibia) tilts inward. If the tibia tilts outward, a child will toe-out. When the thighbone, or femur, is tilted, the tibia will also turn and give the appearance of in-toeing or out-toeing. The medical term for this is femoral anteversion. In-toeing can also be caused by metatarsus adductus, a curvature of the foot that causes toes to point inward.

Why some kids develop gait abnormalities and others don't is unclear, but many experts think that a family history of in-toeing or out-toeing plays a role. So, if you toed-in or -out as a child, there's a chance that your child could develop the same tendency.

Also, being cramped in the womb during pregnancy can contribute to a child in-toeing or out-toeing. As a fetus grows, some of the bones have to rotate slightly to fit into the small space of the uterus. In many cases, these bones are still rotated to some degree for the first few years of life. Often this is most noticeable when a child learns to walk because if the tibia or femur tilt at an angle, the feet will too.

Does Walking Improve?

As most kids get older, their bones very gradually rotate to a normal angle. Walking, like other skills, improves with experience, so kids will become better able to control their muscles and foot position.

In-toeing and out-toeing gets better over time, but this happens very gradually and is hard to notice. So doctors often recommend using video clips to help parents track improvement. Parents can record their child walking, and then wait about a year to take another video. This usually makes it easy to see if the gait abnormality has improved over time. In most cases, it has. If not, parents should speak with their child's doctor to discuss whether treatment is necessary.

In the past, special shoes and braces were used to treat gait abnormalities. But doctors found that these didn't make in-toeing or out-toeing disappear any faster, so they're rarely used now.

If Walking Does Not Improve

Speak with your doctor if you're concerned about the way your child walks. For a small number of kids, gait abnormalities can be associated with other problems. For example, out-toeing could signal a neuromuscular condition in rare cases.

Have your child evaluated by a doctor if you notice:

- in-toeing or out-toeing that doesn't improve by age 3
- limping or complaints of pain
- one foot that turns out more than the other

- developmental delays, such as not learning to talk as expected
- gait abnormalities that worsen instead of improve

The doctor can then decide if more specialized exams or testing should be done to make sure that your child gets the proper care.

Section 26.5

Juvenile Idiopathic (Rheumatoid) Arthritis

This section includes text excerpted from "Questions and Answers about Juvenile Arthritis," National Institute of Arthritis and Musculoskeletal and Skin Diseases (NIAMS), June 2015.

What Is Juvenile Idiopathic Arthritis?

Juvenile arthritis (JA) is a term often used to describe arthritis in children. Children can develop almost all types of arthritis that affect adults, but the most common type that affects children is juvenile idiopathic arthritis.

Both juvenile idiopathic arthritis (JIA) and juvenile rheumatoid arthritis (JRA) are classification systems for chronic arthritis in children. The juvenile rheumatoid arthritis classification system was developed decades ago and had three different subtypes: polyarticular, pauciarticular, and systemic-onset. More recently, pediatric rheumatologists throughout the world developed the juvenile idiopathic arthritis classification system, which includes more types of chronic arthritis that affect children. This classification system also provides a more accurate separation of the three juvenile rheumatoid arthritis subtypes.

Prevalence statistics for juvenile arthritis vary, but according to a report from the National Arthritis Data Workgroup, about 294,000 children age 0 to 17 are affected with arthritis or other rheumatic conditions.

What Causes Juvenile Arthritis?

Most forms of juvenile arthritis are autoimmune disorders, which means that the body's immune system—which normally helps to fight off bacteria or viruses—mistakenly attacks some of its own healthy cells and tissues. The result is inflammation, marked by redness, heat, pain, and swelling. Inflammation can cause joint damage. Doctors do not know why the immune system attacks healthy tissues in children who develop juvenile arthritis. Scientists suspect that it is a two-step process. First, something in a child's genetic makeup gives him or her a tendency to develop juvenile arthritis; then an environmental factor, such as a virus, triggers the development of the disease.

Not all cases of juvenile arthritis are autoimmune, however. Recent research has demonstrated that some people, such as many with systemic arthritis, have what is more accurately called an autoinflammatory condition. Although the two terms sound somewhat similar, the disease processes behind autoimmune and autoinflammatory disorders are different.

When the immune system is working properly, foreign invaders such as bacteria and viruses provoke the body to produce proteins called antibodies. Antibodies attach to these invaders so that they can be recognized and destroyed. In an autoimmune reaction, the antibodies attach to the body's own healthy tissues by mistake, signaling the body to attack them. Because they target the self, these proteins are called autoantibodies.

Like autoimmune disorders, autoinflammatory conditions also cause inflammation. And like autoimmune disorders, they also involve an overactive immune system. However, autoinflammation is not caused by autoantibodies. Instead, autoinflammation involves a more primitive part of the immune system that in healthy people causes white blood cells to destroy harmful substances. When this system goes awry, it causes inflammation for unknown reasons. In addition to inflammation, autoinflammatory diseases often cause fever and rashes.

What Are Its Symptoms and Signs?

The most common symptom of all types of juvenile arthritis is persistent joint swelling, pain, and stiffness that is typically worse in the morning or after a nap. The pain may limit movement of the affected joint, although many children, especially younger ones, will not complain of pain. Juvenile arthritis commonly affects the knees and the joints in the hands and feet. One of the earliest signs of juvenile arthritis may be limping in the morning because of an affected knee. Besides joint symptoms, children with systemic juvenile arthritis have a high fever and a skin rash. The rash and fever may appear and disappear very quickly. Systemic arthritis also may cause the lymph nodes located in the neck and other parts of the body to swell. In some cases (fewer than half), internal organs including the heart and (very rarely) the lungs, may be involved.

Eye inflammation is a potentially severe complication that commonly occurs in children with oligoarthritis but can also be seen in other types of juvenile arthritis. All children with juvenile arthritis need to have regular eye exams, including a special exam called a slit lamp exam. Eye diseases such as iritis or uveitis can be present at the beginning of arthritis but often develop some time after a child first develops juvenile arthritis. Very commonly, juvenile arthritis-associated eye inflammation does not cause any symptoms and is found only by performing eye exams.

Typically, there are periods when the symptoms of juvenile arthritis are better or disappear (remissions) and times when symptoms "flare," or get worse. Juvenile arthritis is different in each child; some may have just one or two flares and never have symptoms again, while others may experience many flares or even have symptoms that never go away.

Some children with juvenile arthritis have growth problems. Depending on the severity of the disease and the joints involved, bone growth at the affected joints may be too fast or too slow, causing one leg or arm to be longer than the other, for example, or resulting in a small or misshapen chin. Overall growth also may be slowed. Doctors are exploring the use of growth hormone to treat this problem. Juvenile arthritis may also cause joints to grow unevenly.

How Is It Diagnosed?

To be classified as juvenile arthritis, symptoms must have started before age 16. Doctors usually suspect juvenile arthritis, along with several other possible conditions, when they see children with persistent joint pain or swelling, unexplained skin rashes, and fever associated with swelling of lymph nodes or inflammation of internal organs. A diagnosis of juvenile arthritis also is considered in children with an unexplained limp or excessive clumsiness.

No single test can be used to diagnose juvenile arthritis. A doctor diagnoses juvenile arthritis by carefully examining the patient and considering his or her medical history and the results of tests that help confirm juvenile arthritis or rule out other conditions. Specific findings or problems that relate to the joints are the main factors that go into making a juvenile arthritis diagnosis.

Who Treats It?

Treating juvenile arthritis often requires a team approach, encompassing the child and his or her family and a number of different health professionals. Ideally, the child's care should be managed by a pediatric rheumatologist, who is a doctor who has been specially trained to treat the rheumatic diseases in children. However, many pediatricians and "adult" rheumatologists also treat children with juvenile arthritis. Because there are relatively few pediatric rheumatologists and they are mainly concentrated at major medical centers in metropolitan areas, children who live in smaller towns and rural areas may benefit from having a doctor in their town coordinate care through a pediatric rheumatologist. Many large centers now conduct outreach clinics, in which doctors and a supporting team travel from large cities to smaller towns for 1 or 2 days to treat local patients.

Other members of your child's healthcare team may include:

- **Physical therapist.** This health professional can work with your child to develop a plan of exercises that will improve joint function and strengthen muscles without causing further harm to affected joints.
- **Occupational therapist.** This health professional can teach ways to protect joints, minimize pain, conserve energy, and exercise. Occupational therapists specialize in the upper extremities (hands, wrists, elbows, arms, shoulders, and neck).
- **Counselor or psychologist.** Being a child or adolescent with a chronic disease isn't easy, for the child or his or her family. Some children may benefit from sorting out their feelings with a psychologist or counselor trained to help children in this situation. Members of the child's family may benefit from counseling as well.
- **Ophthalmologist.** If your child's medications or form of arthritis can affect the eyes, catching problems early can help keep them from becoming serious. All children with juvenile arthritis need to have regular exams by an ophthalmologist (eye doctor) to detect eye inflammation.
- **Dentist and orthodontist.** Dental care can be difficult if a child's hands are so affected by arthritis that thorough brushing and flossing of the teeth becomes difficult. In addition, children with involvement of the jaw may have difficulty opening the mouth for proper brushing. Therefore, regular dental exams are

important. Because juvenile arthritis can affect the alignment of the jaw, it is important for children with this disease to be evaluated by an orthodontist.

- **Orthopaedic surgeon.** For some children, surgery is necessary to help minimize or repair the effects of their disease. Orthopaedic surgeons are doctors who perform surgery on the joints and bones.
- **Dietitian.** For children with chronic diseases, good nutrition is particularly important. A dietitian can help design a nutritious diet that will benefit the whole family.
- **Pharmacist.** A pharmacist is a good source of information about medications, including possible side effects and drugs that have the potential to interact with one another. If a child has trouble swallowing large pills or taking other medication, the pharmacist may have suggestions for different ways to take the medication or may be able to formulate or help you get kid-friendly versions of some medications.
- **Social worker.** A social worker can help a child and his or her family deal with life and lifestyle changes caused by arthritis. A social worker also can help you identify helpful resources for your child.
- **Rheumatology nurse.** A rheumatology nurse likely will be intimately involved in a child's care, serving as the main point of contact with the doctor's office concerning appointments, tests, medications, and instructions.
- **School nurse.** For a school-age child, the school nurse also may be considered a member of the treatment team, particularly if the child is required to take medications regularly during school hours.

How Is It Treated?

The main goals of treatment are to preserve a high level of physical and social functioning and maintain a good quality of life. To achieve these goals, doctors recommend treatments to reduce swelling, maintain full movement in the affected joints, relieve pain, and prevent, identify, and treat complications. Most children with juvenile arthritis need a combination of medication and non medication treatments to reach these goals.

How Can the Family Help a Child Live Well with Juvenile Arthritis?

Juvenile arthritis affects the entire family, all of whom must cope with the special challenges of this disease. Juvenile arthritis can strain a child's participation in social and after-school activities and make schoolwork more difficult. Family members can do several things to help the child physically and emotionally.

- **Get the best care possible.** Ensure that the child receives appropriate medical care and follows the doctor's instructions. If possible, have a pediatric rheumatologist manage your child's care. If such a specialist is not close by, consider having your child see one yearly or twice a year. A pediatric rheumatologist can devise a treatment plan and consult with your child's doctor, who will help you carry it out and monitor your child's progress.
- **Learn as much as you can about your child's disease and its treatment.** Many treatment options are available, and because juvenile arthritis is different in each child, what works for one may not work for another. If the medications that the doctor prescribes do not relieve symptoms or if they cause unpleasant side effects, you and your child should discuss other choices with the doctor. A person with juvenile arthritis can be more active when symptoms are controlled.
- **Consider joining a support group.** Try to find other parents and kids who face similar experiences. It can help you—and your child—to know you're not alone. Some organizations have support groups for people with juvenile arthritis and their families.
- **Treat the child as normally as possible.** Try not to cut your child too much slack just because he or she has arthritis. Too much coddling can keep your child from being responsible and independent and can cause resentment in siblings.
- **Encourage exercise and physical therapy for the child.** For many young people, exercise and physical therapy play important roles in managing juvenile arthritis. Parents can arrange for children to participate in activities that the doctor recommends. During symptom-free periods, many doctors suggest playing team sports or doing other activities. The goal is to help keep the joints strong and flexible, to provide play time with other children, and to encourage appropriate social development.

- **Work closely with your child's school.** Help your child's school to develop a suitable lesson plan, and educate your child's teacher and classmates about juvenile arthritis. Some children with juvenile arthritis may be absent from school for prolonged periods and need to have the teacher send assignments home. Some minor changes—such as having an extra set of books or leaving class a few minutes early to get to the next class on time—can be a great help. With proper attention, most children progress normally through school.
- **Talk with your child.** Explain that getting juvenile arthritis is nobody's fault. Some children believe that juvenile arthritis is a punishment for something they did. Let your child know you are always available to listen, and help him or her in any way you can.
- **Work with therapists or social workers.** They can help you and your child adapt more easily to the lifestyle changes juvenile arthritis may bring.

Section 26.6

Legg-Calvé-Perthes Disease

This section contains text excerpted from the following sources: Text beginning with the heading "Legg-Calvé-Perthes" is excerpted from "Legg-Calvé-Perthes disease," Genetics Home Reference (GHR), National Institutes of Health (NIH), September 28, 2016; Text under the heading "Treatment" is excerpted from "Legg-Calve-Perthes disease," Genetic and Rare Diseases (GARD) Information Center, National Institutes of Health (NIH), July 28, 2016.

Legg-Calvé-Perthes

Legg-Calvé-Perthes disease is a bone disorder that affects the hips. Usually, only one hip is involved, but in about 10 percent of cases, both hips are affected. Legg-Calvé-Perthes disease begins in childhood, typically between ages 4 and 8, and affects boys more frequently than girls.

In this condition, the upper end of the thigh bone, known as the femoral head, breaks down. As a result, the femoral head is no longer round and does not move easily in the hip socket, which leads to hip pain, limping, and restricted leg movement. The bone eventually begins to heal itself through a normal process called bone remodeling, by which old bone is removed and new bone is created to replace it. This cycle of breakdown and healing can recur multiple times. Affected individuals are often shorter than their peers due to the bone abnormalities. Many people with Legg-Calvé-Perthes disease go on to develop a painful joint disorder called osteoarthritis in the hips at an early age.

Frequency

The incidence of Legg-Calvé-Perthes disease varies by population. The condition is most common in white populations, in which it affects an estimated 1 to 3 in 20,000 children under age 15.

Genetic Changes

Legg-Calvé-Perthes disease is usually not caused by genetic factors. The cause in these cases is unknown. In a small percentage of cases, mutations in the *COL2A1* gene cause the bone abnormalities characteristic of Legg-Calvé-Perthes disease. *The COL2A1* gene provides instructions for making a protein that forms type II collagen. This type of collagen is found mostly in cartilage, a tough but flexible tissue that makes up much of the skeleton during early development. Most cartilage is later converted to bone, except for the cartilage that continues to cover and protect the ends of bones and is present in the nose and external ears. Type II collagen is essential for the normal development of bones and other connective tissues that form the body's supportive framework.

COL2A1 gene mutations involved in Legg-Calvé-Perthes disease lead to production of an altered protein; collagen that contains this protein may be less stable than normal. Researchers speculate that the breakdown of bone characteristic of Legg-Calvé-Perthes disease is caused by impaired blood flow to the femoral head, which leads to death of the bone tissue (osteonecrosis); however it is unclear how abnormal type II collagen is involved in this process or why the hips are specifically affected.

Treatment

Treatment aims to keep the thigh bone inside the hip socket. Treatment options may include rest or medication for pain; physical therapy; using a brace; or surgery

Prognosis

The prognosis for people with Legg-Calve-Perthes disease (LCPD) depends on the extent and severity of bone involvement, and residual deformity. Overall, the prognosis for recovery and sports participation after treatment is very good for most people. Generally, a younger age at diagnosis is associated with a better outcome.

For people who are younger than age 5 when LCPD develops, the incidence of degenerative arthritis later in life is reportedly very low. The more deformed the femoral head is during healing, the greater the risk of osteoarthritis of the hip later in life. The risk is also higher for those with metaphyseal defects (where the shaft of the bone flares out); and for those who develop LCPD late in childhood (at age 10 or older). Nearly 100% of people with complex involvement of the femoral head and residual deformity will develop degenerative arthritis. Total hip replacement in early adulthood may be needed in some cases.

Section 26.7

Marfan Syndrome

This section includes text excerpted from "Learning about Marfan Syndrome," National Human Genome Research Institute (NHGRI), April 21, 2014.

What Is Marfan Syndrome?

Marfan syndrome is one of the most common inherited disorders of connective tissue. It is an autosomal dominant condition occurring once in every 10,000 to 20,000 individuals. There is a wide variability in clinical symptoms in Marfan syndrome with the most notable occurring in eye, skeleton, connective tissue and cardiovascular systems.

Marfan syndrome is caused by mutations in the FBN1 gene. FBN1 mutations are associated with a broad continuum of physical features ranging from isolated features of Marfan syndrome to a severe and rapidly progressive form in newborns.

What Are the Symptoms of Marfan Syndrome?

The most common symptom of Marfan syndrome is myopia (nearsightedness from the increased curve of the retina due to connective tissue changes in the globe of the eye). About 60 percent of individuals who have Marfan syndrome have lens displacement from the center of the pupil (ectopia lentis). Individuals who have Marfan syndrome also have an increased risk for retinal detachment, glaucoma and early cataract formation.

Other common symptoms of Marfan syndrome involve the skeleton and connective tissue systems. These include bone overgrowth and loose joints (joint laxity). Individuals who have Marfan syndrome have long thin arms and legs (dolichostenomelia). Overgrowth of the ribs can cause the chest bone (sternum) to bend inward (pectus excavatum or funnel chest) or push outward (pectus carinatum or pigeon breast). Curvature of the spine (scoliosis) is another common skeletal symptom that can be mild or severe and progressively worsen with age. Scoliosis shortens the trunk also contributes to the arms and legs appearing too long.

Cardiovascular malformations are the most life threatening symptom of Marfan syndrome. They include dilated aorta just as it leaves the heart (at the level of the sinuses of Valsalva), mitral valve prolapse, tricuspid valve prolapse, enlargement of the proximal pulmonary artery, and a high risk for aortic tear and rupture(aortic dissection).

How Is Marfan Syndrome Diagnosed?

The diagnosis of Marfan syndrome is a clinical diagnosis that is based on family history and the presence of characteristic clinical findings in ocular, skeletal and cardiovascular systems. There are four major clinical diagnostic features:

1. Dilatation or dissection of the aorta at the level of the sinuses of Valsava.
2. Ectopia lentis (dislocated lens of the eye).
3. Lumbosacral dural ectasia determined by CT scan or magnetic resonance imaging (MRI).
4. Four of the eight typical skeletal features.

Major criteria for establishing the diagnosis in a family member also include having a parent, child, or sibling who meets major criteria independently, the presence of an FBN-1 mutation known to cause the syndrome, or a haplotype around FBN-1 inherited by descent and identified in a familial Marfan patient (also known as genetic linkage to the gene).

The FBN1 gene is the gene associated with the true Marfan syndrome. Genetic testing of the FBN1 gene identifies 70–93 percent of the mutations and is available in clinical laboratories. However patients negative for the test for gene mutation should be considered for evaluation for other conditions that have similar features of Marfan syndrome such as Dietz syndrome, Ehlers Danlos syndrome, and homocystinuria. To unequivocally establish the diagnosis in the absence of a family history requires a major manifestation from two systems and involvement of a third system. If a mutation known to cause Marfan syndrome is identified, the diagnosis requires one major criterion and involvement of a second organ system.

To establish the diagnosis in a relative of a patient known to have Marfan Syndrome (index case) requires the presence of a major criterion in the family history and one major criterion in an organ system with involvement of a second organ system.

What Is the Treatment for Marfan Syndrome?

Individuals who have Marfan syndrome are treated by a multidisciplinary medical team that includes a geneticist, cardiologist, ophthalmologist, orthopedist and cardiothoracic surgeon.

Eye problems are generally treated with eyeglasses. When lens dislocation interferes with vision or causes glaucoma, surgery can be performed and an artificial lens implanted.

Skeletal problems such as scoliosis and pectus excavatum may require surgery. For those individuals who have pes planus (flat feet) arch supports and orthotics can be used to decrease leg fatigue and muscle cramps.

Medication, such as beta blockers, is used to decrease the stress on the aorta at the time of diagnosis or when there is progressive aortic dilatation. Surgery to repair the aorta is done when the aortic diameter is greater than 5 cm in adults and older children, when the aortic diameter increases by 1.0 cm per year, or when there is progressive aortic regurgitation.

Cardiovascular surveillance includes yearly echocardiograms to monitor the status of the aorta. Currently the use of beta blocker medications has delayed but not prevented the need to eventually perform aortic surgery.

Recent work on Angiotensin II receptor blockers, another blood pressure medication like beta blockers, has shown additional promise to protect the aorta from dilatation. Clinical trials will be starting soon to see if this drug can prevent the need for surgery better than beta blockers have.

Individuals who have Marfan syndrome are advised to avoid contact and competitive sports and isometric exercise like weightlifting and other static forms of exercise. They can participate in aerobic exercises like swimming. They are also advised to avoid medications such as decongestants and foods that contain caffeine which can lead to chronic increases in blood pressure and stretch the connective tissue in the cardiovascular system.

Is Marfan Syndrome Inherited?

Marfan syndrome is inherited in families in an autosomal dominant manner. Approximately seventy-five percent of individuals who have Marfan syndrome have a parent who also has the condition (inherited). Approximately 25 percent of individuals who have Marfan syndrome, have the condition as a result of a new (de novo) mutation. When a parent has Marfan syndrome, each of his or her children has a 50 percent chance (1 chance in 2) to inherit the FBN1 gene. While Marfan syndrome is not always inherited, it is always heritable.

When a child with Marfan syndrome is born to parents who do not show features of the Marfan syndrome, it is likely the child has a new mutation. In this family situation, the chance for future siblings (brothers and sisters of the child with Marfan syndrome) to be born with Marfan syndrome is less than 50 percent. But the risk is still greater than the general population risk of 1 in 10,000. The risk is higher for siblings because there are rare families where a Marfan gene mutation is in some percentage of the germline cells of one of the parents (testes or ovaries).

Prenatal testing for Marfan syndrome is available when the gene mutation is known, and also using a technique called linkage analysis (tracking the gene for Marfan syndrome in a family using genetic markers).

Section 26.8

Muscular Dystrophy

This section includes text excerpted from "Muscular Dystrophy: Hope through Research," National Institute of Neurological Disorders and Stroke (NINDS), March 4, 2016.

What Is Muscular Dystrophy?

Muscular dystrophy (MD) refers to a group of more than 30 genetic diseases that cause progressive weakness and degeneration of skeletal muscles used during voluntary movement. The word dystrophy is derived from the Greek dys, which means "difficult" or "faulty," and troph, or "nourish." These disorders vary in age of onset, severity, and pattern of affected muscles. All forms of MD grow worse as muscles progressively degenerate and weaken. Many individuals eventually lose the ability to walk.

Some types of MD also affect the heart, gastrointestinal system, endocrine glands, spine, eyes, brain, and other organs. Respiratory and cardiac diseases may occur, and some people may develop a swallowing disorder. MD is not contagious and cannot be brought on by injury or activity.

What Causes MD?

All of the muscular dystrophies are inherited and involve a mutation in one of the thousands of genes that program proteins critical to muscle integrity. The body's cells don't work properly when a protein is altered or produced in insufficient quantity (or sometimes missing completely). Many cases of MD occur from spontaneous mutations that are not found in the genes of either parent, and this defect can be passed to the next generation.

How Many People Have MD?

MD occurs worldwide, affecting all races. Its incidence varies, as some forms are more common than others. Its most common form in children, Duchenne muscular dystrophy, affects approximately 1 in every 3,500 to 6,000 male births each year in the United States. Some types of MD are more prevalent in certain countries and regions of the world. Many muscular dystrophies are familial, meaning there is some family history of the disease. Duchenne cases often have no prior family history. This is likely due to the large size of the dystrophin gene that is implicated in the disorder, making it a target for spontaneous mutations.

How Does MD Affect Muscles?

Muscles are made up of thousands of muscle fibers. Each fiber is actually a number of individual cells that have joined together during development and are encased by an outer membrane. Muscle fibers that make up individual muscles are bound together by connective tissue.

Muscles are activated when an impulse, or signal, is sent from the brain through the spinal cord and peripheral nerves (nerves that connect the central nervous system to sensory organs and muscles) to the neuromuscular junction (the space between the nerve fiber and the muscle it activates). There, a release of the chemical acetylcholine triggers a series of events that cause the muscle to contract.

The muscle fiber membrane contains a group of proteins—called the dystrophin-glycoprotein complex—which prevents damage as muscle fibers contract and relax. When this protective membrane is damaged, muscle fibers begin to leak the protein creatine kinase (needed for the chemical reactions that produce energy for muscle contractions) and take on excess calcium, which causes further harm. Affected muscle fibers eventually die from this damage, leading to progressive muscle degeneration.

Although MD can affect several body tissues and organs, it most prominently affects the integrity of muscle fibers. The disease causes muscle degeneration, progressive weakness, fiber death, fiber branching and splitting, phagocytosis (in which muscle fiber material is broken down and destroyed by scavenger cells), and, in some cases, chronic or permanent shortening of tendons and muscles. Also, overall muscle strength and tendon reflexes are usually lessened or lost due to replacement of muscle by connective tissue and fat.

How Are the Muscular Dystrophies Diagnosed?

Both the individual's medical history and a complete family history should be thoroughly reviewed to determine if the muscle disease is secondary to a disease affecting other tissues or organs or is an inherited condition. It is also important to rule out any muscle weakness resulting from prior surgery, exposure to toxins, or current medications that may affect the person's functional status or rule out many acquired muscle diseases. Thorough clinical and neurological exams can rule out disorders of the central and/or peripheral nervous systems, identify any patterns of muscle weakness and atrophy, test reflex responses and coordination, and look for contractions.

How Do the Muscular Dystrophies Differ?

There are nine major groups of the muscular dystrophies. The disorders are classified by the extent and distribution of muscle weakness, age of onset, rate of progression, severity of symptoms, and family history (including any pattern of inheritance). Although some forms of MD become apparent in infancy or childhood, others may not appear until middle age or later. Overall, incidence rates and severity vary, but each of the dystrophies causes progressive skeletal muscle deterioration, and some types affect cardiac muscle.

Duchenne MD is the most common childhood form of MD, as well as the most common of the muscular dystrophies overall, accounting for approximately 50 percent of all cases. Because inheritance is X-linked recessive (caused by a mutation on the X, or sex, chromosome), Duchenne MD primarily affects boys, although girls and women who carry the defective gene may show some symptoms. About one-third of the cases reflect new mutations and the rest run in families. Sisters of boys with Duchenne MD have a 50 percent chance of carrying the defective gene.

Duchenne MD usually becomes apparent during the toddler years, sometimes soon after an affected child begins to walk. Progressive weakness and muscle wasting (a decrease in muscle strength and size) caused by degenerating muscle fibers begins in the upper legs and pelvis before spreading into the upper arms. Other symptoms include loss of some reflexes, a waddling gait, frequent falls and clumsiness (especially when running), difficulty when rising from a sitting or lying position or when climbing stairs, changes to overall posture, impaired breathing, lung weakness, and cardiomyopathy. Many children are unable to run or jump. The wasting muscles, in particular the calf muscles (and, less commonly, muscles in the buttocks, shoulders, and arms), may be enlarged by an accumulation of fat and connective tissue, causing them to look larger and healthier than they actually are (called pseudohypertrophy). As the disease progresses, the muscles in the diaphragm that assist in breathing and coughing may weaken. Affected individuals may experience breathing difficulties, respiratory infections, and swallowing problems. Bone thinning and scoliosis (curving of the spine) are common. Some affected children have varying degrees of cognitive and behavioral impairments. Between ages 3 and 6, children may show brief periods of physical improvement followed later on by progressive muscle degeneration. Children with Duchenne MD typically lose the ability to walk by early adolescence. Without aggressive care, they usually die in their late teens or early twenties from progressive weakness of the heart muscle, respiratory complications, or infection. However, improvements in multidisciplinary care have extended the life expectancy and improved the quality of life significantly for these children; numerous individuals with Duchenne muscular dystrophy now survive into their 30s, and some even into their 40s.

Duchenne MD results from an absence of the muscle protein dystrophin. Dystrophin is a protein found in muscle that helps muscles stay healthy and strong. Blood tests of children with Duchenne MD show an abnormally high level of creatine kinase; this finding is apparent from birth.

Becker MD is less severe than but closely related to Duchenne MD. People with Becker MD have partial but insufficient function of the protein dystrophin. There is greater variability in the clinical course of Becker MD compared to Duchenne MD. The disorder usually appears around age 11 but may occur as late as age 25, and affected individuals generally live into middle age or later. The rate of progressive, symmetric (on both sides of the body) muscle atrophy and weakness varies greatly among affected individuals. Many individuals are able to walk until they are in their mid-thirties or later, while others are unable to walk past their teens. Some affected individuals never need to use a wheelchair. As in Duchenne MD, muscle weakness in Becker MD is typically noticed first in the upper arms and shoulders, upper legs, and pelvis.

Early symptoms of Becker MD include walking on one's toes, frequent falls, and difficulty rising from the floor. Calf muscles may appear large and healthy as deteriorating muscle fibers are replaced by fat, and muscle activity may cause cramps in some people. Cardiac complications are not as consistently present in Becker MD compared to Duchenne MD, but may be as severe in some cases. Cognitive and behavioral impairments are not as common or severe as in Duchenne MD, but they do occur.

Congenital MD refers to a group of autosomal recessive muscular dystrophies that are either present at birth or become evident before age 2. They affect both boys and girls. The degree and progression of muscle weakness and degeneration vary with the type of disorder. Weakness may be first noted when children fail to meet landmarks in motor function and muscle control. Muscle degeneration may be mild or severe and is restricted primarily to skeletal muscle. The majority of individuals are unable to sit or stand without support, and some affected children may never learn to walk. There are three groups of congenital MD:

- merosin-negative disorders, where the protein merosin (found in the connective tissue that surrounds muscle fibers) is missing;
- merosin-positive disorders, in which merosin is present but other needed proteins are missing; and
- neuronal migration disorders, in which very early in the development of the fetal nervous system the migration of nerve cells (neurons) to their proper location is disrupted.

Defects in the protein merosin cause nearly half of all cases of congenital MD.

People with congenital MD may develop contractures (chronic shortening of muscles or tendons around joints, which prevents the joints from moving freely), scoliosis, respiratory and swallowing difficulties, and foot deformities. Some individuals have normal intellectual development while others become severely impaired. Weakness in diaphragm muscles may lead to respiratory failure. Congenital MD may also affect the central nervous system, causing vision and speech problems, seizures, and structural changes in the brain. Some children with the disorders die in infancy while others may live into adulthood with only minimal disability.

Distal MD, also called distal myopathy, describes a group of at least six specific muscle diseases that primarily affect distal muscles (those farthest away from the shoulders and hips) in the forearms, hands, lower legs, and feet. Distal dystrophies are typically less severe, progress more slowly, and involve fewer muscles than other forms of MD, although they can spread to other muscles, including the proximal ones later in the course of the disease. Distal MD can affect the heart and respiratory muscles, and individuals may eventually require the use of a ventilator. Affected individuals may not be able to perform fine hand movement and have difficulty extending the fingers. As leg muscles become affected, walking and climbing stairs become difficult and some people may be unable to hop or stand on their heels. Onset of distal MD, which affects both men and women, is typically between the ages of 40 and 60 years. In one form of distal MD, a muscle membrane protein complex called dysferlin is known to be lacking.

Although distal MD is primarily an autosomal dominant disorder, autosomal recessive forms have been reported in young adults. Symptoms are similar to those of Duchenne MD but with a different pattern of muscle damage. An infantile-onset form of autosomal recessive distal MD has also been reported. Slow but progressive weakness is often first noticed around age 1, when the child begins to walk, and continues to progress very slowly throughout adult life.

Emery-Dreifuss MD primarily affects boys. The disorder has two forms: one is X-linked recessive and the other is autosomal dominant.

Onset of Emery-Dreifuss MD is usually apparent by age 10, but symptoms can appear as late as the mid-twenties. This disease causes slow but progressive wasting of the upper arm and lower leg muscles and symmetric weakness. Contractures in the spine, ankles, knees, elbows, and back of the neck usually precede significant muscle weakness, which is less severe than in Duchenne MD. Contractures may cause elbows to become locked in a flexed position. The entire spine may become rigid as the disease progresses. Other symptoms include shoulder deterioration, toe-walking, and mild facial weakness. Serum creatine kinase levels may be moderately elevated. Nearly all people with Emery-Dreifuss MD have some form of heart problem by age 30, often requiring a pacemaker or other assistive device. Female carriers of the disorder often have cardiac complications without muscle weakness. Affected individuals often die in mid-adulthood from progressive pulmonary or cardiac failure. In some cases, the cardiac symptoms may be the earliest and most significant symptom of the disease, and may appear years before muscle weakness does.

Facioscapulohumeral MD (FSHD) initially affects muscles of the face (facio), shoulders (scapulo), and upper arms (humera) with progressive weakness. Also known as Landouzy-Dejerine disease, this third most common form of MD is an autosomal dominant disorder. Most individuals have a normal life span, but some individuals become severely disabled. Disease progression is typically very slow, with intermittent spurts of rapid muscle deterioration. Onset is usually in the teenage years but may occur as early as childhood or as late as age 40. One hallmark of FSHD is that it commonly causes asymmetric weakness. Muscles around the eyes and mouth are often affected first, followed by weakness around the shoulders, chest, and upper arms. A particular pattern of muscle wasting causes the shoulders to appear to be slanted and the shoulder blades to appear winged. Muscles in the lower extremities may also become weakened. Reflexes are diminished, typically in the same distribution as the weakness. Changes in facial appearance may include the development of a crooked smile, a pouting look, flattened facial features, or a mask-like appearance. Some individuals cannot pucker their lips or whistle and may have difficulty swallowing, chewing, or speaking. In some individuals, muscle weakness can spread to the diaphragm, causing respiratory problems. Other symptoms may include hearing loss (particularly at high frequencies) and lordosis, an abnormal swayback curve in the spine. Contractures are rare. Some people with FSHD feel severe pain in the affected limb. Cardiac muscles are not usually affected, and significant weakness of the pelvic girdle is less common than in other forms of MD. An infant-onset form of FSHD can also cause retinal disease and some hearing loss.

Limb-girdle MD (LGMD) refers to more than 20 inherited conditions marked by progressive loss of muscle bulk and symmetrical weakening of voluntary muscles, primarily those in the shoulders and around the hips. At least 5 forms of autosomal dominant limb-girdle MD (known as type 1) and 17 forms of autosomal recessive limb-girdle MD (known as type 2) have been identified. Some autosomal recessive forms of the disorder are now known to be due to a deficiency of any of four dystrophin-glycoprotein complex proteins called the sarcoglycans. Deficiencies in dystroglycan, classically associated with congenital muscular dystrophies, may also cause LGMD.

The recessive LGMDs occur more frequently than the dominant forms, usually begin in childhood or the teenage years, and show dramatically increased levels of serum creatine kinase. The dominant LGMDs usually begin in adulthood. In general, the earlier the clinical signs appear, the more rapid the rate of disease progression. Limb-girdle MD affects both males and females. Some forms of the disease progress rapidly, resulting in serious muscle damage and loss of the ability to walk, while others advance very slowly over many years and cause minimal disability, allowing a normal life expectancy. In some cases, the disorder appears to halt temporarily, but progression then resumes.

The pattern of muscle weakness is similar to that of Duchenne MD and Becker MD. Weakness is typically noticed first around the hips before spreading to the shoulders, legs, and neck. Individuals develop a waddling gait and have difficulty when rising from chairs, climbing stairs, or carrying heavy objects. They fall frequently and are unable to run. Contractures at the elbows and knees are rare but individuals may develop contractures in the back muscles, which gives them the appearance of a rigid spine. Proximal reflexes (closest to the center of the body) are often impaired. Some individuals also experience cardiomyopathy and respiratory complications, depending in part on the specific subtype. Intelligence remains normal in most cases, though exceptions do occur. Many individuals with limb-girdle MD become severely disabled within 20 years of disease onset.

Myotonic dystrophy (DM1), also known as Steinert disease and dystrophia myotonica, is another common form of MD. Myotonia, or an inability to relax muscles following a sudden contraction, is found only in this form of MD, but is also found in other non-dystrophic muscle diseases. People with DM1 can live a long life, with variable but slowly progressive disability. Typical disease onset is between ages 20 and 30, but childhood onset and congenital onset are well-documented. Muscles in the face and the front of the neck are usually first to show weakness and may produce a haggard, "hatchet" face and a thin, swan-like neck. Wasting and weakness noticeably affect forearm muscles. DM1 affects the central nervous system and other body systems, including the heart, adrenal glands and thyroid, eyes, and gastrointestinal tract. Other symptoms include cardiac complications, difficulty swallowing, droopy eyelids (called ptosis), cataracts, poor vision, early frontal baldness, weight loss, impotence, testicular atrophy, mild mental impairment, and increased sweating. Individuals may also feel drowsy and have an excess need to sleep. There is a second form of the disease that is similar to the classic form, but usually affects proximal muscles more significantly. This form is known as myotonic dystrophy type 2 (DM2).

This autosomal dominant disease affects both men and women. Females may have irregular menstrual periods and are sometimes infertile. The disease may occur earlier and be more severe in successive generations. A childhood-onset form of myotonic MD may become apparent between ages 5 and 10. Symptoms include general muscle weakness (particularly in the face and distal muscles), lack of muscle tone, and mental impairment.

A woman with DM1 can give birth to an infant with a rare congenital form of the disorder. Symptoms at birth may include difficulty swallowing or sucking, impaired breathing, absence of reflexes, skeletal deformities and contractures (such as club feet), and muscle weakness, especially in the face. Children with congenital myotonic MD may also experience mental impairment and delayed motor development. This severe infantile form of myotonic MD occurs almost exclusively in children who have inherited the defective gene from their mother, whose symptoms may be so mild that she is sometimes not aware that she has the disease until she has an affected child.

The inherited gene defect that causes DM1 is an abnormally long repetition of a three-letter “word” in the genetic code. In unaffected people, the word is repeated a number of times, but in people with DM1, it is repeated many more times. This triplet repeat gets longer with each successive generation. The triplet repeat mechanism has now been implicated in at least 15 other disorders, including Huntington’s disease and the spinocerebellar ataxias.

Oculopharyngeal MD (OPMD) generally begins in a person’s forties or fifties and affects both men and women. In the United States, the disease is most common in families of French-Canadian descent and among Hispanic residents of northern New Mexico. People first report drooping eyelids, followed by weakness in the facial muscles and pharyngeal muscles in the throat, causing difficulty swallowing. The tongue may atrophy and changes to the voice may occur. Eyelids may droop so dramatically that some individuals compensate by tilting back their heads. Affected individuals may have double vision and problems with upper gaze, and others may have retinitis pigmentosa (progressive degeneration of the retina that affects night vision and peripheral vision) and cardiac irregularities. Muscle weakness and wasting in the neck and shoulder region is common. Limb muscles may also be affected. Persons with OPMD may find it difficult to walk, climb stairs, kneel, or bend. Those persons most severely affected will eventually lose the ability to walk.

How Are the Muscular Dystrophies Treated?

There is no specific treatment that can stop or reverse the progression of any form of MD. All forms of MD are genetic and cannot be prevented at this time, aside from the use of prenatal screening interventions. However, available treatments are aimed at keeping the person independent for as long as possible and prevent complications that result from weakness, reduced mobility, and cardiac and respiratory difficulties. Treatment may involve a combination of approaches, including physical therapy, drug therapy, and surgery. The available treatments are sometimes quite effective and can have a significant impact on life expectancy and quality of life.

What Is the Prognosis?

The prognosis varies according to the type of MD and the speed of progression. Some types are mild and progress very slowly, allowing normal life expectancy, while others are more severe and result in functional disability and loss of ambulation. Life expectancy often depends on the degree of muscle weakness, as well as the presence and severity of respiratory and/or cardiac complications.

Section 26.9

Tendon Injuries: Osgood-Schlatter Disease and Jumper's Knee

This section contains text excerpted from the following sources: Text beginning with the heading "Osgood-Schlatter Disease" is excerpted from "Questions and Answers about Knee Problems," National Institute of Arthritis and Musculoskeletal and Skin Diseases (NIAMS), March 2016; Text under the heading "Tendons and Tendinitis" is excerpted from "Tendinitis," MedlinePlus, U.S. Department of Health and Human Services (HHS), August 2, 2014; Text beginning with the heading "Knee Tendinitis or Jumper's Knee" is excerpted from "What Are Bursitis and Tendinitis?" National Institute of Arthritis and Musculoskeletal and Skin Diseases (NIAMS), November 1, 2014.

Osgood-Schlatter Disease

Osgood-Schlatter disease is a condition caused by repetitive stress or tension on part of the growth area of the upper tibia (the apophysis). It is characterized by inflammation of the patellar tendon and surrounding soft tissues at the point where the tendon attaches to the tibia. The disease may also be associated with an injury in which the tendon is stretched so much that it tears away from the tibia and takes a fragment of bone with it. The disease most commonly affects active young people, particularly boys between the ages of 10 and 15, who play games or sports that include frequent running and jumping.

Symptoms

People with this disease experience pain just below the knee joint that usually worsens with activity and is relieved by rest. A bony bump that is particularly painful when pressed may appear on the upper edge of the tibia (below the kneecap). Usually, the motion of the knee is not affected. Pain may last a few months and may recur until the child's growth is completed.

Diagnosis

Osgood-Schlatter disease is most often diagnosed by the symptoms. An X-ray may be normal, or show an injury, or, more typically, show that the growth area is in fragments.

Treatment

Osgood-Schlatter disease is temporary and the pain usually goes away without treatment. Applying ice to the knee when pain begins helps relieve inflammation and is sometimes used along with stretching and strengthening exercises. The doctor may advise you to limit participation in vigorous sports. Children who wish to continue moderate or less stressful sports activities may need to wear knee pads for protection and apply ice to the knee after activity. If there is a great deal of pain, sports activities may be limited until the discomfort becomes tolerable.

Tendons and Tendinitis

Tendons are flexible bands of tissue that connect muscles to bones. They help your muscles move your bones. Tendinitis is the severe swelling of a tendon.

Tendinitis usually happens after repeated injury to an area such as the wrist or ankle. It causes pain and soreness around a joint. Some common forms of tendinitis are named after the sports that increase their risk. They include tennis elbow, golfer's elbow, pitcher's shoulder, swimmer's shoulder, and jumper's knee. Doctors diagnose tendinitis with your medical history, a physical exam, and imaging tests.

Knee Tendinitis or Jumper's Knee

If you overuse a tendon during activities such as dancing, bicycling, or running, it may become stretched, torn, and swollen. Trying to break a fall can also damage tendons around the kneecap. This type of injury often happens to older people whose tendons may be weaker and less flexible. Pain in the tendons around the knee is sometimes called jumper's knee. This is because it often happens to young people who play sports like basketball. The overuse of the muscles and force of hitting the ground after a jump can strain the tendon. After repeated stress from jumping, the tendon may swell or tear.

People with tendinitis of the knee may feel pain while running, jumping, or walking quickly. Knee tendinitis can increase the risk for large tears to the tendon.

Treatment for Tendinitis

The focus of treatment is to heal the injured tendon. The first step is to reduce pain and swelling. This can be done with rest, tightly wrapping or elevating the affected area, or taking drugs that bring down the swelling. Aspirin, naproxen, and ibuprofen all serve that purpose. Ice may be helpful in recent, severe injuries, but is of little or no use in long-term cases. When ice is needed, an ice pack can be held on the affected area for 15 to 20 minutes every 4 to 6 hours for 3 to 5 days. A healthcare provider may suggest longer use of ice and a stretching program. Your healthcare provider may also suggest limiting activities that involve the affected joint.

Other treatments may include:

- Ultrasound, which are gentle sound-wave vibrations that warm deep tissues and improve blood flow
- An electrical current that pushes a corticosteroid drug through the skin directly over the swollen bursa or tendon
- Gentle stretching and strengthening exercises
- Massage of the soft tissue

If there is no improvement, your doctor may inject a drug into the area around the swollen bursa or tendon. If the joint still does not improve after 6 to 12 months, the doctor may perform surgery to repair damage and relieve pressure on the tendons.

Section 26.10

Upper and Lower Limb Reduction Defects

This section includes text excerpted from "Facts about Upper and Lower Limb Reduction Defects," Centers for Disease Control and Prevention (CDC), July 18, 2016.

Facts about Upper and Lower Limb Reduction Defects

Upper and lower limb reduction defects occur when a part of or the entire arm (upper limb) or leg (lower limb) of a fetus fails to form completely during pregnancy. The defect is referred to as a "limb reduction" because a limb is reduced from its normal size or is missing.

How Often Does Limb Reduction Defects Occur?

Centers for Disease Control and Prevention (CDC) estimates that each year about 1,500 babies in the United States are born with upper limb reductions and about 750 are born with lower limb reductions. In other words, each year about 4 out of every 10,000 babies will have upper limb reductions and about 2 out of every 10,000 babies will have lower limb reductions. Some of these babies will have both upper and lower limb reduction defects.

What Problems Do Children with Limb Reduction Defects Have?

Babies and children with limb reduction defects will face various issues and difficulties, but the extent of these will depend on the location and size of the reduction. Some potential difficulties and problems include:

- Difficulties with normal development such as motor skills
- Needing assistance with daily activities such as self-care
- Limitations with certain movements, sports, or activities
- Potential emotional and social issues because of physical appearance

Specific treatment for limb reduction defects will be determined by the child's doctor, based on things like the child's age, the extent and type of defect, and the child's tolerance for certain medications, procedures, and therapies.

The overall goal for treatment of limb reduction defects is to provide the child with a limb that has proper function and appearance. Treatment can vary for each child. Potential treatments include:

- Prosthetics (artificial limbs)
- Orthotics (splints or braces)
- Surgery
- Rehabilitation (physical or occupational therapy)

It is important to remember that some babies and children with limb reductions will have some difficulties and limitations throughout life, but with proper treatment and care they can live long, healthy, and productive lives.

What Causes Limb Reduction Defects?

The cause of limb reduction defects is unknown. However, research has shown that certain behaviors or exposures during pregnancy can increase the risk of having a baby with a limb reduction defect. These include:

- Exposure of the mother to certain chemicals or viruses while she is pregnant
- Exposure of the mother to certain medications
- Possible exposure of the mother to tobacco smoking (although more research is needed)

CDC works with many researchers to study risk factors that can increase the chance of having a baby with limb reduction defects, as well as outcomes of babies with the defect. Following are examples of what this research has found:

- A woman taking multivitamins before she gets pregnant might decrease her risk for having a baby with limb reduction defects, although more research is needed.
- Certain sets of limb reduction defects might be associated with other birth defects, such as heart defects, omphalocele, and gastroschisis.

Can Limb Reduction Defects Be Prevented?

There is no known way to prevent this type of defect, but some of the problems experienced later in life by a person born with a limb reduction defect can be prevented or screened if the defect is treated early.

Even so, mothers can take steps before and during pregnancy to have a healthy pregnancy. Steps include taking a daily multivitamin with folic acid (400 micrograms), not smoking, and not drinking alcohol during pregnancy.

Section 26.11

Scoliosis

This section includes text excerpted from "Scoliosis in Children and Adolescents," National Institute of Arthritis and Musculoskeletal and Skin Diseases (NIAMS), December 2015.

What Is Scoliosis?

Scoliosis is a musculoskeletal disorder in which there is a sideways curvature of the spine, or backbone. The bones that make up the spine are called vertebrae. Some people who have scoliosis require treatment. Other people, who have milder curves, may need to visit their doctor for periodic observation only.

Who Gets Scoliosis?

People of all ages can have scoliosis, but this publication focuses on children and adolescents. Adolescent idiopathic scoliosis (scoliosis of unknown cause) is the most common type and typically occurs after the age of 10. Girls are more likely than boys to have this type of scoliosis. Because scoliosis can run in families, a child who has a parent, brother, or sister with idiopathic scoliosis should be checked regularly for scoliosis by the family doctor.

What Causes Scoliosis?

In most cases, the cause of scoliosis is unknown; this is called idiopathic scoliosis. Before concluding that a person has idiopathic scoliosis, the doctor looks for other possible causes, such as injury or infection. Causes of curves are classified as either nonstructural or structural.

- **Nonstructural (functional) scoliosis.** A structurally normal spine that appears curved. This is a temporary, changing curve. It is caused by an underlying condition such as a difference in leg length, muscle spasms, or inflammatory conditions such as appendicitis. Doctors treat this type of scoliosis by correcting the underlying problem.
- **Structural scoliosis.** A fixed curve that doctors treat case by case. Sometimes structural scoliosis is one part of a syndrome or disease, such as Marfan syndrome, an inherited connective tissue disorder. In other cases, it occurs by itself. Structural scoliosis can be caused by neuromuscular diseases (such as cerebral palsy, poliomyelitis, or muscular dystrophy), birth defects (such as hemivertebra, in which one side of a vertebra fails to form normally before birth), injury, certain infections, tumors (such as those caused by neurofibromatosis, a birth defect sometimes associated with benign tumors on the spinal column), metabolic diseases, connective tissue disorders, rheumatic diseases, or unknown factors (idiopathic scoliosis).

How Is Scoliosis Diagnosed?

Doctors take the following steps to evaluate patients for scoliosis:

- **Medical history.** The doctor talks to the patient and the patient's parent(s) and reviews the patient's records to look for medical problems that might be causing the spine to curve, for example, birth defects, trauma, or other disorders that can be associated with scoliosis.
- **Physical examination.** The doctor looks at the patient's back, chest, pelvis, legs, feet, and skin. The doctor checks if the patient's shoulders are level, whether the head is centered, and whether opposite sides of the body look level. The doctor also examines the back muscles while the patient is bending forward to see if one side of the rib cage is higher than the other.

- **X-ray evaluation.** An X-ray of the spine can confirm the diagnosis of scoliosis. The doctor measures the curve on the X-ray image. He or she finds the vertebrae at the beginning and end of the curve and measures the angle of the curve.

Doctors group curves of the spine by their location, shape, pattern, and cause. They use this information to decide how best to treat the scoliosis.

Location. To identify a curve's location, doctors find the apex of the curve (the vertebra within the curve that is the most off-center); the location of the apex is the "location" of the curve. A thoracic curve has its apex in the thoracic area (the part of the spine to which the ribs attach). A lumbar curve has its apex in the lower back. A thoracolumbar curve has its apex where the thoracic and lumbar vertebrae join.

Shape. The curve usually is s- or c-shaped.

Pattern. Curves frequently follow patterns that have been studied in previous patients. The larger the curve is, the more likely it will progress(depending on the amount of growth remaining).

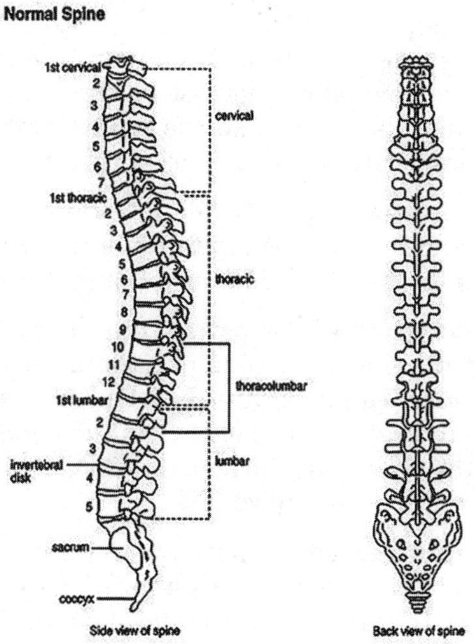

Figure 26.1. *Normal Spine*

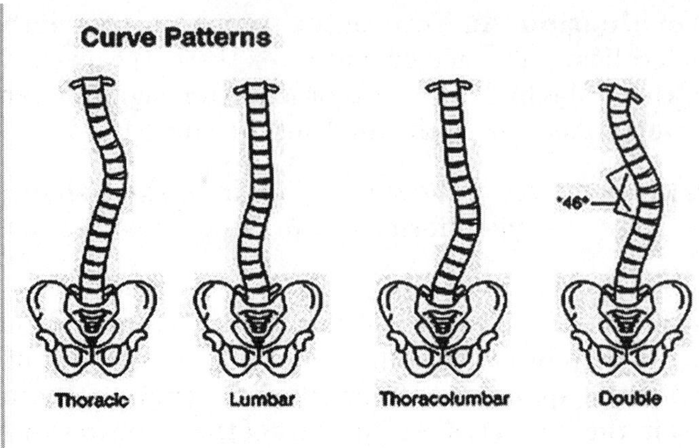

Figure 26.2. *Curved Spine*

Does Scoliosis Have to Be Treated? What Are the Treatments?

Many children who are sent to the doctor by a school scoliosis screening program have very mild spinal curves that do not need treatment. When treatment is needed, the doctor may send the child to an orthopaedic spine specialist.

The doctor will suggest the best treatment for each patient based on the patient's age, how much more he or she is likely to grow, the degree and pattern of the curve, and the type of scoliosis. The doctor may recommend observation, bracing, or surgery.

- **Observation.** Doctors typically follow patients without treatment and re-examine them every few months when the patient is still growing (is skeletally immature) and the curve is mild.
- **Bracing.** Doctors may advise patients to wear a brace to stop a curve from getting any worse in patients who are still growing with moderate spinal curvature. As a child nears the end of growth, the indications for bracing will depend on how the curve affects the child's appearance, whether the curve is getting worse, and the size of the curve.
- **Surgery.** Doctors may advise patients to have surgery to correct a curve or stop it from worsening when the patient is still growing, has a curve that is severe, and has a curve that is getting worse.

Chapter 27

Neurological Disorders in Children

Chapter Contents

Section 27.1

Brain Tumors

This section includes text excerpted from "Childhood Brain and Spinal Cord Tumors Treatment Overview (PDQ®)—Patient Version," National Cancer Institute (NCI), August 26, 2016.

What Is a Childhood Brain or Spinal Cord Tumor?

A childhood brain or spinal cord tumor is a disease in which abnormal cells form in the tissues of the brain or spinal cord.

Types of Childhood Brain and Spinal Cord Tumors

There are many types of childhood brain and spinal cord tumors. The tumors are formed by the abnormal growth of cells and may begin in different areas of the brain or spinal cord.

The tumors may be benign (not cancer) or malignant (cancer). Benign brain tumors grow and press on nearby areas of the brain. They rarely spread into other tissues. Malignant brain tumors are likely to grow quickly and spread into other brain tissue. When a tumor grows into or presses on an area of the brain, it may stop that part of the brain from working the way it should. Both benign and malignant brain tumors can cause signs or symptoms and need treatment.

Signs and Symptoms of Childhood Brain and Spinal Cord Tumors

Signs and symptoms depend on the following:

- Where the tumor forms in the brain or spinal cord.
- The size of the tumor.
- How fast the tumor grows.
- The child's age and development.

Signs and symptoms may be caused by childhood brain and spinal cord tumors or by other conditions, including cancer that has spread to the brain. Check with your child's doctor if your child has any of the following:

Brain Tumor Signs and Symptoms

- Morning headache or headache that goes away after vomiting.
- Frequent nausea and vomiting.
- Vision, hearing, and speech problems.
- Loss of balance and trouble walking.
- Unusual sleepiness or change in activity level.
- Unusual changes in personality or behavior.
- Seizures.
- Increase in the head size (in infants).

Spinal Cord Tumor Signs and Symptoms

- Back pain or pain that spreads from the back towards the arms or legs.
- A change in bowel habits or trouble urinating.
- Weakness in the legs.
- Trouble walking.

In addition to these signs and symptoms of brain and spinal cord tumors, some children are unable to reach certain growth and development milestones such as sitting up, walking, and talking in sentences.

Tests to Detect (Find) Childhood Brain and Spinal Cord Tumors

The following tests and procedures may be used:

- **Physical exam and history:** An exam of the body to check general signs of health, including checking for signs of disease, such as lumps or anything else that seems unusual. A history of the patient's health habits and past illnesses and treatments will also be taken.
- **Neurological exam:** A series of questions and tests to check the brain, spinal cord, and nerve function. The exam checks a

person's mental status, coordination, and ability to walk normally, and how well the muscles, senses, and reflexes work. This may also be called a neuro exam or a neurologic exam.

- **MRI (magnetic resonance imaging) with gadolinium:** A procedure that uses a magnet, radio waves, and a computer to make a series of detailed pictures of the brain and spinal cord. A substance called gadolinium is injected into a vein. The gadolinium collects around the cancer cells so they show up brighter in the picture. This procedure is also called nuclear magnetic resonance imaging (NMRI).
- **Serum tumor marker test:** A procedure in which a sample of blood is examined to measure the amounts of certain substances released into the blood by organs, tissues, or tumor cells in the body. Certain substances are linked to specific types of cancer when found in increased levels in the blood. These are called tumor markers.

Most childhood brain tumors are diagnosed and removed in surgery.

If doctors think there might be a brain tumor, a biopsy may be done to remove a sample of tissue. For tumors in the brain, the biopsy is done by removing part of the skull and using a needle to remove a sample of tissue. A pathologist views the tissue under a microscope to look for cancer cells. If cancer cells are found, the doctor may remove as much tumor as safely possible during the same surgery. The pathologist checks the cancer cells to find out the type and grade of brain tumor. The grade of the tumor is based on how abnormal the cancer cells look under a microscope and how quickly the tumor is likely to grow and spread.

Craniotomy: An opening is made in the skull and a piece of the skull is removed to show part of the brain.

The following test may be done on the sample of tissue that is removed:

- Immunohistochemistry: A test that uses antibodies to check for certain antigens in a sample of tissue. The antibody is usually linked to a radioactive substance or a dye that causes the tissue to light up under a microscope. This type of test may be used to tell the difference between different types of cancer.

Some childhood brain and spinal cord tumors are diagnosed by imaging tests.

Sometimes a biopsy or surgery cannot be done safely because of where the tumor formed in the brain or spinal cord. These tumors are diagnosed based on the results of imaging tests and other procedures.

Certain factors affect prognosis (chance of recovery).

The prognosis (chance of recovery) depends on the following:

- Whether there are any cancer cells left after surgery.
- The type of tumor.
- Where the tumor is in the body.
- The child's age.
- Whether the tumor has just been diagnosed or has recurred (come back).

Staging Childhood Brain and Spinal Cord Tumors

Staging is the process used to find how much cancer there is and if cancer has spread within the brain, spinal cord, or to other parts of the body. It is important to know the stage in order to plan cancer treatment.

In childhood brain and spinal cord tumors, there is no standard staging system. Instead, the plan for cancer treatment depends on several factors:

- The type of tumor and where the tumor formed in the brain.
- Whether the tumor is newly diagnosed or recurrent. A newly diagnosed brain or spinal cord tumor is one that has never been treated. A recurrent childhood brain or spinal cord tumor is one that has recurred (come back) after it has been treated. Childhood brain and spinal cord tumors may come back in the same place or in another part of the brain, or spinal cord. Sometimes they come back in another part of the body. The tumor may come back many years after first being treated. Tests and procedures, including biopsy, that were done to diagnose and stage the tumor may be done to find out if the tumor has recurred.
- The grade of the tumor. The grade of the tumor is based on how abnormal the cancer cells look under a microscope and how quickly the tumor is likely to grow and spread. It is important to know the grade of the tumor and if there were any cancer cells remaining after surgery in order to plan treatment. The grade of

the tumor is not used to plan treatment for all types of brain and spinal cord tumors.

- The tumor risk group. Risk groups are either average risk and poor risk or low, intermediate, and high risk. The risk groups are based on the amount of tumor remaining after surgery, the spread of cancer cells within the brain and spinal cord or to other parts of the body, where the tumor has formed, and the age of the child. The risk group is not used to plan treatment for all types of brain and spinal cord tumors.

Three Types of Standard Treatment Are Used

Surgery

Surgery may be used to diagnose and treat childhood brain and spinal cord tumors.

Radiation Therapy

Radiation therapy is a cancer treatment that uses high-energy X-rays or other types of radiation to kill cancer cells or keep them from growing. There are two types of radiation therapy:

- External radiation therapy uses a machine outside the body to send radiation toward the cancer.
- Internal radiation therapy uses a radioactive substance sealed in needles, seeds, wires, or catheters that are placed directly into or near the cancer.

The way the radiation therapy is given depends on the type of cancer being treated. External radiation therapy is used to treat childhood brain and spinal cord tumors.

Chemotherapy

Chemotherapy is a cancer treatment that uses drugs to stop the growth of cancer cells, either by killing the cells or by stopping them from dividing. When chemotherapy is taken by mouth or injected into a vein or muscle, the drugs enter the bloodstream and can reach cancer cells throughout the body (systemic chemotherapy). When chemotherapy is placed directly in the cerebrospinal fluid, an organ, or a body cavity such as the abdomen, the drugs mainly affect cancer cells in those areas (regional chemotherapy). The way the chemotherapy is given depends on the type and stage of the cancer being treated.

Anticancer drugs given by mouth or vein to treat brain and spinal cord tumors cannot cross the blood-brain barrier and enter the fluid that surrounds the brain and spinal cord. Instead, an anticancer drug is injected into the fluid-filled space to kill cancer cells there. This is called intrathecal chemotherapy.

New Types of Treatment Are Being Tested in Clinical Trials

This section describes treatments that are being studied in clinical trials. It may not mention every new treatment being studied.

High-Dose Chemotherapy with Stem Cell Transplant

High-dose chemotherapy with stem cell transplant is a way of giving high doses of chemotherapy and replacing blood forming cells destroyed by the cancer treatment. Stem cells (immature blood cells) are removed from the blood or bone marrow of the patient or a donor and are frozen and stored. After the chemotherapy is completed, the stored stem cells are thawed and given back to the patient through an infusion. These reinfused stem cells grow into (and restore) the body's blood cells.

Patients May Want to Think about Taking Part in a Clinical Trial

For some patients, taking part in a clinical trial may be the best treatment choice. Clinical trials are part of the cancer research process. Clinical trials are done to find out if new cancer treatments are safe and effective or better than the standard treatment.

Many of today's standard treatments for cancer are based on earlier clinical trials. Patients who take part in a clinical trial may receive the standard treatment or be among the first to receive a new treatment.

Patients who take part in clinical trials also help improve the way cancer will be treated in the future. Even when clinical trials do not lead to effective new treatments, they often answer important questions and help move research forward.

Patients Can Enter Clinical Trials before, during, or after Starting Their Cancer Treatment

Some clinical trials only include patients who have not yet received treatment. Other trials test treatments for patients whose cancer has not gotten better. There are also clinical trials that test new ways to stop cancer from recurring (coming back) or reduce the side effects of cancer treatment.

Clinical trials are taking place in many parts of the country.

Follow-Up Tests May Be Needed

Some of the tests that were done to diagnose the cancer or to find out the stage of the cancer may be repeated. Some tests will be repeated in order to see how well the treatment is working. Decisions about whether to continue, change, or stop treatment may be based on the results of these tests.

Some of the tests will continue to be done from time to time after treatment has ended. The results of these tests can show if your child's condition has changed or if the cancer has recurred (come back). These tests are sometimes called follow-up tests or check-ups.

Section 27.2

Cerebral Palsy

This section includes text excerpted from "Cerebral Palsy: Hope Through Research," National Institute of Neurological Disorders and Stroke (NINDS), March 15, 2016.

What Is Cerebral Palsy?

Cerebral palsy refers to a group of neurological disorders that appear in infancy or early childhood and permanently affect body movement and muscle coordination Cerebral palsy (CP) is caused by damage to or abnormalities inside the developing brain that disrupt the brain's ability to control movement and maintain posture and balance. The term cerebral refers to the brain; palsy refers to the loss or impairment of motor function.

Cerebral palsy affects the motor area of the brain's outer layer (called the cerebral cortex), the part of the brain that directs muscle movement.

In some cases, the cerebral motor cortex hasn't developed normally during fetal growth. In others, the damage is a result of injury to the brain either before, during, or after birth. In either case, the damage is not repairable and the disabilities that result are permanent.

Children with CP exhibit a wide variety of symptoms, including:

- lack of muscle coordination when performing voluntary movements (ataxia);
- stiff or tight muscles and exaggerated reflexes (spasticity);
- weakness in one or more arm or leg;
- walking on the toes, a crouched gait, or a "scissored" gait;
- variations in muscle tone, either too stiff or too floppy;
- excessive drooling or difficulties swallowing or speaking;
- shaking (tremor) or random involuntary movements;
- delays in reaching motor skill milestones; and
- difficulty with precise movements such as writing or buttoning a shirt.

The symptoms of CP differ in type and severity from one person to the next, and may even change in an individual over time. Symptoms may vary greatly among individuals, depending on which parts of the brain have been injured. All people with cerebral palsy have problems with movement and posture, and some also have some level of intellectual disability, seizures, and abnormal physical sensations or perceptions, as well as other medical disorders. People with CP also may have impaired vision or hearing, and language, and speech problems.

CP is the leading cause of childhood disabilities, but it doesn't always cause profound disabilities. While one child with severe CP might be unable to walk and need extensive, lifelong care, another child with mild CP might be only slightly awkward and require no special assistance. The disorder isn't progressive, meaning it doesn't get worse over time. However, as the child gets older, certain symptoms may become more or less evident.

A study by the Centers for Disease Control and Prevention shows the average prevalence of cerebral palsy is 3.3 children per 1,000 live births.

There is no cure for cerebral palsy, but supportive treatments, medications, and surgery can help many individuals improve their motor skills and ability to communicate with the world.

What Are the Early Signs?

The signs of cerebral palsy usually appear in the early months of life, although specific diagnosis may be delayed until age two years or later. Infants with CP frequently have developmental delay, in which they are slow to reach developmental milestones such as learning to roll over, sit, crawl, or walk. Some infants with CP have abnormal muscle tone. Decreased muscle tone (hypotonia) can make them appear relaxed, even floppy. Increased muscle tone (hypertonia) can make them seem stiff or rigid. In some cases, an early period of hypotonia will progress to hypertonia after the first 2 to 3 months of life. Children with CP may also have unusual posture or favor one side of the body when they reach, crawl, or move. It is important to note that some children without CP also might have some of these signs.

Some early warning signs:

In a Baby Younger than 6 Months of Age

- His head lags when you pick him up while he's lying on his back
- He feels stiff
- He feels floppy
- When you pick him up, his legs get stiff and they cross or scissor

In a Baby Older than 6 Months of Age

- She doesn't roll over in either direction
- She cannot bring her hands together
- She has difficulty bringing her hands to her mouth
- She reaches out with only one hand while keeping the other fisted

In a Baby Older than 10 Months of Age

- He crawls in a lopsided manner, pushing off with one hand and leg while dragging the opposite hand and leg
- He cannot stand holding onto support

What Causes Cerebral Palsy?

Cerebral palsy is caused by abnormal development of part of the brain or by damage to parts of the brain that control movement. This damage can occur before, during, or shortly after birth. The majority of children have congenital cerebral palsy CP (that is, they were born with it), although it may not be detected until months or years later. A small number of children have acquired cerebral palsy, which means the disorder begins after birth. Some causes of acquired cerebral palsy include brain damage in the first few months or years of life, brain infections such as bacterial meningitis or viral encephalitis, problems with blood flow to the brain, or head injury from a motor vehicle accident, a fall, or child abuse.

What Are the Risk Factors?

There are some medical conditions or events that can happen during pregnancy and delivery that may increase a baby's risk of being born with cerebral palsy. These risks include:

Low birthweight and premature birth. Premature babies (born less than 37 weeks into pregnancy) and babies weighing less than 5 ½ pounds at birth have a much higher risk of developing cerebral palsy than full-term, heavier weight babies. Tiny babies born at very early gestational ages are especially at risk.

Multiple births. Twins, triplets, and other multiple births—even those born at term—are linked to an increased risk of cerebral palsy. The death of a baby's twin or triplet further increases the risk.

Infections during pregnancy. Infections such as toxoplasmosis, rubella (German measles), cytomegalovirus, and herpes, can infect the womb and placenta. Inflammation triggered by infection may then go on to damage the developing nervous system in an unborn baby. Maternal fever during pregnancy or delivery can also set off this kind of inflammatory response.

Blood type incompatibility between mother and child. *Rh incompatibility* is a condition that develops when a mother's Rh blood type (either positive or negative) is different from the blood type of her baby. The mother's system doesn't tolerate the baby's different blood type and her body will begin to make antibodies that will attack and kill her baby's blood cells, which can cause brain damage.

Exposure to toxic substances. Mothers who have been exposed to toxic substances during pregnancy, such as methyl mercury, are at a heightened risk of having a baby with cerebral palsy.

Mothers with thyroid abnormalities, intellectual disability, excess protein in the urine, or seizures. Mothers with any of these conditions are slightly more likely to have a child with CP.

There are also medical conditions during labor and delivery, and immediately after delivery that act as warning signs for an increased risk of CP. However, most of these children will not develop CP. Warning signs include:

Breech presentation. Babies with cerebral palsy are more likely to be in a breech position (feet first) instead of head first at the beginning of labor. Babies who are unusually floppy as fetuses are more likely to be born in the breech position.

Complicated labor and delivery. A baby who has vascular or respiratory problems during labor and delivery may already have suffered brain damage or abnormalities.

Small for gestational age. Babies born smaller than normal for their gestational age are at risk for cerebral palsy because of factors that kept them from growing naturally in the womb.

Low *Apgar* score. The Apgar score is a numbered rating that reflects a newborn's physical health. Doctors periodically score a baby's heart rate, breathing, muscle tone, reflexes, and skin color during the first minutes after birth. A low score at 10–20 minutes after delivery is often considered an important sign of potential problems such as CP.

Jaundice. More than 50 percent of newborns develop jaundice (a yellowing of the skin or whites of the eyes) after birth when *bilirubin*, a substance normally found in bile, builds up faster than their livers can break it down and pass it from the body. Severe, untreated jaundice can kill brain cells and can cause deafness and CP.

Seizures. An infant who has seizures faces a higher risk of being diagnosed later in childhood with CP.

Can Cerebral Palsy Be Prevented?

Cerebral palsy related to genetic abnormalities cannot be prevented, but a few of the risk factors for congenital cerebral palsy can be managed or avoided. For example, *rubella*, or German measles, is preventable if women are vaccinated against the disease before becoming pregnant. Rh incompatibilities can also be managed early in pregnancy. Acquired cerebral palsy, often due to head injury, is often preventable using common safety tactics, such as using car seats for infants and toddlers.

What Are the Different Forms?

The specific forms of cerebral palsy are determined by the extent, type, and location of a child's abnormalities. Doctors classify CP according to the type of movement disorder involved—spastic (stiff muscles), athetoid (writhing movements), or ataxic (poor balance and coordination)—plus any additional symptoms, such weakness (paresis) or paralysis (plegia). For example, hemiparesis (hemi = half) indicates that only one side of the body is weakened. Quadriplegia (quad = four) means all four limbs are affected.

How Is Cerebral Palsy Diagnosed?

Most children with cerebral palsy are diagnosed during the first 2 years of life. But if a child's symptoms are mild, it can be difficult for a doctor to make a reliable diagnosis before the age of 4 or 5.

Doctors will order a series of tests to evaluate the child's motor skills. During regular visits, the doctor will monitor the child's development, growth, muscle tone, age-appropriate motor control, hearing and vision, posture, and coordination, in order to rule out other disorders that could cause similar symptoms. Although symptoms may change over time, CP is not progressive. If a child is continuously losing motor skills, the problem more likely is a condition other than CP—such as a genetic or muscle disease, metabolism disorder, or tumors in the nervous system.

Lab tests can identify other conditions that may cause symptoms similar to those associated with CP.

Neuroimaging techniques that allow doctors to look into the brain (such as an MRI scan) can detect abnormalities that indicate a potentially treatable movement disorder.

Another test, an **electroencephalogram,** uses a series of electrodes that are either taped or temporarily pasted to the scalp to detect electrical activity in the brain. Changes in the normal electrical pattern may help to identify epilepsy.

Some metabolic disorders can masquerade as CP. Most of the childhood metabolic disorders have characteristic brain abnormalities or malformations that will show up on an MRI.

How Is Cerebral Palsy Treated?

Cerebral palsy can't be cured, but treatment will often improve a child's capabilities. Many children go on to enjoy near-normal adult lives if their disabilities are properly managed. In general, the earlier treatment begins, the better chance children have of overcoming developmental disabilities or learning new ways to accomplish the tasks that challenge them.

There is no standard therapy that works for every individual with cerebral palsy. Once the diagnosis is made, and the type of CP is determined, a team of healthcare professionals will work with a child and his or her parents to identify specific impairments and needs, and then develop an appropriate plan to tackle the core disabilities that affect the child's quality of life.

Physical therapy, usually begun in the first few years of life or soon after the diagnosis is made, is a cornerstone of CP treatment. Specific sets of exercises (such as resistive, or strength training programs) and activities can maintain or improve muscle strength, balance, and motor skills, and prevent contractures. Special braces (called orthotic devices) may be used to improve mobility and stretch spastic muscles.

Occupational therapy focuses on optimizing upper body function, improving posture, and making the most of a child's mobility. Occupational therapists help individuals address new ways to meet everyday activities such as dressing, going to school, and participating in day-to-day activities.

Recreation therapy encourages participation in art and cultural programs, sports, and other events that help an individual expand physical and cognitive skills and abilities. Parents of children who participate in recreational therapies usually notice an improvement in their child's speech, self-esteem, and emotional well-being.

Speech and language therapy can improve a child's ability to speak, more clearly, help with swallowing disorders, and learn new ways to communicate—using sign language and/or special communication devices such as a computer with a voice synthesizer, or a special board covered with symbols of everyday objects and activities to which a child can point to indicate his or her wishes.

Treatments for problems with eating and drooling are often necessary when children with CP have difficulty eating and drinking because they have little control over the muscles that move their mouth, jaw, and tongue. They are also at risk for breathing food or fluid into the lungs, as well as for malnutrition, recurrent lung infections, and progressive lung disease.

Drug Treatments

Oral medications such as diazepam, baclofen, dantrolene sodium, and tizanidine are usually used as the first line of treatment to relax stiff, contracted, or overactive muscles. Some drugs have some risk side effects such as drowsiness, changes in blood pressure, and risk of liver damage that require continuous monitoring. Oral medications are most appropriate for children who need only mild reduction in muscle tone or who have widespread spasticity.

Botulinum toxin (BT-A), injected locally, has become a standard treatment for overactive muscles in children with spastic movement disorders such as CP. BT-A relaxes contracted muscles by keeping nerve cells from over-activating muscle. The relaxing effect of a BT-A injection lasts approximately 3 months. Undesirable side effects are mild and short-lived, consisting of pain upon injection and occasionally mild flu-like symptoms. BT-A injections are most effective when followed by a stretching program including physical therapy and splinting. BT-A injections work best for children who have some control over their motor movements and have a limited number of muscles to treat, none of which is fixed or rigid.

Intrathecal baclofen therapy uses an implantable pump to deliver baclofen, a muscle relaxant, into the fluid surrounding the spinal cord. Baclofen decreases the excitability of nerve cells in the spinal cord, which then reduces muscle spasticity throughout the body. The pump can be adjusted if muscle tone is worse at certain times of the day or night. The baclofen pump is most appropriate for individuals with chronic, severe stiffness or uncontrolled muscle movement throughout the body.

Surgery

Orthopedic surgery is often recommended when spasticity and stiffness are severe enough to make walking and moving about difficult or painful. For many people with CP, improving the appearance of how they walk – their gait – is also important. Surgeons can lengthen muscles and tendons that are proportionately too short, which can improve mobility and lessen pain. Tendon surgery may help the symptoms for some children with CP but could also have negative long-term consequences. Orthopedic surgeries may be staggered at times appropriate to a child's age and level of motor development. Surgery can also correct or greatly improve spinal deformities in people with CP. Surgery may not be indicated for all gait abnormalities and the surgeon may request a quantitative gait analysis before surgery.

Surgery to cut nerves. Selective dorsal rhizotomy (SDR) is a surgical procedure recommended for cases of severe spasticity when all of the more conservative treatments – physical therapy, oral medications, and intrathecal baclofen -- have failed to reduce spasticity or chronic pain. A surgeon locates and selectively severs overactivated nerves at the base of the spinal column. SDR is most commonly used to relax muscles and decrease chronic pain in one or both of the lower or upper limbs. It is also sometimes used to correct an overactive bladder. Potential side effects include sensory loss, numbness, or uncomfortable sensations in limb areas once supplied by the severed nerve.

Assistive devices

Assistive devices such devices as computers, computer software, voice synthesizers, and picture books can greatly help some individuals with CP improve communications skills. Other devices around the home or workplace make it easier for people with CP to adapt to activities of daily living.

Orthotic devices help to compensate for muscle imbalance and increase independent mobility. Braces and splints use external force to correct muscle abnormalities and improve function such as sitting or walking. Other orthotics help stretch muscles or the positioning of a joint. Braces, wedges, special chairs, and other devices can help people sit more comfortably and make it easier to perform daily functions. Wheelchairs, rolling walkers, and powered scooters can help individuals who are not independently mobile. Vision aids include glasses, magnifiers, and large-print books and computer typeface. Some individuals with CP may need surgery to correct vision problems. Hearing aids and telephone amplifiers may help people hear more clearly.

Complementary and Alternative Therapies

Many children and adolescents with CP use some form of complementary or alternative medicine. Controlled clinical trials involving some of the therapies have been inconclusive or showed no benefit and the therapies have not been accepted in mainstream clinical practice.

Although there are anecdotal reports of some benefit in some children with CP, these therapies have not been approved by the U.S. Food and Drug Administration for the treatment of CP. Such therapies include hyperbaric oxygen therapy, special clothing worn during resistance exercise training, certain forms of electrical stimulation, assisting children in completing certain motions several times a day, and specialized learning strategies. Also, dietary supplements, including herbal products, may interact with other products or medications a child with CP may be taking or have unwanted side effects on their own. Families of children with CP should discuss all therapies with their doctor.

Stem cell therapy is being investigated as a treatment for cerebral palsy, but research is in early stages and large-scale clinical trials are needed to learn if stem cell therapy is safe and effective in humans. Stem cells are capable of becoming other cell types in the body. Scientists are hopeful that stem cells may be able to repair damaged nerves and brain tissues. Studies in the U.S. are examining the safety and tolerability of umbilical cord blood stem cell infusion in children with CP.

Section 27.3

Epilepsy

This section includes text excerpted from "Epilepsy," Center for Parent Information and Resources (CPIR), July 2015.

Definition of Epilepsy

Epilepsy is a seizure disorder. According to the Epilepsy Foundation of America, a seizure happens when a brief, strong surge of electrical activity affects part or all of the brain. Seizures can last from a few seconds to a few minutes. They can have different symptoms, too, from convulsions and loss of consciousness, to signs such as blank staring, lip smacking, or jerking movements of arms and legs.

Some people can have a seizure and yet not have epilepsy. For example, many young children have convulsions from fevers. Other types of seizures not classified as epilepsy include those caused by an imbalance of body fluids or chemicals or by alcohol or drug withdrawal. Thus, a single seizure does not mean that the person has epilepsy. Generally speaking, the diagnosis of epilepsy is made when a person has two or more unprovoked seizures.

Incidence

About three million Americans have epilepsy. Of the 200,000 new cases diagnosed each year, nearly 45,000 are children and adolescents. Epilepsy affects people in all nations and of all races. Its incidence is greater in African American and socially disadvantaged populations.

Characteristics

Although the symptoms listed below do not necessarily mean that a person has epilepsy, it is wise to consult a doctor if you or a member of your family experiences one or more of them:

- "Blackouts" or periods of confused memory;
- Episodes of staring or unexplained periods of unresponsiveness;
- Involuntary movement of arms and legs;
- "Fainting spells" with incontinence or followed by excessive fatigue; or
- Odd sounds, distorted perceptions, or episodic feelings of fear that cannot be explained.

Doctors have described more than 30 different types of seizures. These are divided into two major categories—generalized seizures and partial seizures (also known as focal seizures).

Generalized Seizures: This type of seizure involves both sides of the brain from the beginning of the seizure. The best known subtype of generalized seizures is the grand mal seizure. In a grand mal seizure, the person's arms and legs stiffen (the tonic phase), and then begin to jerk (the clonic phase). That's why the grand mal seizure is also known as a generalized tonic clonic seizure.

Grand mal seizures typically last 1–2 minutes and are followed by a period of confusion and then deep sleep. The person will not remember what happened during the seizure.

You may also have heard of the petit mal seizure, which is an older term for another type of generalized seizure. It's now called an absence seizure, because during the seizure, the person stares blankly off into space and doesn't seem to be aware of his or her surroundings. The person may also blink rapidly and seem to chew. Absence seizures typically last from 2–15 seconds and may not be noticed by others. Afterwards, the person will resume whatever he or she was doing at the time of the seizure, without any memory of the event.

Partial Seizures: Partial seizures are so named because they involve only one hemisphere of the brain. They may be simple partial seizures (in which the person jerks and may have odd sensations and perceptions, but doesn't lose consciousness) or complex partial seizures (in which consciousness is impaired or lost). Complex partial seizures often involve periods of "automatic behavior" and altered consciousness. This is typified by purposeful-looking behavior, such as buttoning or unbuttoning a shirt. Such behavior, however, is unconscious, may be repetitive, and is usually not remembered afterwards.

Diagnosis

Diagnosing epilepsy is a multi-step process. According to the Epilepsy Foundation of America:

"...the doctor's main tool...is a careful medical history with as much information as possible about what the seizures looked like and what happened just before they began. The doctor will also perform a thorough physical examination, especially of the nervous system, as well as analysis of blood and other bodily fluids."

The doctor may also order an electroencephalograph (EEG) of the patient's brain activity, which may show patterns that help the doctor decide whether or not someone has epilepsy. Other tests may also be used—such as the computerized tomography (CT) or magnetic resonance imaging (MRI)—in order to look for any growths, scars, or other physical conditions in the brain that may be causing the seizures. Which tests and how many of them are ordered may vary, depending on how much each test reveals.

Treatment

Anti-epileptic medication is the most common treatment for epilepsy. It's effective in stopping seizures in 70% of patients. Interestingly, it's not uncommon for doctors to wait a while before prescribing an anti-seizure medication, especially if the patient is a young child. Unless the EEG of the patient's brain is clearly abnormal, doctors may suggest waiting until a second or even third seizure occurs. Why? Because studies show that an otherwise normal child who has had a single seizure has a relatively low (15%) risk of a second one.

When anti-epileptic medications are not effective in stopping a person's seizures, other treatment options may be discussed. These include:

- surgery to remove the areas of the brain that are producing the seizures;
- stimulation of the vagus nerve (a large nerve in the neck), where short bursts of electrical energy are directed into the brain via the vagus nerve; and
- a ketogenic diet (one that is very high in fats and low in carbohydrates), which makes the body burn fat for energy instead of glucose.

According to the Epilepsy Foundation of America, 10% of new patients cannot bring their seizures disorder under control despite optimal medical management.

Educational and Developmental Considerations

It's not unusual for seizures to interfere with a child's development and learning. For example, if a student has the type of seizure characterized by periods of fixed staring, he or she is likely to miss parts of what the teacher is saying. If teachers—or other caregivers such as babysitters, daycare providers, preschool teachers, K-12 personnel—observe such an episode, it's important that they document and report it promptly to parents (and the school nurse, if appropriate).

Because epilepsy can affect a child's learning and development (even babies), families will want to learn more about the systems of help that are available. Much of that help comes from the nation's special education law, the Individuals with Disabilities Education Act (IDEA), which makes available these two sets of services:

- **Early intervention:** A system of services to help infants and toddlers with disabilities (before their 3rd birthday) and their families.
- **Special education and related services:** Services available through the public school system for school-aged children, including preschoolers (ages 3–21).

In both of these systems, eligible children receive special services designed to address the developmental, functional, and educational needs resulting from their disability.

To access early intervention services for a child up to his or her 3rd birthday, ask your child's pediatrician for a referral. You can also call the local hospital's maternity ward or pediatric ward, and ask for the contact information of the local early intervention program.

To access special education services for a school-aged child, get in touch with your local public school system. Calling the elementary school in your neighborhood is an excellent place to start. Ask to have your child evaluated to see if he or she is eligible for services.

Section 27.4

Headache

This section includes text excerpted from "Headache: Hope Through Research," National Institute of Neurological Disorders and Stroke (NINDS), August 5, 2016.

Children and Headache

Headaches are common in children. Headaches that begin early in life can develop into migraines as the child grows older. Migraines in children or adolescents can develop into tension-type headaches at any time. In contrast to adults with migraine, young children often feel migraine pain on both sides of the head and have headaches that usually last less than 2 hours. Children may look pale and appear restless or irritable before and during an attack. Other children may become nauseous, lose their appetite, or feel pain elsewhere in the body during the headache.

Headaches in children can be caused by a number of factors, including emotional problems such as tension between family members, stress from school activities, weather changes, irregular eating and sleep, dehydration, and certain foods and drinks. Of special concern among children are headaches that occur after head injury or those accompanied by rash, fever, or sleepiness.

It may be difficult to identify the type of headache because children often have problems describing where it hurts, how often the headaches occur, and how long they last. Asking a child with a headache to draw a picture of where the pain is and how it feels can make it easier for the doctor to determine the proper treatment.

Migraine in particular is often misdiagnosed in children. Parents and caretakers sometimes have to be detectives to help determine that a child has migraine. Clues to watch for include sensitivity to light and noise, which may be suspected when a child refuses to watch television or use the computer, or when the child stops playing to lie down in a dark room. Observe whether or not a child is able to eat during a headache. Very young children may seem cranky or irritable and complain of abdominal pain (abdominal migraine).

Headache treatment in children and teens usually includes rest, fluids, and over-the-counter pain relief medicines. The U.S. Food and Drug Administration (FDA) has approved the drug almotriptan as a treatment for migraine pain in children age 12 and older, and the drug topiramate for migraine prevention in children ages 12 to 17. Always consult with a physician before giving headache medicines to a child. Most tension-type headaches in children can be treated with over-the-counter medicines that are marked for children with usage guidelines based on the child's age and weight. Headaches in some children may also be treated effectively using relaxation/behavioral therapy. Children with cluster headache may be treated with oxygen therapy early in the initial phase of the attacks.

A variety of headache education and drug and/or behavioral management approaches are now under development to improve headache treatment and prevention in children and adolescents. In 2015 the National Institute of Neurological Disorders and Stroke launched a project to develop a phone app to help pre-teen and adolescent children better manage their headaches by creating and following a headache log, monitoring medications, and noting changes they can share with their healthcare practitioner.

Why Headaches Hurt

Information about touch, pain, temperature, and vibration in the head and neck is sent to the brain by the trigeminal nerve, one of the 12 cranial nerves that start at the base of the brain.

The nerve has three branches that relay sensations from the scalp, the blood vessels inside and outside of the skull, the lining around the brain (the meninges), and the face, mouth, neck, ears, eyes, and throat.

Brain tissue itself lacks pain-sensitive nerves and does not feel pain. Headaches occur when pain-sensitive nerve endings called nociceptors are activated in response to things that may bring on a headache (such as stress, certain foods or odors, or use of medicines). The nociceptors send messages through the trigeminal nerve to the brain stem and then to the thalamus, the brain's "relay station" for pain sensation from all over the body, and then onto the parts of the cortex (the brain's outer layer) involved in sensory and emotional processing. Other parts of the brain may also be part of the process, causing nausea, vomiting, diarrhea, trouble concentrating, and other neurological symptoms.

When to See a Doctor

Not all headaches require a physician's attention. People who experience uncontrolled recurring headaches, however, should be seen by a doctor. This is even more important in children. Most headaches are benign, but headaches can signal a more serious disorder that requires prompt medical care. Immediately call or see a physician if you or someone you're with experience any of these symptoms:

- Very sudden, severe headache that may be accompanied by a stiff neck.
- Severe headache accompanied by fever, nausea, or vomiting that is not related to another illness.
- Sudden "worst" headache, often accompanied by confusion, weakness, double vision, or loss of consciousness (called a "thunderclap" headache because it occurs suddenly and severely).
- Headache that worsens over days or weeks or has changed in pattern or behavior.
- Headache following a head injury.
- Headache occurring with a loss of sensation or weakness in any part of the body, which could be a sign of a stroke.
- Headache associated with convulsions.
- Headache associated with shortness of breath.
- New onset of two or more headaches a week.
- Persistent headache in someone who has been previously headache-free, particularly someone over age 50.

- New headaches in someone with a history of cancer immune suppression or human immunodeficiency virus (HIV)/ Acquired immune deficiency syndrome (AIDS).
- Headache that occurs with upright position and goes away when lying flat.

Diagnosing Your Headache

The circumstances under which a person experiences a headache can be key to diagnosing its cause. Keeping a headache journal can help a physician better diagnose your type of headache and determine the best treatment. After each headache, note the time of day when it occurred; its intensity and duration; any increased sensitivity to light, sound, or odors; nausea or vomiting; activity immediately prior to the headache; use of prescription and nonprescription over-the-counter medicines; amount of sleep the previous night; any stressful or emotional conditions; any influence from weather or daily activity; foods and fluids consumed in the past 24 hours; and any known health conditions at that time. Women should record the days of their menstrual cycles. Include notes about other family members who have a history of headache or other disorder. A pattern may emerge that can be helpful to reducing or preventing headaches.

Once the doctor has reviewed the individual's medical and headache history and conducted a physical and neurological exam, lab screening and diagnostic tests can help rule out or identify conditions that might be the cause of the headaches. Blood tests and urinalysis can diagnose brain or spinal cord infections, blood vessel damage, and toxins that affect the nervous system. Testing a sample of the fluid that surrounds the brain and spinal cord (obtained through a procedure called a lumbar puncture) can detect infections, bleeding in the brain (called a brain hemorrhage), and measure any buildup of pressure within the skull. Diagnostic imaging, such as with computed tomography (CT) and magnetic resonance imaging (MRI), can detect irregularities in blood vessels and bones, certain brain tumors and cysts, brain damage from head injury, brain hemorrhage, inflammation, infection, and other disorders. Neuroimaging also gives research doctors a way to see what's happening in the brain during headache attacks. An electroencephalogram (EEG) measures brain wave activity and can help diagnose brain tumors, seizures, head injury, and inflammation that may lead to headaches.

Headache Types and Their Treatment

The International Classification of Headache Disorders, published by the International Headache Society, is used to classify more than 150 types of primary and secondary headache disorders. The major types are discussed below.

Primary Headache Disorders, including Migraine

Primary headaches occur independently and are not caused by another medical condition. It's uncertain what sets the process of a primary headache in motion. A cascade of events that affect blood vessels and nerves inside and outside the head sends pain signals to the brain. Brain chemicals and inflammatory molecules are involved in creating head pain, as are changes in nerve cell activity (called cortical spreading depression in the case of migraine headaches).

Primary headache disorders are divided into four main groups: migraine, tension-type headache, cluster headache and trigeminal autonomic cephalgias (a group of short-lasting but severe headaches), and a miscellaneous group.

Migraine

If you suffer from migraine headaches, you're not alone. About 12 percent of the United States population experience migraines, one form of *vascular* headaches. Migraine headaches are characterized by a buildup of throbbing and pulsating pain caused by the activation of nerve fibers within the wall of brain blood vessels of the meninges. Migraine headaches are recurrent attacks of moderate to severe pain that is throbbing or pulsing and often strikes one side of the head. Untreated attacks last from 4 to 72 hours. Other common symptoms are increased sensitivity to light, noise, and odor; as well as nausea and vomiting. Routine physical activity, movement, or even coughing or sneezing can worsen migraine pain.

Migraines occur most frequently in the morning, especially upon waking. Some people have migraines at predictable times, such as before menstruation or on weekends following a stressful week of work. Many people feel exhausted or weak following a migraine but are usually symptom-free between attacks.

A number of factors can increase the risk of having a migraine and trigger the headache process. Although migraine triggers vary from person to person and include sudden changes in weather or environment, too much or not enough sleep, strong odors or fumes, emotion, stress, overexertion, loud or sudden noises, motion sickness, low blood sugar, skipped meals, tobacco, depression, anxiety, head trauma, hangover, some medications, hormonal changes, and bright or flashing lights. Overusing analgesic medication or missing doses of preventive medications may also cause headaches. In some 50 percent of migraine sufferers, foods or ingredients can induce headaches. These include aspartame, caffeine (or caffeine withdrawal), wine and other types of alcohol, chocolate, aged cheeses, monosodium glutamate, some fruits and nuts, fermented or pickled goods, yeast, and cured or processed meats. Keeping a diet journal can help identify food triggers.

Who Gets Migraines?

Migraines occur in both children and adults, but affect adult women three times more often than men (perhaps due to hormonal triggers). There is evidence that migraines are genetic, with most migraine sufferers having a family history of the disorder. They also frequently occur in people who have other medical conditions. Depression, anxiety, bipolar disorder, sleep disorders, and epilepsy are more common in individuals with migraine than in the general population. Migraine sufferers—in particular those individuals who have pre-migraine symptoms referred to as aura—have a slightly increased risk of having a stroke.

Migraine in women often relates to changes in hormones. The headaches may begin at the start of the first menstrual cycle or during pregnancy. Most women see improvement after menopause, although surgical removal of the ovaries usually worsens migraines. Women with migraine who take oral contraceptives may experience changes in the frequency and severity of attacks, while women who do not suffer from headaches may develop migraines as a side effect of oral contraceptives.

Phases of Migraine

A migraine is divided into four phases, all of which may or may not be present during the attack:

- Premonitory symptoms occur up to 48 hours prior to developing a migraine. These include food cravings, unexplained mood changes (depression or euphoria), uncontrollable yawning, fluid retention, or increased urination.

- Aura. Some people will see flashing or bright lights or what looks like heat waves 10–12 minutes prior to or during the migraine, while others may experience muscle weakness or the sensation of being touched or grabbed.
- Headache. Headache pain usually starts gradually and builds in intensity. It is associated with increased sensitivity to light and/or noise. It is possible, however, to have migraine without a headache.
- Postdrome (following the headache). Individuals are often exhausted or confused following a migraine. The postdrome period may last up to a day before people feel healthy.

Types of Migraine

The two major types of migraine are:

Migraine with aura, previously called classic migraine, includes visual disturbances and other neurological symptoms that appear about 10 to 60 minutes before the actual headache and usually last no more than an hour. Individuals may temporarily lose part or all of their vision. Other classic symptoms include trouble speaking; an abnormal sensation, numbness, or muscle weakness on one side of the body; a tingling sensation in the hands or face, and confusion. Nausea, vertigo, loss of appetite, and increased sensitivity to light, sound, or noise may precede the headache.

Migraine without aura, or common migraine, is the more frequent form of migraine. Symptoms include headache pain that occurs without warning and is usually felt on one side of the head, along with fatigue and associated symptoms seem in classic migraine.

Section 27.5

Neurofibromatosis

This section includes text excerpted from "Neurofibromatosis Fact Sheet," National Institute of Neurological Disorders and Stroke (NINDS), February 3, 2016.

What Are the Neurofibromatoses?

The neurofibromatoses are a group of three genetically distinct disorders that cause tumors to grow in the nervous system. Tumors begin in the supporting cells that make up the nerve and the myelin sheath (the thin membrane that envelops and protects the nerves), rather than the cells that actually transmit information. The type of tumor that develops depends on the type of supporting cells involved.

Scientists have classified the disorders as neurofibromatosis type 1 (NF1, also called von Recklinghaus disease), neurofibromatosis type 2 (NF2), and a type that was once considered to be a variation of NF2 but is now called schwannomatosis. An estimated 100,000 Americans have a neurofibromatosis disorder, which occurs in both sexes and in all races and ethnic groups.

The most common nerve-associated tumors in NF1 are neurofibromas (tumors of the peripheral nerves), whereas schwannomas (tumors that begin in Schwann cells that help form the myelin sheath) are most common in NF2 and schwannomatosis. Most tumors are benign, although occasionally they may become cancerous.

Why these tumors occur still isn't completely known, but it appears to be related mainly to mutations in genes that play key roles in suppressing cell growth in the nervous system. These mutations keep the genes—identified as NF1, NF2 and *SMARCB1/INI1*—from making normal proteins that control cell production. Without the normal function of these proteins, cells multiply out of control and form tumors.

What Is NF1?

NF1 is the most common neurofibromatosis, occurring in 1 in 3,000 to 4,000 individuals in the United States. Although many affected people inherit the disorder, between 30 and 50 percent of new cases result from a spontaneous genetic mutation of unknown cause. Once this mutation has taken place, the mutant gene can be passed to succeeding generations.

What Are the Signs and Symptoms of NF1?

To diagnose NF1, a doctor looks for two or more of the following:

- six or more light brown spots on the skin (often called "café-au-lait" spots), measuring more than 5 millimeters in diameter in children or more than 15 millimeters across in adolescents and adults;
- two or more neurofibromas, or one plexiform neurofibroma (a neurofibroma that involves many nerves);
- freckling in the area of the armpit or the groin;
- two or more growths on the iris of the eye (known as Lisch nodules or iris hamartomas);
- a tumor on the optic nerve (called an optic nerve glioma)
- abnormal development of the spine (scoliosis), the temple (sphenoid) bone of the skull, or the tibia (one of the long bones of the shin);
- a parent, sibling, or child with NF1.

What Other Symptoms or Conditions Are Associated with NF1?

Many children with NF1 have larger than normal head circumference and are shorter than average. Hydrocephalus, the abnormal buildup of fluid in the brain, is a possible complication of the disorder. Headache and epilepsy are also more likely in individuals with NF1 than in the healthy population. Cardiovascular complications associated with NF1 include congenital heart defects, high blood pressure (hypertension), and constricted, blocked, or damaged blood vessels (vasculopathy). Children with NF1 may have poor language and visual-spatial skills, and perform less well on academic achievement tests, including those that measure reading, spelling, and math skills. Learning disabilities, such as attention deficit hyperactivity disorder (ADHD), are common in children with NF1. An estimated 3 to 5 percent of tumors may become cancerous, requiring aggressive treatment. These tumors are called malignant peripheral nerve sheath tumors.

When Do Symptoms Appear?

Symptoms, particularly the most common skin abnormalities-café-au-lait spots, neurofibromas, Lisch nodules, and freckling in the armpit and groin-are often evident at birth or shortly afterwards, and almost always by the time a child is 10 years old. Because many features of these disorders are age dependent, a definitive diagnosis may take several years.

What Is the Prognosis for Someone with NF1?

NF1 is a progressive disorder, which means most symptoms will worsen over time, although a small number of people may have symptoms that remain constant. It isn't possible to predict the course of an individual's disorder. In general, most people with NF1 will develop mild to moderate symptoms. Most people with NF1 have a normal life expectancy. Neurofibromas on or under the skin can increase with age and cause cosmetic and psychological issues.

How Is NF1 Treated?

Scientists don't know how to prevent neurofibromas from growing. Surgery is often recommended to remove tumors that become symptomatic and may become cancerous, as well as for tumors that cause significant cosmetic disfigurement. Several surgical options exist, but there is no general agreement among doctors about when surgery should be performed or which surgical option is best. Individuals considering surgery should carefully weigh the risks and benefits of all their options to determine which treatment is right for them. Treatment for neurofibromas that become malignant may include surgery, radiation, or chemotherapy. Surgery, radiation and/or chemotherapy may also be used to control or reduce the size of optic nerve gliomas when vision is threatened. Some bone malformations, such as scoliosis, can be corrected surgically.

Treatments for other conditions associated with NF1 are aimed at controlling or relieving symptoms. Headache and seizures are treated with medications. Since children with NF1 have a higher than average risk for learning disabilities, they should undergo a detailed neurological exam before they enter school. Once these children are in school, teachers or parents who suspect there is evidence of one or more learning disabilities should request an evaluation that includes an IQ test and the standard range of tests to evaluate verbal and spatial skills.

What Is NF2?

This rare disorder affects about 1 in 25,000 people. Approximately 50 percent of affected people inherit the disorder; in others the disorder is caused by a spontaneous genetic mutation of unknown cause. The hallmark finding in NF2 is the presence of slow-growing tumors on the eighth cranial nerves. These nerves have two branches: the acoustic branch helps people hear by transmitting sound sensations to the brain; and the vestibular branch helps people maintain their balance. The characteristic tumors of NF2 are called vestibular schwannomas because of their location and the types of cells involved. As these tumors grow, they may press against and damage nearby structures such as other cranial nerves and the brain stem, the latter which can cause serious disability. Schwannomas in NF2 may occur along any nerve in the body, including the spinal nerves, other cranial nerves, and peripheral nerves in the body. These tumors may be seen as bumps under the skin (when the nerves involved are just under the skin surface) or can also be seen on the skin surface as small (less than 1 inch), dark, rough areas of hairy skin. In children, tumors may be smoother, less pigmented, and less hairy.

Although individuals with NF2 may have schwannomas that resemble small, flesh-colored skin flaps, they rarely have the café-au-lait spots that are seen in NF1.

Individuals with NF2 are at risk for developing other types of nervous system tumors, such as ependymomas and gliomas (two tumor types that grow in the spinal cord) and meningiomas (tumors that grow along the protective layers surrounding the brain and spinal cord). Affected individuals may develop cataracts at an earlier age or changes in the retina that may affect vision. Individuals with NF2 may also develop problems with nerve function independent of tumors, usually symmetric numbness and weakness in the extremities, due to the development of a peripheral neuropathy.

What Are the Signs and Symptoms of NF2?

To diagnose NF2, a doctor looks for the following:

- bilateral vestibular schwannomas; or
- a family history of NF2 (parent, sibling, or child) plus a unilateral vestibular schwannoma before age 30; or
- any two of the following:
- glioma;

- meningioma,
- schwannoma; or
- juvenile posterior subcapsular/lenticular opacity (cataract) or juvenile cortical cataract.

When Do Symptoms Appear?

Signs of NF2 may be present in childhood but are so subtle that they can be overlooked, especially in children who don't have a family history of the disorder. Typically, symptoms of NF2 are noticed between 18 and 22 years of age. The most frequent first symptom is hearing loss or ringing in the ears (tinnitus). Less often, the first visit to a doctor will be because of disturbances in balance, visual impairment (such as vision loss from cataracts), weakness in an arm or leg, seizures, or skin tumors.

What Is the Prognosis for Someone with NF2?

Because NF2 is so rare, few studies have been done to look at the natural progression of the disorder. The course of NF2 varies greatly among individuals, although inherited NF2 appears to run a similar course among affected family members. Generally, vestibular schwannomas grow slowly, and balance and hearing deteriorate over a period of years. A recent study suggests that an earlier age of onset and the presence of meningiomas are associated with greater mortality risk.

How Is NF2 Treated?

NF2 is best managed at a specialty clinic with an initial screening and annual follow-up evaluations (more frequent if the disease is severe). Improved diagnostic technologies, such as magnetic resonance imaging (MRI), can reveal tumors of the vestibular nerve as small as a few millimeters in diameter. Vestibular schwannomas grow slowly, but they can grow large enough to engulf one of the eighth cranial nerves and cause brain stem compression and damage to surrounding cranial nerves. Surgical options depend on tumor size and the extent of hearing loss. There is no general agreement among doctors about when surgery should be performed or which surgical option is best. Individuals considering surgery should carefully weigh the risks and benefits of all options to determine which treatment is right for them. Surgery to remove the entire tumor while it's still small might help preserve hearing. If hearing is lost during this surgery, but the auditory nerve is maintained, the surgical placement of a cochlear implant (a device placed in the inner ear, or cochlea, that processes electronic signals from sound waves to the auditory nerve) may be an option to improve hearing. As tumors grow larger, it becomes harder to surgically preserve hearing and the auditory nerve. The development of the penetrating auditory brain stem implant (a device that stimulates the hearing portions of the brain) can restore some hearing in individuals who have completely lost hearing and do not have an auditory nerve present. Surgery for other tumors associated with NF2 is aimed at controlling or relieving symptoms. Surgery also can correct cataracts and retinal abnormalities.

Are There Prenatal Tests for the Neurofibromatoses?

Clinical genetic testing can confirm the presence of a mutation in the NF1 gene. Prenatal testing for the NF1 mutation is also possible using amniocentesis or chorionic villus sampling procedures. Genetic testing for the NF2 mutation is sometimes available, but is accurate only in about 65 percent of those individuals tested. Prenatal or genetic testing for schwannomatosis currently does not exist.

Section 27.6

Tourette Syndrome

This section includes text excerpted from "Tourette Syndrome Fact Sheet," National Institute of Neurological Disorders and Stroke (NINDS), April 16, 2014.

What Is Tourette Syndrome?

Tourette syndrome (TS) is a neurological disorder characterized by repetitive, stereotyped, involuntary movements and vocalizations called tics. The disorder is named for Dr. Georges Gilles de la Tourette, the pioneering French neurologist who in 1885 first described the condition in an 86-year-old French noblewoman.

The early symptoms of TS are typically noticed first in childhood, with the average onset between the ages of 3 and 9 years. TS occurs in people from all ethnic groups; males are affected about three to four times more often than females. It is estimated that 200,000 Americans have the most severe form of TS, and as many as one in 100 exhibit milder and less complex symptoms such as chronic motor or vocal tics. Although TS can be a chronic condition with symptoms lasting a lifetime, most people with the condition experience their worst tic symptoms in their early teens, with improvement occurring in the late teens and continuing into adulthood.

What Are the Symptoms?

Tics are classified as either simple or complex. Simple motor tics are sudden, brief, repetitive movements that involve a limited number of muscle groups. Some of the more common simple tics include eye blinking and other eye movements, facial grimacing, shoulder shrugging, and head or shoulder jerking. Simple vocalizations might include repetitive throat-clearing, sniffing, or grunting sounds. Complex tics are distinct, coordinated patterns of movements involving several muscle groups. Complex motor tics might include facial grimacing combined with a head twist and a shoulder shrug. Other complex motor tics may actually appear purposeful, including sniffing or touching objects, hopping, jumping, bending, or twisting. Simple vocal tics may include throat-clearing, sniffing/snorting, grunting, or barking. More complex vocal tics include words or phrases. Perhaps the most dramatic and disabling tics include motor movements that result in self-harm such as punching oneself in the face or vocal tics including coprolalia (uttering socially inappropriate words such as swearing) or echolalia (repeating the words or phrases of others). However, coprolalia is only present in a small number (10 to 15 percent) of individuals with TS. Some tics are preceded by an urge or sensation in the affected muscle group, commonly called a premonitory urge. Some with TS will describe a need to complete a tic in a certain way or a certain number of times in order to relieve the urge or decrease the sensation.

Tics are often worse with excitement or anxiety and better during calm, focused activities. Certain physical experiences can trigger or worsen tics, for example tight collars may trigger neck tics, or hearing another person sniff or throat-clear may trigger similar sounds. Tics do not go away during sleep but are often significantly diminished.

What Is the Course of TS?

Tics come and go over time, varying in type, frequency, location, and severity. The first symptoms usually occur in the head and neck area and may progress to include muscles of the trunk and extremities. Motor tics generally precede the development of vocal tics and simple tics often precede complex tics. Most patients experience peak tic severity before the mid-teen years with improvement for the majority of patients in the late teen years and early adulthood. Approximately 10–15 percent of those affected have a progressive or disabling course that lasts into adulthood.

Can People with TS Control Their Tics?

Although the symptoms of TS are involuntary, some people can sometimes suppress, camouflage, or otherwise manage their tics in an effort to minimize their impact on functioning. However, people with TS often report a substantial buildup in tension when suppressing their tics to the point where they feel that the tic must be expressed (against their will). Tics in response to an environmental trigger can appear to be voluntary or purposeful but are not.

What Causes TS?

Although the cause of TS is unknown, current research points to abnormalities in certain brain regions (including the basal ganglia, frontal lobes, and cortex), the circuits that interconnect these regions, and the neurotransmitters (dopamine, serotonin, and norepinephrine) responsible for communication among nerve cells. Given the often complex presentation of TS, the cause of the disorder is likely to be equally complex.

What Disorders Are Associated with TS?

Many individuals with TS experience additional neurobehavioral problems that often cause more impairment than the tics themselves. These include inattention, hyperactivity and impulsivity attention deficit hyperactivity disorder (ADHD); problems with reading, writing, and arithmetic; and obsessive-compulsive symptoms such as intrusive thoughts/worries and repetitive behaviors. For example, worries about dirt and germs may be associated with repetitive hand-washing, and concerns about bad things happening may be associated with ritualistic behaviors such as counting, repeating, or ordering and arranging.

People with TS have also reported problems with depression or anxiety disorders, as well as other difficulties with living, that may or may not be directly related to TS. In addition, although most individuals with TS experience a significant decline in motor and vocal tics in late adolescence and early adulthood, the associated neurobehavioral conditions may persist. Given the range of potential complications, people with TS are best served by receiving medical care that provides a comprehensive treatment plan.

How Is TS Diagnosed?

TS is a diagnosis that doctors make after verifying that the patient has had both motor and vocal tics for at least 1 year. The existence of other neurological or psychiatric conditions can also help doctors arrive at a diagnosis. Common tics are not often misdiagnosed by knowledgeable clinicians. However, atypical symptoms or atypical presentations (for example, onset of symptoms in adulthood) may require specific specialty expertise for diagnosis. There are no blood, laboratory, or imaging tests needed for diagnosis. In rare cases, neuroimaging studies, such as magnetic resonance imaging (MRI) or computerized tomography (CT), electroencephalogram (EEG) studies, or certain blood tests may be used to rule out other conditions that might be confused with TS when the history or clinical examination is atypical.

It is not uncommon for patients to obtain a formal diagnosis of TS only after symptoms have been present for some time. The reasons for this are many. For families and physicians unfamiliar with TS, mild and even moderate tic symptoms may be considered inconsequential, part of a developmental phase, or the result of another condition. For example, parents may think that eye blinking is related to vision problems or that sniffing is related to seasonal allergies. Many patients are self-diagnosed after they, their parents, other relatives, or friends read or hear about TS from others.

How Is TS Treated?

Because tic symptoms often do not cause impairment, the majority of people with TS require no medication for tic suppression. However, effective medications are available for those whose symptoms interfere with functioning. Neuroleptics (drugs that may be used to treat psychotic and non-psychotic disorders) are the most consistently useful medications for tic suppression; a number are available but some are more effective than others (for example, haloperidol and pimozide).

Unfortunately, there is no one medication that is helpful to all people with TS, nor does any medication completely eliminate symptoms. In addition, all medications have side effects. Many neuroleptic side effects can be managed by initiating treatment slowly and reducing the dose when side effects occur. The most common side effects of neuroleptics include sedation, weight gain, and cognitive dulling. Neurological side effects such as tremor, dystonic reactions (twisting movements or postures), parkinsonian-like symptoms, and other dyskinetic (involuntary) movements are less common and are readily managed with dose reduction.

Discontinuing neuroleptics after long-term use must be done slowly to avoid rebound increases in tics and withdrawal dyskinesias. One form of dyskinesia called tardive dyskinesia is a movement disorder distinct from TS that may result from the chronic use of neuroleptics. The risk of this side effect can be reduced by using lower doses of neuroleptics for shorter periods of time.

Other medications may also be useful for reducing tic severity, but most have not been as extensively studied or shown to be as consistently useful as neuroleptics. Additional medications with demonstrated efficacy include alpha-adrenergic agonists such as clonidine and guanfacine. These medications are used primarily for hypertension but are also used in the treatment of tics. The most common side effect from these medications that precludes their use is sedation. However, given the lower side effect risk associated with these medications, they are often used as first-line agents before proceeding to treatment with neuroleptics.

Effective medications are also available to treat some of the associated neurobehavioral disorders that can occur in patients with TS. Recent research shows that stimulant medications such as methylphenidate and dextroamphetamine can lessen ADHD symptoms in people with TS without causing tics to become more severe. However, the product labeling for stimulants currently contraindicates the use of these drugs in children with tics/TS and those with a family history of tics. Scientists hope that future studies will include a thorough discussion of the risks and benefits of stimulants in those with TS or a family history of TS and will clarify this issue. For obsessive-compulsive symptoms that significantly disrupt daily functioning, the serotonin reuptake inhibitors (clomipramine, fluoxetine, fluvoxamine, paroxetine, and sertraline) have been proven effective in some patients.

Behavioral treatments such as awareness training and competing response training can also be used to reduce tics. A recent National Institutes of Health (NIH)-funded, multi-center randomized control trial called Cognitive Behavioral Intervention for Tics, or CBIT, showed that training to voluntarily move in response to a premonitory urge can reduce tic symptoms. Other behavioral therapies, such as biofeedback or supportive therapy, have not been shown to reduce tic symptoms. However, supportive therapy can help a person with TS better cope with the disorder and deal with the secondary social and emotional problems that sometimes occur.

Is TS Inherited?

Evidence from twin and family studies suggests that TS is an inherited disorder. Although early family studies suggested an autosomal dominant mode of inheritance (an autosomal dominant disorder is one in which only one copy of the defective gene, inherited from one parent, is necessary to produce the disorder), more recent studies suggest that the pattern of inheritance is much more complex. Although there may be a few genes with substantial effects, it is also possible that many genes with smaller effects and environmental factors may play a role in the development of TS.

Genetic studies also suggest that some forms of attention deficit hyperactivity disorder (ADHD) and obsessive-compulsive behaviors (OCD) are genetically related to TS, but there is less evidence for a genetic relationship between TS and other neurobehavioral problems that commonly co-occur with TS. It is important for families to understand that genetic predisposition may not necessarily result in full-blown TS; instead, it may express itself as a milder tic disorder or as obsessive-compulsive behaviors. It is also possible that the gene-carrying offspring will not develop any TS symptoms.

The gender of the person also plays an important role in TS gene expression. At-risk males are more likely to have tics and at-risk females are more likely to have obsessive-compulsive symptoms.

Genetic counseling of individuals with TS should include a full review of all potentially hereditary conditions in the family.

What Is the Prognosis?

Although there is no cure for TS, the condition in many individuals improves in the late teens and early 20s. As a result, some may actually become symptom-free or no longer need medication for tic suppression. Although the disorder is generally lifelong and chronic, it is not a degenerative condition. Individuals with TS have a normal life expectancy. TS does not impair intelligence. Although tic symptoms tend to decrease with age, it is possible that neurobehavioral disorders such as ADHD, OCD, depression, generalized anxiety, panic attacks, and mood swings can persist and cause impairment in adult life.

What Is the Best Educational Setting for Children with TS?

Although students with TS often function well in the regular classroom, ADHD, learning disabilities, obsessive-compulsive symptoms, and frequent tics can greatly interfere with academic performance or social adjustment. After a comprehensive assessment, students should be placed in an educational setting that meets their individual needs. Students may require tutoring, smaller or special classes, and in some cases special schools.

All students with TS need a tolerant and compassionate setting that both encourages them to work to their full potential and is flexible enough to accommodate their special needs. This setting may include a private study area, exams outside the regular classroom, or even oral exams when the child's symptoms interfere with his or her ability to write. Untimed testing reduces stress for students with TS.

Chapter 28

Respiratory and Lung Conditions in Children

Chapter Contents

Section 28.1

Asthma

This section includes text excerpted from "What Is Asthma?" National Heart, Lung, and Blood Institute (NHLBI), August 4, 2014.

What Is Asthma?

Asthma is a chronic (long-term) lung disease that inflames and narrows the airways. Asthma causes recurring periods of wheezing (a whistling sound when you breathe), chest tightness, shortness of breath, and coughing. The coughing often occurs at night or early in the morning.

Asthma affects people of all ages, but it most often starts during childhood. In the United States, more than 25 million people are known to have asthma. About 7 million of these people are children.

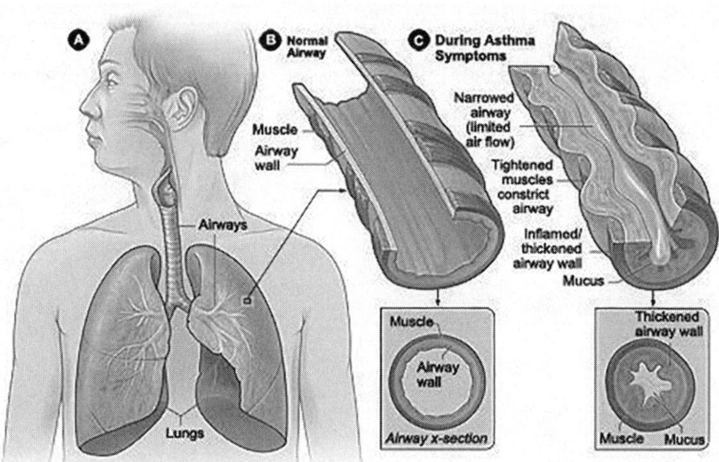

Figure 28.1. *Asthma*

Figure A shows the location of the lungs and airways in the body. Figure B shows a cross-section of a normal airway. Figure C shows a cross-section of an airway during asthma symptoms.

What Causes Asthma?

The exact cause of asthma isn't known. Researchers think some genetic and environmental factors interact to cause asthma, most often early in life. These factors include:

- An inherited tendency to develop allergies, called atopy
- Parents who have asthma
- Certain respiratory infections during childhood
- Contact with some airborne allergens or exposure to some viral infections in infancy or in early childhood when the immune system is developing

If asthma or atopy runs in your family, exposure to irritants (for example, tobacco smoke) may make your airways more reactive to substances in the air.

Some factors may be more likely to cause asthma in some people than in others. Researchers continue to explore what causes asthma.

The "Hygiene Hypothesis"

One theory researchers have for what causes asthma is the "hygiene hypothesis." They believe that our Western lifestyle—with its emphasis on hygiene and sanitation—has resulted in changes in our living conditions and an overall decline in infections in early childhood.

Many young children no longer have the same types of environmental exposures and infections as children did in the past. This affects the way that young children's immune systems develop during very early childhood, and it may increase their risk for atopy and asthma. This is especially true for children who have close family members with one or both of these conditions.

Who Is at Risk for Asthma?

Asthma affects people of all ages, but it most often starts during childhood. In the United States, more than 22 million people are known to have asthma. Nearly 6 million of these people are children.

Young children who often wheeze and have respiratory infections—as well as certain other risk factors—are at highest risk of developing asthma that continues beyond 6 years of age. The other risk factors include having allergies, eczema (an allergic skin condition), or parents who have asthma.

Among children, more boys have asthma than girls. But among adults, more women have the disease than men. It's not clear whether or how sex and sex hormones play a role in causing asthma.

Most, but not all, people who have asthma have allergies.

Some people develop asthma because of contact with certain chemical irritants or industrial dusts in the workplace. This type of asthma is called occupational asthma.

What Are the Signs and Symptoms of Asthma?

Common signs and symptoms of asthma include:

- Coughing. Coughing from asthma often is worse at night or early in the morning, making it hard to sleep.
- Wheezing. Wheezing is a whistling or squeaky sound that occurs when you breathe.
- Chest tightness. This may feel like something is squeezing or sitting on your chest.
- Shortness of breath. Some people who have asthma say they can't catch their breath or they feel out of breath. You may feel like you can't get air out of your lungs.

Not all people who have asthma have these symptoms. Likewise, having these symptoms doesn't always mean that you have asthma. The best way to diagnose asthma for certain is to use a lung function test, a medical history (including type and frequency of symptoms), and a physical exam.

The types of asthma symptoms you have, how often they occur, and how severe they are may vary over time. Sometimes your symptoms may just annoy you. Other times, they may be troublesome enough to limit your daily routine.

Severe symptoms can be fatal. It's important to treat symptoms when you first notice them so they don't become severe.

With proper treatment, most people who have asthma can expect to have few, if any, symptoms either during the day or at night.

How Is Asthma Diagnosed?

Your primary care doctor will diagnose asthma based on your medical and family histories, a physical exam, and test results.

Your doctor also will figure out the severity of your asthma—that is, whether it's intermittent, mild, moderate, or severe. The level of severity will determine what treatment you'll start on.

You may need to see an asthma specialist if:

- You need special tests to help diagnose asthma
- You've had a life-threatening asthma attack
- You need more than one kind of medicine or higher doses of medicine to control your asthma, or if you have overall problems getting your asthma well controlled
- You're thinking about getting allergy treatments

Diagnosing Asthma in Young Children

Most children who have asthma develop their first symptoms before 5 years of age. However, asthma in young children (aged 0 to 5 years) can be hard to diagnose.

Sometimes it's hard to tell whether a child has asthma or another childhood condition. This is because the symptoms of asthma also occur with other conditions.

Also, many young children who wheeze when they get colds or respiratory infections don't go on to have asthma after they're 6 years old.

A child may wheeze because he or she has small airways that become even narrower during colds or respiratory infections. The airways grow as the child grows older, so wheezing no longer occurs when the child gets colds.

A young child who has frequent wheezing with colds or respiratory infections is more likely to have asthma if:

- One or both parents have asthma
- The child has signs of allergies, including the allergic skin condition eczema
- The child has allergic reactions to pollens or other airborne allergens
- The child wheezes even when he or she doesn't have a cold or other infection

The most certain way to diagnose asthma is with a lung function test, a medical history, and a physical exam. However, it's hard to do lung function tests in children younger than 5 years. Thus, doctors must rely on children's medical histories, signs and symptoms, and physical exams to make a diagnosis.

Doctors also may use a 4–6 week trial of asthma medicines to see how well a child responds.

How Is Asthma Treated and Controlled?

Asthma is a long-term disease that has no cure. The goal of asthma treatment is to control the disease. Good asthma control will:

- Prevent chronic and troublesome symptoms, such as coughing and shortness of breath
- Reduce your need for quick-relief medicines
- Help you maintain good lung function
- Let you maintain your normal activity level and sleep through the night
- Prevent asthma attacks that could result in an emergency room visit or hospital stay

Follow an Asthma Action Plan

You can work with your doctor to create a personal asthma action plan. The plan will describe your daily treatments, such as which medicines to take and when to take them. The plan also will explain when to call your doctor or go to the emergency room.

If your child has asthma, all of the people who care for him or her should know about the child's asthma action plan. This includes babysitters and workers at daycare centers, schools, and camps. These caretakers can help your child follow his or her action plan.

Asthma Treatment for Special Groups

The treatments described above generally apply to all people who have asthma. However, some aspects of treatment differ for people in certain age groups and those who have special needs.

Children

It's hard to diagnose asthma in children younger than 5 years. Thus, it's hard to know whether young children who wheeze or have other asthma symptoms will benefit from long-term control medicines. (Quick-relief medicines tend to relieve wheezing in young children whether they have asthma or not.)

Doctors will treat infants and young children who have asthma symptoms with long-term control medicines if, after assessing a child, they feel that the symptoms are persistent and likely to continue after 6 years of age.

Inhaled corticosteroids are the preferred treatment for young children. Montelukast and cromolyn are other options. Treatment might be given for a trial period of 1 month to 6 weeks. Treatment usually is stopped if benefits aren't seen during that time and the doctor and parents are confident the medicine was used properly.

Inhaled corticosteroids can possibly slow the growth of children of all ages. Slowed growth usually is apparent in the first several months of treatment, is generally small, and doesn't get worse over time. Poorly controlled asthma also may reduce a child's growth rate.

Many experts think the benefits of inhaled corticosteroids for children who need them to control their asthma far outweigh the risk of slowed growth.

Section 28.2

Bronchitis

This section includes text excerpted from "Bronchitis (Chest Cold)," Centers for Disease Control and Prevention (CDC), April 17, 2015.

Overview

Antibiotics are almost never needed for bronchitis, a condition that occurs when the airways in the lungs swell and produce mucus, which causes a person to cough. While there are many different types of bronchitis, the following information is specific to one of the most common types—acute bronchitis.

Causes

Acute bronchitis, or chest cold, often occurs after an upper respiratory infection like a cold, and is usually caused by a viral infection. The most common viruses that cause acute bronchitis include:

- Respiratory syncytial virus (RSV)

- Adenovirus
- Influenza viruses
- Parainfluenza

Risk Factors

There are many things that can increase your risk for acute bronchitis, including:

- Contact with another person with bronchitis
- Exposure to secondhand smoke, chemicals, dust, or air pollution
- A weakened immune system or taking drugs that weaken the immune system

Signs and Symptoms

Signs and symptoms of acute bronchitis include:

- Coughing that produces mucus (you may not see mucus during the first few days you are sick)
- Soreness in the chest
- Fatigue (being tired)
- Mild headache
- Mild body aches
- Fever (usually less than 101 °F)
- Watery eyes
- Sore throat

Most symptoms of acute bronchitis last for up to 2 weeks, but the cough can last up to 8 weeks in some people.

When to Seek Medical Care

See a healthcare professional if you or your child has any of the following:

- Temperature higher than 100.4 °F
- A fever and cough with thick or bloody mucus

- Shortness of breath or trouble breathing
- Symptoms that last more than 3 weeks
- Repeated episodes of bronchitis

In addition, people with chronic heart or lung problems should see a healthcare professional if they experience any new symptoms of acute bronchitis.

If your child is younger than three months of age and has a fever, it's important to always call your healthcare professional right away.

Diagnosis and Treatment

Acute bronchitis is diagnosed based on the signs and symptoms a patient has when they visit their healthcare professional.

Acute bronchitis almost always gets better on its own and is almost never caused by bacteria, so antibiotics are not needed. Antibiotic treatment in these cases may even cause harm in both children and adults. Your healthcare professional may prescribe other medicine or give you tips to help with symptoms like sore throat and coughing.

If your healthcare professional diagnoses you or your child with another type of respiratory infection, such as pneumonia or whooping cough (pertussis), antibiotics will most likely be prescribed.

Symptom Relief

Rest, over-the-counter medicines and other self-care methods may help you or your child feel better. Remember, always use over-the-counter products as directed. Many over-the-counter products are not recommended for children of certain ages.

Prevention

There are several steps you can take to help prevent bronchitis, including:

- Avoid smoking and avoid exposure to secondhand smoke
- Practice good hand hygiene
- Keep you and your child up to date with recommended immunizations

Section 28.3

Cystic Fibrosis

This section includes text excerpted from "What Is Cystic Fibrosis?" National Heart, Lung, and Blood Institute (NHLBI), December 26, 2013.

What Is Cystic Fibrosis?

Cystic fibrosis, or CF, is an inherited disease of the secretory glands. Secretory glands include glands that make mucus and sweat.

"Inherited" means the disease is passed from parents to children through genes. People who have CF inherit two faulty genes for the disease—one from each parent. The parents likely don't have the disease themselves.

CF mainly affects the lungs, pancreas, liver, intestines, sinuses, and sex organs.

What Causes Cystic Fibrosis?

A defect in the cystic fibrosis transmembrane conductance regulator (CFTR) gene causes cystic fibrosis (CF). This gene makes a protein that controls the movement of salt and water in and out of your body's cells. In people who have CF, the gene makes a protein that doesn't work well. This causes thick, sticky mucus and very salty sweat.

Research suggests that the CFTR protein also affects the body in other ways. This may help explain other symptoms and complications of CF.

More than a thousand known defects can affect the CFTR gene. The type of defect you or your child has may affect the severity of CF. Other genes also may play a role in the severity of the disease.

How Is Cystic Fibrosis Inherited?

Every person inherits two CFTR genes—one from each parent. Children who inherit a faulty CFTR gene from each parent will have CF.

Children who inherit one faulty CFTR gene and one normal CFTR gene are "CF carriers." CF carriers usually have no symptoms of CF and live normal lives. However, they can pass the faulty CFTR gene to their children.

The image below shows how two parents who are both CF carriers can pass the faulty CFTR gene to their children.

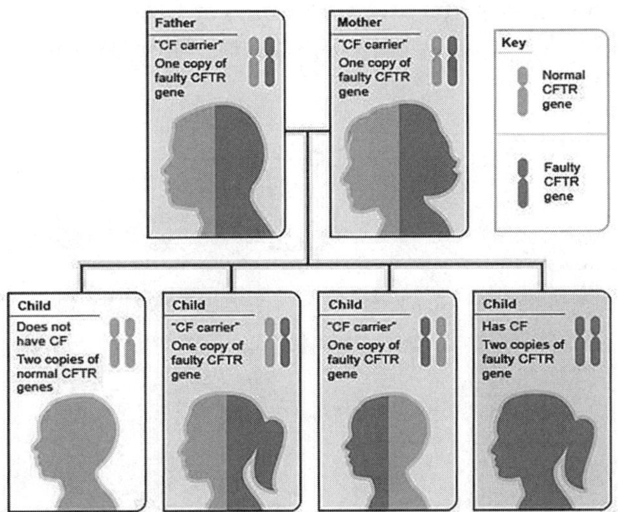

Figure 28.2. *Example of an Inheritance Pattern for Cystic Fibrosis*

The image shows how CFTR genes are inherited. A person inherits two copies of the CFTR gene—one from each parent. If each parent has a normal CFTR gene and a faulty CFTR gene, each child has a 25 percent chance of inheriting two normal genes; a 50 percent chance of inheriting one normal gene and one faulty gene; and a 25 percent chance of inheriting two faulty genes.

Who Is at Risk for Cystic Fibrosis?

Cystic fibrosis (CF) affects both males and females and people from all racial and ethnic groups. However, the disease is most common among Caucasians of Northern European descent.

CF also is common among Latinos and American Indians, especially the Pueblo and Zuni. The disease is less common among African Americans and Asian Americans.

More than 10 million Americans are carriers of a faulty CF gene. Many of them don't know that they're CF carriers.

What Are the Signs and Symptoms of Cystic Fibrosis?

The signs and symptoms of cystic fibrosis (CF) vary from person to person and over time. Sometimes you'll have few symptoms. Other times, your symptoms may become more severe.

One of the first signs of CF that parents may notice is that their baby's skin tastes salty when kissed, or the baby doesn't pass stool when first born.

Most of the other signs and symptoms of CF happen later. They're related to how CF affects the respiratory, digestive, or reproductive systems of the body.

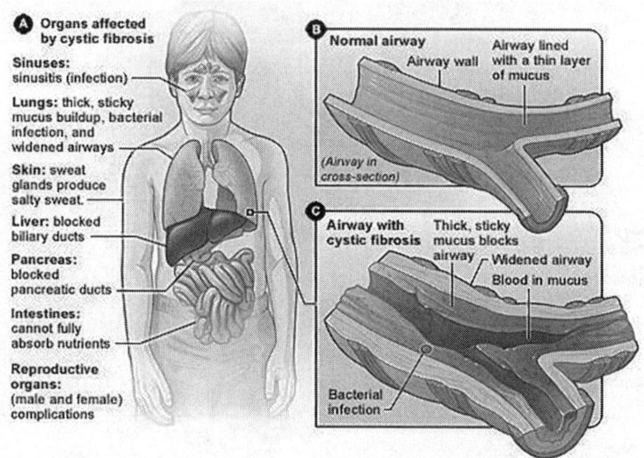

Figure 28.3. *Cystic Fibrosis*

Figure A shows the organs that cystic fibrosis can affect. Figure B shows a cross-section of a normal airway. Figure C shows an airway with cystic fibrosis. The widened airway is blocked by thick, sticky mucus that contains blood and bacteria.

How Is Cystic Fibrosis Diagnosed?

Doctors diagnose cystic fibrosis (CF) based on the results from various tests.

Newborn Screening

All States screen newborns for CF using a genetic test or a blood test. The genetic test shows whether a newborn has faulty CFTR genes. The blood test shows whether a newborn's pancreas is working properly.

Sweat Test

If a genetic test or blood test suggests CF, a doctor will confirm the diagnosis using a sweat test. This test is the most useful test for diagnosing CF. A sweat test measures the amount of salt in sweat.

For this test, the doctor triggers sweating on a small patch of skin on an arm or leg. He or she rubs the skin with a sweat-producing chemical and then uses an electrode to provide a mild electrical current. This may cause a tingling or warm feeling.

Sweat is collected on a pad or paper and then analyzed. The sweat test usually is done twice. High salt levels confirm a diagnosis of CF.

Other Tests

If you or your child has CF, your doctor may recommend other tests, such as:

- Genetic tests
- Chest X-ray
- Sinus X-ray
- Lung function tests
- Sputum culture

Prenatal Screening

If you're pregnant, prenatal genetic tests can show whether your fetus has CF. These tests include amniocentesis and chorionic villus sampling (CVS).

Cystic Fibrosis Carrier Testing

People who have one normal CFTR gene and one faulty CFTR gene are CF carriers. CF carriers usually have no symptoms of CF and live normal lives. However, carriers can pass faulty CFTR genes on to their children.

If you have a family history of CF or a partner who has CF (or a family history of it) and you're planning a pregnancy, you may want to find out whether you're a CF carrier.

A genetics counselor can test a blood or saliva sample to find out whether you have a faulty CF gene. This type of testing can detect faulty CF genes in 9 out of 10 cases.

How Is Cystic Fibrosis Treated?

Cystic fibrosis (CF) has no cure. However, treatments have greatly improved in recent years. The goals of CF treatment include:

- Preventing and controlling lung infections

- Loosening and removing thick, sticky mucus from the lungs
- Preventing or treating blockages in the intestines
- Providing enough nutrition
- Preventing dehydration (a lack of fluid in the body)

Depending on the severity of CF, you or your child may be treated in a hospital.

Chapter 29

Skin Conditions in Children

Chapter Contents

Section 29.1

Eczema (Atopic Dermatitis)

This section includes text excerpted from "Eczema (Atopic Dermatitis)," National Institute of Allergy and Infectious Diseases (NIAID), June 28, 2016.

What Is Eczema (Atopic Dermatitis)?

Atopic dermatitis, also known as eczema, is a non-contagious inflammatory skin condition. It is a chronic disease characterized by dry, itchy skin that can weep clear fluid when scratched. People with eczema also may be particularly susceptible to bacterial, viral, and fungal skin infections.

Eczema (Atopic Dermatitis) Causes

A combination of genetic and environmental factors appears to be involved in the development of eczema. The condition often is associated with other allergic diseases such as asthma, hay fever, and food allergy. Children whose parents have asthma and allergies are more likely to develop atopic dermatitis than children of parents without allergic diseases. Approximately 30 percent of children with atopic dermatitis have food allergies, and many develop asthma or respiratory allergies. People who live in cities or drier climates also appear more likely to develop the disease.

The condition tends to worsen when a person is exposed to certain triggers, such as

- Pollen, mold, dust mites, animals, and certain foods (for allergic individuals)
- Cold and dry air
- Colds or the flu
- Skin contact with irritating chemicals
- Skin contact with rough materials such as wool

- Emotional factors such as stress
- Fragrances or dyes added to skin lotions or soaps.

Taking too many baths or showers and not moisturizing the skin properly afterward may also make eczema worse.

Eczema (Atopic Dermatitis) Treatment

Skin Care at Home

You and your doctor should discuss the best treatment plan and medications for your atopic dermatitis. But taking care of your skin at home may reduce the need for prescription medications. Some recommendations include

- Avoid scratching the rash or skin.
- Relieve the itch by using a moisturizer or topical steroids. Take antihistamines to reduce severe itching.
- Keep your fingernails cut short. Consider light gloves if nighttime scratching is a problem.
- Lubricate or moisturize the skin two to three times a day using ointments such as petroleum jelly. Moisturizers should be free of alcohol, scents, dyes, fragrances, and other skin-irritating chemicals. A humidifier in the home also can help.
- Avoid anything that worsens symptoms, including
- Irritants such as wool and lanolin (an oily substance derived from sheep wool used in some moisturizers and cosmetics)
- Strong soaps or detergents
- Sudden changes in body temperature and stress, which may cause sweating
- When washing or bathing
- Keep water contact as brief as possible and use gentle body washes and cleansers instead of regular soaps. Lukewarm baths are better than long, hot baths.
- Do not scrub or dry the skin too hard or for too long.
- After bathing, apply lubricating ointments to damp skin. This will help trap moisture in the skin.

Wet Wrap Therapy

Researchers at NIAID and other institutions are studying an innovative treatment for severe eczema called wet wrap therapy. It includes three lukewarm baths a day, each followed by an application of topical medicines and moisturizer that is sealed in by a wrap of wet gauze.

Eczema (Atopic Dermatitis) Complications

The skin of people with atopic dermatitis lacks infection-fighting proteins, making them susceptible to skin infections caused by bacteria and viruses. Fungal infections also are common in people with atopic dermatitis.

Bacterial Infections

A major health risk associated with atopic dermatitis is skin colonization or infection by bacteria such as *Staphylococcus aureus*. Sixty to 90 percent of people with atopic dermatitis are likely to have staph bacteria on their skin. Many eventually develop infection, which worsens the atopic dermatitis.

Viral Infections

People with atopic dermatitis are highly vulnerable to certain viral infections of the skin. For example, if infected with herpes simplex virus, they can develop a severe skin condition called atopic dermatitis with eczema herpeticum.

Those with atopic dermatitis should not receive the currently licensed smallpox vaccine, even if their disease is in remission, because they are at risk of developing a severe infection called eczema vaccinatum. This infection is caused when the live vaccinia virus in the smallpox vaccine reproduces and spreads throughout the body. Furthermore, those in close contact with people who have atopic dermatitis or a history of the disease should not receive the smallpox vaccine because of the risk of transmitting the live vaccine virus to the person with atopic dermatitis.

Section 29.2

Psoriasis

This section includes text excerpted from "Questions and Answers about Psoriasis," National Institute of Arthritis and Musculoskeletal and Skin Diseases (NIAMS), July 2016.

What Is Psoriasis?

Psoriasis is a chronic (long-lasting) skin disease of scaling and inflammation that affects greater than 3.1 percent of the United States population, or more than 6.7 million adults. Although the disease occurs in all age groups, it primarily affects adults. It appears about equally in males and females.

Psoriasis occurs when skin cells quickly rise from their origin below the surface of the skin and pile up on the surface before they have a chance to mature. Usually this movement (also called turnover) takes about a month, but in psoriasis it may occur in only a few days.

In its typical form, psoriasis results in patches of thick, red (inflamed) skin covered with silvery scales. These patches, which are sometimes referred to as plaques, usually itch or feel sore. They most often occur on the elbows, knees, other parts of the legs, scalp, lower back, face, palms, and soles of the feet, but they can occur on skin anywhere on the body. The disease may also affect the fingernails, the toenails, and the soft tissues of the genitals, and inside the mouth.

How Does Psoriasis Affect Quality of Life?

Individuals with psoriasis may experience significant physical discomfort and some disability. Itching and pain can interfere with basic functions, such as self-care, walking, and sleep. Plaques on hands and feet can prevent individuals from working at certain occupations, playing some sports, and caring for family members or a home. The frequency of medical care is costly and can interfere with an employment or school schedule. People with moderate to severe psoriasis may feel self-conscious about their appearance. Psychological distress can lead to depression and social isolation.

What Causes Psoriasis?

Psoriasis is a skin disorder driven by the immune system, especially involving a type of white blood cell called a T cell. Normally, T cells help protect the body against infection and disease. In the case of psoriasis, T cells are put into action by mistake and become so active that they trigger other immune responses, which lead to inflammation and to rapid turnover of skin cells.

In many cases, there is a family history of psoriasis. Researchers have studied a large number of families affected by psoriasis and identified genes linked to the disease.

People with psoriasis may notice that there are times when their skin worsens, called flares, then improves. Conditions that may cause flares include infections, stress, and changes in climate that dry the skin. Also, certain medicines may trigger an outbreak or worsen the disease. Sometimes people who have psoriasis notice that lesions will appear where the skin has experienced trauma. The trauma could be from a cut, scratch, sunburn, or infection.

How Is Psoriasis Diagnosed?

Occasionally, doctors may find it difficult to diagnose psoriasis, because it often looks like other skin diseases. It may be necessary to confirm a diagnosis by examining a small skin sample under a microscope.

There are several forms of psoriasis. Some of these include:

- **Plaque psoriasis.** Skin lesions are red at the base and covered by silvery scales.
- **Guttate psoriasis**. Small, drop-shaped lesions appear on the trunk, limbs, and scalp. Guttate psoriasis is most often triggered by upper respiratory infections (for example, a sore throat caused by streptococcal bacteria).
- **Pustular psoriasis.** Blisters of noninfectious pus appear on the skin. Attacks of pustular psoriasis may be triggered by medications, infections, stress, or exposure to certain chemicals.
- **Inverse psoriasis.** Smooth, red patches occur in the folds of the skin near the genitals, under the breasts, or in the armpits. The symptoms may be worsened by friction and sweating.
- **Erythrodermic psoriasis.** Widespread reddening and scaling of the skin may be a reaction to severe sunburn or to taking

corticosteroids (cortisone) or other medications. It can also be caused by a prolonged period of increased activity of psoriasis that is poorly controlled. Erythrodermic psoriasis can be very serious and requires immediate medical attention.

Another condition in which people may experience psoriasis is psoriatic arthritis. This is a form of arthritis that produces the joint inflammation common in arthritis and the lesions common in psoriasis. The joint inflammation and the skin lesions don't necessarily have to occur at the same time.

How Is Psoriasis Treated?

Doctors generally treat psoriasis in steps based on the severity of the disease, size of the areas involved, type of psoriasis, where the psoriasis is located, and the patient's response to initial treatments. Treatment can include:

- medicines applied to the skin (topical treatment)
- light treatment (phototherapy)
- medicines by mouth or injection (systemic therapy).

Section 29.3

Warts

Text in this section is excerpted from "What's up with Warts?" © 1995–2016. The Nemours Foundation/KidsHealth®. Reprinted with permission.

A wart is a small area of hardened skin that usually has a bumpy surface. Warts come in many sizes, colors, and shapes. They can appear anywhere on the body. Kids get them most often on the hands, feet, and face.

Anybody can get warts, but kids get them more often than adults do. Lots of kids get warts, although some kids never get any warts at all. Doctors really don't know why some kids get warts. (But they're sure it's not from touching frogs or toads!) It could be that some people's immune systems, which fight infections, make them less likely to get warts.

The good news is that most warts won't make you sick or cause a health problem. And if a wart is bothering you, a doctor can remove it.

Why Do Kids Get Warts?

Viruses cause warts. They're called human papilloma viruses, or HPV for short.

HPV viruses are like other germs. The wart virus loves warm, moist places like small cuts or scratches on your hands or feet. Once the virus finds a nice warm place on the skin, a wart begins to develop. Warts can grow for many months—sometimes a year or more—before they are big enough to see. So if you do get a wart, you may never know where you came into contact with HPV.

If you touch a towel, surface, or anything else someone with a wart has used, you can pick up HPV. Kids who bite their fingernails or pick at hangnails get warts more often than kids who don't. That's why it's important to avoid picking, rubbing, or scratching a wart, whether it's on another person or on your own body.

How Do Warts Look and Feel?

Most warts don't hurt. But a wart can be annoying if it's on a part of your body that gets bumped or touched all the time. Different kinds of warts grow on different parts of the body. Some warts are smooth and flat. Some are big, rough bumps. Others are tiny and grow in clusters.

Here are some types of warts:

- **Common warts** usually grow on fingers, hands, knees, and elbows. A common wart is dome-shaped and is usually grayish-brown. It has a rough surface with black dots.
- **Flat warts** are also called juvenile warts, probably because kids get them more often than adults do. These warts are small and about the size of a pinhead. They're smoother than other kinds of warts and have flat tops. A flat wart may be pink, light brown, or yellow. Most kids who get flat warts have them on their faces, but flat warts can also grow on arms, knees, or hands. There can be as many as 100 flat warts all clustered together.
- Although most warts are painless, a wart on the bottom of the foot—called a **plantar wart**—can really hurt. It can feel like

you have a stone in your shoe. To prevent plantar warts, do not walk barefoot in public places—like a gym locker or at a public pool. Also, change your shoes and socks every day and keep your feet clean and dry.

- You've probably seen **filiform warts.** They're the kind that witches in movies and fairytale books have on their chins or noses. But you don't have to be a witch to get one! A filiform wart has a finger-like shape and usually is flesh-colored. It often grows on or around the mouth, eyes, or nose.

How Warts Are Removed

In general, the treatment for a wart depends on the type of wart a person has. It's a good idea to have a doctor look at a wart before trying to treat it, especially if it is on the bottom of your foot. Corns, calluses, and plantar warts all can form areas of thick, hard skin on feet, and it isn't always easy to tell them apart.

For some kinds of warts, the doctor may even suggest that you don't need medicines to make them go away. In time, these warts will disappear on their own. Warts can be hard to get rid of because the thick layers of skin make it hard for medicine to reach the virus that causes them. There are many ways to treat warts, but treatments can sometimes be tricky. After a wart seems to be removed, it might come right back.

Sometimes, a wart can be treated with medicine you can buy at the drugstore. These medicines contain mild acid that removes the dead skin cells on the wart. A grown-up applies the medicine or you just wear a little medicine patch in that spot. Over time, the wart crumbles away from the healthy skin.

In other cases, you need a doctor to help you get rid of a wart. Here are some common ways to get rid of warts:

Prescription medicine, which your doctor can give you. You and a parent would apply it nightly for a few weeks.

Cryosurgery, in which the doctor uses a special chemical (sometimes containing liquid nitrogen) to freeze the wart, and a scab usually forms as the skin heals. This treatment is usually repeated every 1 to 3 weeks for a few months to fully kill the virus that causes the wart.

Laser treatment may be used for warts that are stubborn and haven't gone away with other kinds of treatment. A tiny laser can be used to zap a plantar wart or other wart. It may need to be repeated a few times to get rid of deep plantar warts.

Surgery is sometimes used to remove a wart. It's not a doctor's first choice because it can leave scar.

With any of the treatments above, the doctor will take steps to prevent you from feeling pain while the wart is being removed. And after it's all over, you can wave goodbye to your wart!

Chapter 30

Vision and Eye Problems in Children

Chapter Contents

Section 30.1

Amblyopia (Lazy Eye)

This section includes text excerpted from "Facts about Amblyopia," National Eye Institute (NEI), September 2013.

What Is Amblyopia?

The brain and the eyes work together to produce vision. The eye focuses light on the back part of the eye known as the retina. Cells of the retina then trigger nerve signals that travel along the optic nerves to the brain. Amblyopia is the medical term used when the vision of one eye is reduced because it fails to work properly with the brain. The eye itself looks normal, but for various reasons the brain favors the other eye. This condition is also sometimes called lazy eye.

How Common Is Amblyopia?

Amblyopia is the most common cause of visual impairment among children, affecting approximately 2 to 3 out of every 100 children. Unless it is successfully treated in early childhood, amblyopia usually persists into adulthood. It is also the most common cause of monocular (one eye) visual impairment among young and middle-aged adults.

What Causes Amblyopia?

Amblyopia can result from any condition that prevents the eye from focusing clearly. Amblyopia can be caused by the misalignment of the two eyes—a condition called strabismus. With strabismus, the eyes can cross in (esotropia) or turn out (exotropia). Occasionally, amblyopia is caused by a clouding of the front part of the eye, a condition called cataract.

A common cause of amblyopia is the inability of one eye to focus as well as the other one. Amblyopia can occur when one eye is more nearsighted, more farsighted, or has more astigmatism. These terms refer to the ability of the eye to focus light on the retina. Farsightedness, or hyperopia, occurs when the distance from the front to the back of the eye is too short. Eyes that are farsighted tend to focus better at a distance but have more difficulty focusing on near objects. Nearsightedness, or myopia, occurs when the eye is too long from front to back. Eyes with nearsightedness tend to focus better on near objects. Eyes with astigmatism have difficulty focusing on far and near objects because of their irregular shape.

How Is Amblyopia Treated in Children?

Treating amblyopia involves forcing the child to use the eye with weaker vision. There are two common ways to treat amblyopia:

Patching

An adhesive patch is worn over the stronger eye for weeks to months. This therapy forces the child to use the eye with amblyopia. Patching stimulates vision in the weaker eye and helps parts of the brain involved in vision develop more completely.

An NEI-funded (National Eye Institute) study showed that patching the unaffected eye of children with moderate amblyopia for two hours daily works as well as patching for six hours daily. Shorter patching time can lead to better compliance with treatment and improved quality of life for children with amblyopia. However, a recent study showed that children whose amblyopia persists despite two hours of daily patching may improve if daily patching is extended to 6 hours.

Previously, eye care professionals thought that treating amblyopia would be of little benefit to older children. However, results from a nationwide clinical trial showed that many children from ages seven to 17 years old benefited from treatment for amblyopia. This study shows that age alone should not be used as a factor to decide whether or not to treat a child for amblyopia.

Atropine

A drop of a drug called atropine is placed in the stronger eye to temporarily blur vision so that the child will use the eye with amblyopia, especially when focusing on near objects. NEI-supported research has shown that atropine eye drops, when placed in the unaffected eye once a day, work as well as eye patching. Atropine eye drops are sometimes easier for parents and children to use.

Section 30.2

Conjunctivitis (Pinkeye)

This section includes text excerpted from "Facts about Pink Eye," National Eye Institute (NEI), November 2015.

Pink eye is one of the most common and treatable eye conditions in children and adults; about 3 million cases of pink eye occur in the United States each year. Treatment is not always needed and the course of treatment depends on the underlying cause.

What Is Pink Eye?

Pink eye, also known as conjunctivitis, involves inflammation of the conjunctiva, the thin, clear tissue that lines the inside of the eyelid and covers the white part of the eye, or sclera. The inflammation makes blood vessels more visible, giving the eye a pink or reddish appearance. The affected eye(s) may be painful, itchy or have a burning sensation. The eyes can also tear or have a discharge that forms a crust during sleep causing the eyes to be "stuck shut" in the morning. Other signs or symptoms that may accompany pink eye include:

- Swelling of the conjunctiva
- Feeling like a foreign body is in the eye(s)
- Sensitivity to bright light
- Enlargement and/or tenderness of the lymph node in front of the ear. This enlargement may feel like a small lump when touched. (Lymph nodes act as filters in the body, collecting and destroying viruses and bacteria.)
- Contact lenses that do not stay in place on the eye and/or feel uncomfortable due to bumps that may form under the eyelid

What Causes Pink Eye?

Pink eye is most often caused by bacterial or viral infections. Allergic reactions or exposure to irritants can also cause pink eye. Pinpointing the cause may be difficult because the signs and symptoms tend to be similar regardless of the underlying cause.

Viral conjunctivitis is caused by a wide variety of viruses, but adenovirus and herpesvirus are the most common viruses that cause pink eye. Viral conjunctivitis may also occur along with an upper respiratory tract infection, cold, or sore throat.

Bacterial conjunctivitis is caused by infection of the eye with bacteria such as *Staphylococcus aureus*, *Streptococcus pneumonia*, or *Haemophilus*. It is a common reason for children to stay home sick from day care or school.

Allergic conjunctivitis can be caused by allergies to pollen, dust mites, molds, or animal dander.

Irritants such as contact lenses and lens solutions, chlorine in a swimming pool, smog or cosmetics may also be an underlying cause of conjunctivitis.

How Is Pink Eye Diagnosed?

Conjunctivitis can be diagnosed with an eye examination by a healthcare provider. In some cases, the type of conjunctivitis can be determined by assessing the person's signs, symptoms, and recent health history (such as whether the person has recently been exposed to someone with conjunctivitis or has a pattern of seasonal allergy). Most cases resolve with time, and there is usually no need for treatment or laboratory tests, unless the person's history suggests bacterial conjunctivitis.

How Is Pink Eye Treated?

Most cases of pink eye are mild and will resolve on their own without prescription treatment. In many cases, symptom relief can be achieved by using artificial tears for the dryness and cold packs for the inflammation. (Artificial tears can be purchased without a doctor's prescription.)

However, you should seek medical attention if you have any of following symptoms:

- Moderate to severe pain in the eye(s)
- Vision problems, such as sensitivity to light or blurred vision, that do not improve when any discharge present is wiped from the eye(s)
- Intense redness in the eye(s)

- Symptoms that become worse or persist when severe viral conjunctivitis is suspected

What Steps Can I Take to Prevent Pink Eye?

Viral and bacterial conjunctivitis are highly contagious and can be easily spread from person to person. Allergic conjunctivitis is not contagious.

If you or someone around you has infectious (viral or bacterial) conjunctivitis, limit its spread by following these steps:

- Wash your hands often with soap and warm water. And wash up immediately if you've touched an affected person's eyes, linens or clothes (for example, when caring for a child who has pink eye). If soap and water are not available, use an alcohol-based hand sanitizer that contains at least 60 percent alcohol.
- Avoid touching or rubbing your eyes.
- If you have conjunctivitis, wash any discharge from around the eyes several times a day.
- Do not use the same eye drop dispenser/bottle for infected and non-infected eyes—even for the same person.
- Avoid sharing articles like towels, blankets, and pillowcases.
- Clean your eyeglasses.
- Clean, store, and replace your contact lenses as instructed by your eye health professional.
- Do not share eye makeup, face makeup, makeup brushes, contact lenses or containers, or eyeglasses.

There are also steps you can take to avoid re-infection once the infection goes away:

- Throw away any eye or face makeup or applicators you used while infected.
- Throw away contact lens solutions you used while infected.
- Throw away contact lenses and cases you used.
- Clean your eyeglasses and cases.

Can Newborns Get Pink Eye?

Newborns can develop pink eye, which is called neonatal conjunctivitis, or less commonly, ophthalmia neonatorum. Common symptoms include eye discharge and puffy, red eyelids within one day to two weeks after birth. Newborn conjunctivitis may be caused by infection, irritation, or a blocked tear duct. A mother can pass on infectious conjunctivitis to her newborn during childbirth, even she has no symptoms herself, because she may carry bacteria or viruses in the birth canal. When caused by an infection, neonatal conjunctivitis can be very serious. The most common types of neonatal conjunctivitis include:

- Chlamydial (or inclusion) conjunctivitis is caused by the bacterium Chlamydia trachomatis and can cause swelling of the eyelids with purulent (pus) discharge. Symptoms often appear 5–12 days after birth but may present at any time during the first month of life.
- Gonococcal conjunctivitis is caused by Neisseria gonorrhoeae, the bacterium that causes gonorrhea. Gonococcal conjunctivitis causes pus discharge and swelling of eyelids, which may appear 2–4 days after birth.
- Chemical conjunctivitis can be caused by eye drops or ointment given to newborns to help prevent bacterial eye infections. Symptoms include red eyes and eyelid swelling, and usually resolve in 24–36 hours. Most hospitals are required by state law to put drops or ointment in a newborn's eyes to prevent disease. The benefits of preventing a more serious type of conjunctivitis are thought to outweigh the risks of chemical conjunctivitis.
- Other bacteria and viruses can also cause conjunctivitis in a newborn. Bacteria that normally live in a woman's vagina and that are not sexually transmitted can cause neonatal conjunctivitis. The viruses that cause genital and oral herpes can also cause neonatal conjunctivitis and severe eye damage. Such viruses may be passed to the baby during childbirth.

How Is Pink Eye Treated in Newborns?

Bacterial conjunctivitis may be treated with topical antibiotic eye drops and ointments, oral antibiotics, or intravenous (given through a vein) antibiotics.

A combination of topical and oral, or topical and intravenous treatments are sometimes used at the same time. A saline solution may be prescribed for rinsing the baby's eye(s) to remove pus, if necessary.

- **Chlamydial conjunctivitis** in newborns is usually treated with oral antibiotics such as erythromycin. Parents are usually treated as well.

- **Gonococcal conjunctivitis** in newborns is usually treated with intravenous antibiotics. If untreated, this condition can lead to corneal ulcers and blindness.
- **Other types of bacterial and viral conjunctivitis** are usually treated with antibiotic eye drops or ointments. A warm compress to the eye may also help relieve swelling and irritation.
- **Blocked tear ducts** may cause conjunctivitis. If a tear duct is blocked, a gentle warm massage between the eye and nasal area may help. If the blocked tear duct is not cleared by one year of age, surgery may be required.
- **Chemical Conjunctivitis** usually resolves in 24–36 hours without treatment.

Section 30.3

Refractive Disorders

This section includes text excerpted from "Facts about Refractive Errors," National Eye Institute (NEI), October 2010. Reviewed October 2016.

What Are Refractive Errors?

Refractive errors occur when the shape of the eye prevents light from focusing directly on the retina. The length of the eyeball (longer or shorter), changes in the shape of the cornea, or aging of the lens can cause refractive errors.

What Is Refraction?

Refraction is the bending of light as it passes through one object to another. Vision occurs when light rays are bent (refracted) as they pass through the cornea and the lens. The light is then focused on the retina. The retina converts the light-rays into messages that are sent through the optic nerve to the brain. The brain interprets these messages into the images we see.

What Are the Different Types of Refractive Errors?

The most common types of refractive errors are myopia, hyperopia, presbyopia, and astigmatism.

Myopia (nearsightedness) is a condition where objects up close appear clearly, while objects far away appear blurry. With myopia, light comes to focus in front of the retina instead of on the retina.

Hyperopia (farsightedness) is a common type of refractive error where distant objects may be seen more clearly than objects that are near. However, people experience hyperopia differently. Some people may not notice any problems with their vision, especially when they are young. For people with significant hyperopia, vision can be blurry for objects at any distance, near or far.

Astigmatism is a condition in which the eye does not focus light evenly onto the retina, the light-sensitive tissue at the back of the eye. This can cause images to appear blurry and stretched out.

Presbyopia is an age-related condition in which the ability to focus up close becomes more difficult. As the eye ages, the lens can no longer change shape enough to allow the eye to focus close objects clearly.

Who Is at Risk for Refractive Errors?

Presbyopia affects most adults over age 35. Other refractive errors can affect both children and adults. Individuals that have parents with certain refractive errors may be more likely to get one or more refractive errors.

What Are the Signs and Symptoms of Refractive Errors?

Blurred vision is the most common symptom of refractive errors. Other symptoms may include:

- Double vision
- Haziness
- Glare or halos around bright lights
- Squinting
- Headaches
- Eye strain

How Are Refractive Errors Diagnosed?

An eye care professional can diagnose refractive errors during a comprehensive dilated eye examination. People with a refractive error often visit their eye care professional with complaints of visual discomfort or blurred vision. However, some people don't know they aren't seeing as clearly as they could.

How Are Refractive Errors Treated?

Refractive errors can be corrected with eyeglasses, contact lenses, or surgery.

Eyeglasses are the simplest and safest way to correct refractive errors. Your eye care professional can prescribe appropriate lenses to correct your refractive error and give you optimal vision.

Contact Lenses work by becoming the first refractive surface for light rays entering the eye, causing a more precise refraction or focus. In many cases, contact lenses provide clearer vision, a wider field of vision, and greater comfort. They are a safe and effective option if fitted and used properly. It is very important to wash your hands and clean your lenses as instructed in order to reduce the risk of infection.

If you have certain eye conditions you may not be able to wear contact lenses. Discuss this with your eye care professional.

Refractive Surgery aims to change the shape of the cornea permanently. This change in eye shape restores the focusing power of the eye by allowing the light rays to focus precisely on the retina for improved vision. There are many types of refractive surgeries. Your eye care professional can help you decide if surgery is an option for you.

Section 30.4

Retinitis Pigmentosa

This section includes text excerpted from "Facts about Retinitis Pigmentosa," National Eye Institute (NEI), May 2014.

What Is Retinitis Pigmentosa (RP)?

Retinitis pigmentosa (RP) is a group of rare, genetic disorders that involve a breakdown and loss of cells in the retina—which is the light sensitive tissue that lines the back of the eye. Common symptoms include difficulty seeing at night and a loss of side (peripheral) vision.

What Causes RP?

RP is an inherited disorder that results from harmful changes in any one of more than 50 genes. These genes carry the instructions for making proteins that are needed in cells within the retina, called photoreceptors. Some of the changes, or mutations, within genes are so severe that the gene cannot make the required protein, limiting the cellís function. Other mutations produce a protein that is toxic to the cell. Still other mutations lead to an abnormal protein that doesnít function properly. In all three cases, the result is damage to the photoreceptors.

What Are Photoreceptors?

Photoreceptors are cells in the retina that begin the process of seeing. They absorb and convert light into electrical signals. These signals are sent to other cells in the retina and ultimately through the optic nerve to the brain where they are processed into the images we see. There are two general types of photoreceptors, called rods and cones. Rods are in the outer regions of the retina, and allow us to see in dim and dark light. Cones reside mostly in the central portion of the retina, and allow us to perceive fine visual detail and color.

How Does RP Affect Vision?

In the early stages of RP, rods are more severely affected than cones. As the rods die, people experience night blindness and a progressive loss of the visual field, the area of space that is visible at a given instant without moving the eyes. The loss of rods eventually leads to a breakdown and loss of cones. In the late stages of RP, as cones die, people tend to lose more of the visual field, developing ìtunnel vision. They may have difficulty performing essential tasks of daily living such as reading, driving, walking without assistance, or recognizing faces and objects.

How Is RP Inherited?

To understand how RP is inherited, it is important to know a little more about genes and how they are passed from parent to child. Genes are bundled together on structures called chromosomes. Each cell in your body contains 23 pairs of chromosomes. One copy of each chromosome is passed by a parent at conception through egg and sperm cells. The X and Y chromosomes, known as sex chromosomes, determine whether a person is born female (XX) or male (XY). The 22 other paired chromosomes, called autosomes, contain the vast majority of genes that determine non-sex traits. RP can be inherited in one of three ways:

Autosomal recessive Inheritance

In autosomal recessive inheritance, it takes two copies of the mutant gene to give rise to the disorder. An individual with a recessive gene mutation is known as a carrier. When two carriers have a child, there is a:

- 1 in 4 chance the child will have the disorder
- 1 in 2 chance the child will be a carrier
- 1 in 4 chance the child will neither have the disorder nor be a carrier

Autosomal dominant Inheritance

In this inheritance pattern, it takes just one copy of the gene with a disorder-causing mutation to bring about the disorder. When a parent has a dominant gene mutation, there is a 1 in 2 chance that any children will inherit this mutation and the disorder.

X-linked Inheritance

In this form of inheritance, mothers carry the mutated gene on one of their X chromosomes and pass it to their sons. Because females have two X chromosomes, the effect of a mutation on one X chromosome is offset by the normal gene on the other X chromosome. If a mother is a carrier of an X-linked disorder there is a:

- 1 in 2 chance of having a son with the disorder
- 1 in 2 chance of having a daughter who is a carrier

How Common Is RP?

RP is considered a rare disorder. Although current statistics are not available, it is generally estimated that the disorder affects roughly 1 in 4,000 people, both in the United States and worldwide.

How Does RP Progress?

The symptoms of RP typically appear in childhood. Children often have difficulty getting around in the dark. It can also take abnormally long periods of time to adjust to changes in lighting. As their visual field becomes restricted, patients often trip over things and appear clumsy. People with RP often find bright lights uncomfortable, a condition known as photophobia. Because there are many gene mutations that cause the disorder, its progression can differ greatly from person to person. Some people retain central vision and a restricted visual field into their 50s, while others experience significant vision loss in early adulthood. Eventually, most individuals with RP will lose most of their sight.

How Is RP Diagnosed?

RP is diagnosed in part through an examination of the retina. An eye care professional will use an ophthalmoscope, a tool that allows for a wider, clear view of the retina. This typically reveals abnormal, dark pigment deposits that streak the retina. These pigment deposits are in part why the disorder was named retinitis pigmentosa. Other tests for RP include:

- Electroretinogram (ERG)
- Visual field testing
- Genetic testing

Section 30.5

Strabismus (Crossed Eye)

Text in this section is excerpted from "Strabismus," © 1995–2016. The Nemours Foundation/KidsHealth®. Reprinted with permission.

About Strabismus

Strabismus is when eyes don't line up or when one or both eyes wander. The eyes may turn inward (called esotropia or "cross-eyed"), outward (exotropia), up (hypertropia), or down (hypotropia). Sometimes strabismus is noticeable all the time. But other times it's only noticeable when a child is tired or looking at something very closely.

Strabismus can be present at birth or develop in childhood. Often, it's caused by a problem with the muscles that move the eyes, and can run in families.

Most kids with strabismus are diagnosed when they're between 1 and 4 years old. Rarely, a child might develop strabismus after 6 years of age. If this happens, it's important for the child to see a doctor right away to rule out other conditions.

How Vision Is Affected

When eyes don't line up together, the straight or straighter eye becomes more dominant. The vision strength (acuity) of this eye remains normal because the eye and its connection to the brain are working as they should. The misaligned or weaker eye, however, does not focus properly and its connection to the brain is not formed correctly.

If strabismus is not treated, the brain eventually will ignore the visual images of the weaker eye. The vision may be blurry or a child may not be able to see in 3D (called depth perception). This change in vision is called amblyopia or "lazy eye." These problems can be permanent if they're not treated.

Signs and Symptoms

Most kids with strabismus don't complain of eye problems or notice changes in their vision. Usually, it's a family member, teacher, or healthcare provider who notices that the eyes are not straight.

Some kids may complain of double vision (seeing two objects when there's only one in view) or have trouble seeing things in general. Younger children who aren't talking yet may squint a lot and turn or tilt their heads in an attempt to see more clearly.

If your child has any of these signs or symptoms, tell your doctor. He or she can refer you to a pediatric ophthalmologist for care, if needed.

Treatment

Treatment for strabismus may include:

- eyeglasses
- eye patching
- eye drops
- eye muscle surgery

Sometimes, wearing eyeglasses is enough to straighten out the eyes. If not, a child might be given an eye patch to wear over the straight eye for a few hours a day. This patch makes the weaker eye do the "seeing" work. Over time, the muscles and vision in the weaker eye become stronger.

For parents of babies and toddlers, using an eye patch can be challenging. But most kids get used to the patch and wearing it just becomes part of their daily routine, like getting dressed in the morning.

Sometimes, though, a child will refuse to wear an eye patch. In these cases, eye drops (called atropine drops) might be used instead. Just as eye patching blocks the vision in the straight eye, the atropine drops temporarily blur out vision in that eye. This makes the weaker eye work harder so that eye muscles and vision becomes stronger.

If eyeglasses, eye patching, and/or atropine drops do not fix a child's strabismus, eye muscle surgery may be recommended. Surgery involves loosening or tightening the muscles that cause the eye to wander. Most kids can go home the same day of surgery.

Outlook

Kids with strabismus usually won't have permanent vision loss if the condition is treated early. This is important because key connections form between the eyes and the brain by about 8 years old.

The earlier strabismus is diagnosed and treated, the better a child's chances are of having straight eyes and developing good vision and proper depth perception. Studies show, however, that older kids and teens (and even many adults with strabismus) can still benefit from treatment.

The social aspect to strabismus also should not be overlooked. Aligned eyes are important for a healthy self-image in adults and kids.

Part Four

Developmental and Pediatric Mental Health Concerns

Chapter 31

Autism Spectrum Disorders

What Is Autism Spectrum Disorder (ASD)?

Autism spectrum disorder (ASD) is a term for a group of developmental disorders described by:

- Lasting problems with social communication and social interaction in different settings
- Repetitive behaviors and/or not wanting any change in daily routines
- Symptoms that begin in early childhood, usually in the first 2 years of life
- Symptoms that cause the person to need help in his or her daily life

The term "spectrum" refers to the wide range of symptoms, strengths, and levels of impairment that people with ASD can have. The diagnosis of ASD now includes these other conditions:

- Autistic disorder
- Asperger syndrome

This chapter includes text excerpted from "Autism Spectrum Disorder," National Institute of Mental Health (NIMH), September 15, 2015.

- Pervasive developmental disorder not otherwise specified

Although ASD begins in early development, it can last throughout a person's lifetime.

What Are the Signs and Symptoms of ASD?

Not all people with ASD will show all of these behaviors, but most will show several.

People with ASD may:

- Repeat certain behaviors or have unusual behaviors
- Have overly focused interests, such as with moving objects or parts of objects
- Have a lasting, intense interest in certain topics, such as numbers, details, or facts
- Be upset by a slight change in a routine or being placed in a new or overstimulating setting
- Make little or inconsistent eye contact
- Tend to look and listen less to people in their environment
- Rarely seek to share their enjoyment of objects or activities by pointing or showing things to others
- Respond unusually when others show anger, distress, or affection
- Fail or be slow to respond to their name or other verbal attempts to gain their attention
- Have difficulties with the back and forth of conversations
- Often talk at length about a favorite subject but won't allow anyone else a chance to respond or notice when others react indifferently
- Repeat words or phrases that they hear, a behavior called echolalia
- Use words that seem odd, out of place, or have a special meaning known only to those familiar with that person's way of communicating
- Have facial expressions, movements, and gestures that do not match what they are saying
- Have an unusual tone of voice that may sound sing-song or flat and robot-like

- Have trouble understanding another person's point of view, leaving him or her unable to predict or understand other people's actions

People with ASD may have other difficulties, such as sensory sensitivity (being sensitive to light, noise, textures of clothing, or temperature), sleep problems, digestion problems, and irritability.

People with ASD can also have many strengths and abilities. For instance, people with ASD may:

- Have above-average intelligence
- Be able to learn things in detail and remember information for long periods of time
- Be strong visual and auditory learners
- Excel in math, science, music, and art

How Is ASD Diagnosed?

Doctors diagnose ASD by looking at a child's behavior and development. Young children with ASD can usually be reliably diagnosed by age 2.

Older children and adolescents should be screened for ASD when a parent or teacher raises concerns based on observations of the child's social, communicative, and play behaviors.

Diagnosing ASD in adults is not easy. In adults, some ASD symptoms can overlap with symptoms of other mental health disorders, such as schizophrenia or attention deficit hyperactivity disorder (ADHD). However, getting a correct diagnosis of ASD as an adult can help a person understand past difficulties, identify his or her strengths, and obtain the right kind of help.

Diagnosis in Young Children

Diagnosis in young children is often a two-stage process:

General Developmental Screening During Well-Child Checkups

Every child should receive well-child check-ups with a pediatrician or an early childhood healthcare provider. Specific ASD screening should be done at the 18- and 24-month visits.

Earlier screening might be needed if a child is at high risk for ASD or developmental problems. Those at high risk include those who:

- Have a sister, brother, or other family member with ASD
- Have some ASD behaviors
- Were born premature, or early, and at a low birth weight

Parents' experiences and concerns are very important in the screening process for young children. Sometimes the doctor will ask parents questions about the child's behaviors and combine this information with his or her observations of the child.

Children who show some developmental problems during this screening process will be referred for another stage of evaluation.

Additional Evaluation

This evaluation is with a team of doctors and other health professionals with a wide range of specialties who are experienced in diagnosing ASD. This team may include:

- A developmental pediatrician—a doctor who has special training in child development
- A child psychologist and/or child psychiatrist—a doctor who knows about brain development and behavior
- A speech-language pathologist—a health professional who has special training in communication difficulties

The evaluation may assess:

- Cognitive level or thinking skills
- Language abilities
- Age-appropriate skills needed to complete daily activities independently, such as eating, dressing, and toileting

Because ASD is a complex disorder that sometimes occurs along with other illnesses or learning disorders, the comprehensive evaluation may include:

- Blood tests
- A hearing test

The outcome of the evaluation will result in recommendations to help plan for treatment.

Diagnosis in Older Children and Adolescents

Older children who begin showing symptoms of ASD after starting school are often first recognized and evaluated by the school's special education team and can be referred to a healthcare professional. Parents may talk with their child's pediatrician about their child's difficulties with social interaction, including problems with subtle communication, such as understanding tone of voice or facial expressions, body language, and lack of understanding of figures of speech, humor, or sarcasm. Parents may also find that their child has trouble forming friendships with peers. At this point, the pediatrician or a child psychologist or psychiatrist who has expertise in ASD can screen the child and refer the family for further evaluation and treatment.

What Are the Treatments for ASD?

Treating ASD early and getting proper care can reduce a person's difficulties and increase his or her ability to maximize strengths and learn new skills. While there is no single best treatment for ASD, working closely with the doctor is an important part of finding the right treatment program.

Medications

There are a few classes of medications that doctors may use to treat some difficulties that are common with ASD. With medication, a person with ASD may have fewer problems with:

- Irritability
- Aggression
- Repetitive behaviors
- Hyperactivity
- Attention problems
- Anxiety and depression

Who Is Affected by ASD?

ASD affects many people, and it has become more commonly diagnosed in recent years. More boys than girls receive an ASD diagnosis.

What Causes ASD?

Scientists don't know the exact causes of ASD, but research suggests that genes and environment play important roles.

- Researchers are starting to identify genes that may increase the risk for ASD.
- ASD occurs more often in people who have certain genetic conditions, such as Fragile X syndrome or tuberous sclerosis.
- Many researchers are focusing on how genes interact with each other and with environmental factors, such as family medical conditions, parental age and other demographic factors, and complications during birth or pregnancy.
- Currently, no scientific studies have linked ASD and vaccines.

Chapter 32

Attention Deficit Hyperactivity Disorder

What Is Attention Deficit Hyperactivity Disorder (ADHD)?

Attention deficit hyperactivity disorder (ADHD) is a brain disorder marked by an ongoing pattern of inattention and/or hyperactivity-impulsivity that interferes with functioning or development.

- **Inattention** means a person wanders off task, lacks persistence, has difficulty sustaining focus, and is disorganized; and these problems are not due to defiance or lack of comprehension.
- **Hyperactivity** means a person seems to move about constantly, including situations in which it is not appropriate when it is not appropriate, excessively fidgets, taps, or talks. In adults, it may be extreme restlessness or wearing others out with their activity.
- **Impulsivity** means a person makes hasty actions that occur in the moment without first thinking about them and that may have high potential for harm; or a desire for immediate rewards or inability to delay gratification. An impulsive person may be socially intrusive and excessively interrupt others or make important decisions without considering the long-term consequences.

This chapter includes text excerpted from "Attention Deficit Hyperactivity Disorder," National Institute of Mental Health (NIMH), March 7, 2016.

Signs and Symptoms of ADHD

Inattention and hyperactivity/impulsivity are the key behaviors of ADHD. Some people with ADHD only have problems with one of the behaviors, while others have both inattention and hyperactivity-impulsivity.Most children have the combined type of ADHD.

In preschool, the most common ADHD symptom is hyperactivity.

It is normal to have some inattention, unfocused motor activity and impulsivity, but for people with ADHD, these behaviors:

- are more severe
- occur more often
- interfere with or reduce the quality of how they functions socially, at school, or in a job

Inattention

People with symptoms of inattention may often:

- Overlook or miss details, make careless mistakes in schoolwork, at work, or during other activities
- Have problems sustaining attention in tasks or play, including conversations, lectures, or lengthy reading
- Not seem to listen when spoken to directly
- Not follow through on instructions and fail to finish schoolwork, chores, or duties in the workplace or start tasks but quickly lose focus and get easily sidetracked
- Have problems organizing tasks and activities, such as what to do in sequence, keeping materials and belongings in order, having messy work and poor time management, and failing to meet deadlines
- Avoid or dislike tasks that require sustained mental effort, such as schoolwork or homework, or for teens and older adults, preparing reports, completing forms or reviewing lengthy papers
- Lose things necessary for tasks or activities, such as school supplies, pencils, books, tools, wallets, keys, paperwork, eyeglasses, and cell phones
- Be easily distracted by unrelated thoughts or stimuli
- Be forgetful in daily activities, such as chores, errands, returning calls, and keeping appointments

Hyperactivity-Impulsivity

People with symptoms of hyperactivity-impulsivity may often:

- Fidget and squirm in their seats
- Leave their seats in situations when staying seated is expected, such as in the classroom or in the office
- Run or dash around or climb in situations where it is inappropriate or, in teens and adults, often feel restless
- Be unable to play or engage in hobbies quietly
- Be constantly in motion or "on the go," or act as if "driven by a motor"
- Talk nonstop
- Blurt out an answer before a question has been completed, finish other people's sentences, or speak without waiting for a turn in conversation
- Have trouble waiting his or her turn
- Interrupt or intrude on others, for example in conversations, games, or activities

Diagnosis of ADHD requires a comprehensive evaluation by a licensed clinician, such as a pediatrician, psychologist, or psychiatrist with expertise in ADHD. For a person to receive a diagnosis of ADHD, the symptoms of inattention and/or hyperactivity-impulsivity must be chronic or long-lasting, impair the person's functioning, and cause the person to fall behind normal development for his or her age. The doctor will also ensure that any ADHD symptoms are not due to another medical or psychiatric condition. Most children with ADHD receive a diagnosis during the elementary school years. For an adolescent or adult to receive a diagnosis of ADHD, the symptoms need to have been present prior to age 12.

ADHD symptoms can appear as early as between the ages of 3 and 6 and can continue through adolescence and adulthood. Symptoms of ADHD can be mistaken for emotional or disciplinary problems or missed entirely in quiet, well-behaved children, leading to a delay in diagnosis. Adults with undiagnosed ADHD may have a history of poor academic performance, problems at work, or difficult or failed relationships.

ADHD symptoms can change over time as a person ages. In young children with ADHD, hyperactivity-impulsivity is the most predominant symptom. As a child reaches elementary school, the symptom of inattention may become more prominent and cause the child to struggle academically. In adolescence, hyperactivity seems to lessen and may show more often as feelings of restlessness or fidgeting, but inattention and impulsivity may remain. Many adolescents with ADHD also struggle with relationships and antisocial behaviors. Inattention, restlessness, and impulsivity tend to persist into adulthood.

Risk Factors

Scientists are not sure what causes ADHD. Like many other illnesses, a number of factors can contribute to ADHD, such as:

- Genes
- Cigarette smoking, alcohol use, or drug use during pregnancy
- Exposure to environmental toxins during pregnancy
- Exposure to environmental toxins, such as high levels of lead, at a young age
- Low birth weight
- Brain injuries

ADHD is more common in males than females, and females with ADHD are more likely to have problems primarily with inattention. Other conditions, such as learning disabilities, anxiety disorder, conduct disorder, depression, and substance abuse, are common in people with ADHD.

Treatment and Therapies

While there is no cure for ADHD, currently available treatments can help reduce symptoms and improve functioning. Treatments include medication, psychotherapy, education or training, or a combination of treatments.

Medication

For many people, ADHD medications reduce hyperactivity and impulsivity and improve their ability to focus, work, and learn. Medication also may improve physical coordination. Sometimes several different medications or dosages must be tried before finding the right one that works for a particular person. Anyone taking medications must be monitored closely and carefully by their prescribing doctor.

Stimulants. The most common type of medication used for treating ADHD is called a "stimulant." Although it may seem unusual to treat ADHD with a medication that is considered a stimulant, it works because it increases the brain chemicals dopamine and norepinephrine, which play essential roles in thinking and attention.

Under medical supervision, stimulant medications are considered safe. However, there are risks and side effects, especially when misused or taken in excess of the prescribed dose.For example, stimulants can raise blood pressure and heart rate and increase anxiety. Therefore, a person with other health problems, including high blood pressure, seizures, heart disease, glaucoma, liver or kidney disease, or an anxiety disorder should tell their doctor before taking a stimulant.

Talk with a doctor if you see any of these side effects while taking stimulants:

- decreased appetite
- sleep problems
- tics (sudden, repetitive movements or sounds);
- personality changes
- increased anxiety and irritability
- stomachaches
- headaches

Non-stimulants. A few other ADHD medications are non-stimulants. These medications take longer to start working than stimulants, but can also improve focus, attention, and impulsivity in a person with ADHD. Doctors may prescribe a non-stimulant: when a person has bothersome side effects from stimulants; when a stimulant was not effective; or in combination with a stimulant to increase effectiveness.

Although not approved by the U.S. Food and Drug Administration (FDA) specifically for the treatment of ADHD, some antidepressants are sometimes used alone or in combination with a stimulant to treat ADHD. Antidepressants may help all of the symptoms of ADHD and can be prescribed if a patient has bothersome side effects from stimulants. Antidepressants can be helpful in combination with stimulants if a patient also has another condition, such as an anxiety disorder, depression, or another mood disorder.

Doctors and patients can work together to find the best medication, dose, or medication combination.

Psychotherapy

Adding psychotherapy to treat ADHD can help patients and their families to better cope with everyday problems.

Behavioral therapy is a type of psychotherapy that aims to help a person change his or her behavior. It might involve practical assistance, such as help organizing tasks or completing schoolwork, or working through emotionally difficult events. Behavioral therapy also teaches a person how to:

- monitor his or her own behavior
- give oneself praise or rewards for acting in a desired way, such as controlling anger or thinking before acting

Parents, teachers, and family members also can give positive or negative feedback for certain behaviors and help establish clear rules, chore lists, and other structured routines to help a person control his or her behavior. Therapists may also teach children social skills, such as how to wait their turn, share toys, ask for help, or respond to teasing. Learning to read facial expressions and the tone of voice in others, and how to respond appropriately can also be part of social skills training.

Cognitive behavioral therapy can also teach a person mindfulness techniques, or meditation. A person learns how to be aware and accepting of one's own thoughts and feelings to improve focus and concentration. The therapist also encourages the person with ADHD to adjust to the life changes that come with treatment, such as thinking before acting, or resisting the urge to take unnecessary risks.

Education and Training

Children and adults with ADHD need guidance and understanding from their parents, families, and teachers to reach their full potential and to succeed. For school-age children, frustration, blame, and anger may have built up within a family before a child is diagnosed. Parents and children may need special help to overcome negative feelings. Mental health professionals can educate parents about ADHD and how it affects a family. They also will help the child and his or her parents develop new skills, attitudes, and ways of relating to each other.

Parenting skills training (behavioral parent management training) teaches parents the skills they need to encourage and reward positive behaviors in their children. It helps parents learn how to use a system of rewards and consequences to change a child's behavior. Parents are taught to give immediate and positive feedback for behaviors they want to encourage, and ignore or redirect behaviors that they want to discourage. They may also learn to structure situations in ways that support desired behavior.

Stress management techniques can benefit parents of children with ADHD by increasing their ability to deal with frustration so that they can respond calmly to their child's behavior.

Support groups can help parents and families connect with others who have similar problems and concerns. Groups often meet regularly to share frustrations and successes, to exchange information about recommended specialists and strategies, and to talk with experts.

Tips to Help Kids with ADHD Stay Organized

Parents and teachers can help kids with ADHD stay organized and follow directions with tools such as:

- Keeping a routine and a schedule. Keep the same routine every day, from wake-up time to bedtime. Include times for homework, outdoor play, and indoor activities. Keep the schedule on the refrigerator or on a bulletin board in the kitchen. Write changes on the schedule as far in advance as possible.
- Organizing everyday items. Have a place for everything, and keep everything in its place. This includes clothing, backpacks, and toys.
- Using homework and notebook organizers. Use organizers for school material and supplies. Stress to your child the importance of writing down assignments and bringing home the necessary books.
- Being clear and consistent. Children with ADHD need consistent rules they can understand and follow.
- Giving praise or rewards when rules are followed. Children with ADHD often receive and expect criticism. Look for good behavior, and praise it.

Chapter 33

Conduct and Oppositional Disorders

Behavior or Conduct Problems

Children sometimes argue, are aggressive, or act angry or defiant around adults. A behavior disorder may be diagnosed when these disruptive behaviors are uncommon for the child's age at the time, persist over time, or are severe. Because behavior disorders involve acting out and showing unwanted behavior towards others they are often called externalizing disorders.

Oppositional Defiant Disorder

When children act out persistently so that it causes serious problems at home, in school, or with peers, they may be diagnosed with Oppositional Defiant Disorder (ODD). ODD usually starts before 8 years of age, but no later than by about 12 years of age. Children with ODD are more likely to act oppositional or defiant around people they know well, such as family members, a regular care provider, or a teacher. Children with ODD show these behaviors more often than other children their age.

This chapter includes text excerpted from "Behavior or Conduct Problems," Centers for Disease Control and Prevention (CDC), April 22, 2016.

Examples of ODD behaviors include:

- Often being angry or losing one's temper
- Often arguing with adults or refusing to comply with adults' rules or requests
- Often resentful or spiteful
- Deliberately annoying others or becoming annoyed with others
- Often blaming other people for one's own mistakes or misbehavior

Conduct Disorder

Conduct Disorder (CD) is diagnosed when children show an ongoing pattern of aggression toward others, and serious violations of rules and social norms at home, in school, and with peers. These rule violations may involve breaking the law and result in arrest. Children with CD are more likely to get injured and may have difficulties getting along with peers.

Examples of CD behaviors include:

- Breaking serious rules, such as running away, staying out at night when told not to, or skipping school
- Being aggressive in a way that causes harm, such as bullying, fighting, or being cruel to animals
- Lying, stealing, or damaging other people's property on purpose

Treatment for Disruptive Behavior Disorders

Starting treatment early is important. Treatment is most effective if it fits the needs of the specific child and family. The first step to treatment is to talk with a healthcare provider. A comprehensive evaluation by a mental health professional may be needed to get the right diagnosis. Some of the signs of behavior problems, such as not following rules in school, could be related to learning problems which may need additional intervention. For younger children, the treatment with the strongest evidence is behavior therapy training for parents, where a therapist helps the parent learn effective ways to strengthen the parent-child relationship and respond to the child's behavior. For school-age children and teens, an often-used effective treatment is a combination of training and therapy that includes the child, the family, and the school.

Get Help Finding Treatment

Here are tools to find a healthcare provider familiar with treatment options:

- Psychologist Locator, a service of the American Psychological Association (APA) Practice Organization.
- Child and Adolescent Psychiatrist Finder, a research tool by the American Academy of Child and Adolescent Psychiatry (AACAP).
- Find a Cognitive Behavioral Therapist, a search tool by the Association for Behavioral and Cognitive Therapies.
- If you need help finding treatment facilities, use the "Treatment Locator" widget.

Prevention of Disruptive Behavior Disorders

It is not known exactly why some children develop disruptive behavior disorders. Many factors may play a role, including biological and social factors. It is known that children are at greater risk when they are exposed to other types of violence and criminal behavior, when they experience maltreatment or harsh or inconsistent parenting, or when their parents have mental health conditions like substance use disorders, depression, or attention-deficit/hyperactivity disorder (ADHD). The quality of early childhood care also can impact whether a child develops behavior problems.

Although these factors appear to increase the risk for disruptive behavior disorders, there are ways to decrease the chance that children experience them.

Chapter 34

Developmental Disorders and Disorders That Affect Learning

Chapter Contents

Section 34.1

Auditory Processing Disorder

Text in this section is excerpted from "Auditory Processing Disorder," © 1995–2016.The Nemours Foundation/KidsHealth®. Reprinted with permission.

Auditory processing disorder (APD), also known as central auditory processing disorder (CAPD), is a hearing problem that affects about 5% of school-aged children.

Kids with this condition can't process what they hear in the same way other kids do because their ears and brain don't fully coordinate. Something interferes with the way the brain recognizes and interprets sounds, especially speech.

With the right therapy, kids with APD can be successful in school and life. Early diagnosis is important, because when the condition isn't caught and treated early, a child can have speech and language delays or problems learning in school.

Trouble Understanding Speech

Kids with APD are thought to hear normally because they can usually hear sounds that are delivered one at a time in a very quiet environment (such as a sound-treated room). The problem is that they usually don't recognize slight differences between sounds in words, even when the sounds are loud and clear enough to be heard.

These kinds of problems usually happen when there is background noise, which is often the case in social situations. So kids with APD can have trouble understanding what is being said to them when they're in noisy places like a playground, sports events, the school cafeteria, and parties.

Symptoms

Symptoms of APD can range from mild to severe and can take many different forms. If you think your child might have a problem processing sounds, ask yourself these questions:

- Is your child easily distracted or unusually bothered by loud or sudden noises?
- Are noisy environments upsetting to your child?
- Does your child's behavior and performance improve in quieter settings?
- Does your child have difficulty following directions, whether simple or complicated?
- Does your child have reading, spelling, writing, or other speech-language difficulties?
- Are verbal (word) math problems difficult for your child?
- Is your child disorganized and forgetful?
- Are conversations hard for your child to follow?

APD is often misunderstood because many of the behaviors noted above also can accompany other problems, like learning disabilities, attention deficit hyperactivity disorder (ADHD), and even depression.

Causes

Often, the cause of a child's APD isn't known. Evidence suggests that head trauma, lead poisoning, and chronic ear infections could play a role. Sometimes, there can be multiple causes.

Diagnosis

If you think your child is having trouble hearing or understanding when people talk, have an audiologist (hearing specialist) exam your child. Only audiologists can diagnose auditory processing disorder.

Audiologists look for five main problem areas in kids with APD:

1. **Auditory figure-ground problems:** This is when a child can't pay attention if there's noise in the background. Noisy, loosely structured classrooms could be very frustrating.
2. **Auditory memory problems:** This is when a child has difficulty remembering information such as directions, lists, or study materials. It can be immediate ("I can't remember it now") and/or delayed ("I can't remember it when I need it for later").
3. **Auditory discrimination problems:** This is when a child has difficulty hearing the difference between words or sounds

that are similar (COAT/BOAT or CH/SH). This can affect following directions and reading, spelling, and writing skills, among others.

4. **Auditory attention problems:** This is when a child can't stay focused on listening long enough to complete a task or requirement (such as listening to a lecture in school). Kids with CAPD often have trouble maintaining attention, although health, motivation, and attitude also can play a role.
5. **Auditory cohesion problems:** This is when higher-level listening tasks are difficult. Auditory cohesion skills — drawing inferences from conversations, understanding riddles, or comprehending verbal math problems — require heightened auditory processing and language levels. They develop best when all the other skills (levels 1 through 4 above) are intact.

Since most of the tests done to check for APD require a child to be at least 7 or 8 years old, many kids aren't diagnosed until then or later.

Helping Your Child

A child's auditory system isn't fully developed until age 15. So, many kids diagnosed with APD can develop better skills over time as their auditory system matures. While there is no known cure, speech-language therapy and assistive listening devices can help kids make sense of sounds and develop good communication skills.

A frequency modulation (FM) system is a type of assistive listening device that reduces background noise and makes a speaker's voice louder so a child can understand it. The speaker wears a tiny microphone and a transmitter, which sends an electrical signal to a wireless receiver that the child wears either on the ear or elsewhere on the body. It's portable and can be helpful in classroom settings.

A crucial part of making the FM system effective is ongoing therapy with a speech-language pathologist, who will help the child develop speaking and hearing skills. The speech-language pathologist or audiologist also may recommend tutoring programs.

Several computer-assisted programs are geared toward children with APD. They mainly help the brain do a better job of processing sounds in a noisy environment. Some schools offer these programs, so if your child has APD, be sure to ask school officials about what may be available.

At Home

Strategies applied at home and school can ease some of the problem behaviors associated with APD.

Kids with APD often have trouble following directions, so these suggestions may help:

- Reduce background noise whenever possible at home and at school.
- Have your child look at you when you're speaking.
- Use simple, expressive sentences.
- Speak at a slightly slower rate and at a mildly increased volume.
- Ask your child to repeat the directions back to you and to keep repeating them aloud (to you or to himself or herself) until the directions are completed.
- For directions that are to be completed later, writing notes, wearing a watch, or maintaining a household routine can help. So can general organization and scheduling.
- It can be frustrating for kids with APD when they're in a noisy setting and they need to listen. Teach your child to notice noisy environments and move to quieter places when listening is necessary.

Other tips that might help:

- Provide your child with a quiet study place (not the kitchen table).
- Maintain a peaceful, organized lifestyle.
- Encourage good eating and sleeping habits.
- Assign regular and realistic chores, including keeping a neat room and desk.
- Build your child's self-esteem.

At School

It's important for the people caring for your child to know about APD. Be sure to tell teachers and other school officials about the APD and how it may affect learning. Kids with APD aren't typically put in special education programs, but you may find that your child is eligible for a 504 plan through the school district that would outline any special needs for the classroom.

Some things that may help:

- changing seating plans so your child can sit in the front of the classroom or with his or her back to the window
- study aids, like a tape recorder or notes that can be viewed online
- computer-assisted programs designed for kids with APD

Keep in regular contact with school officials about your child's progress. One of the most important things that both parents and teachers can do is to acknowledge that APD is real. Its symptoms and behaviors are not something that a child can control. What the child can control is recognizing the problems associated with APD and using the strategies recommended both at home and school.

A positive, realistic attitude and healthy self-esteem in a child with APD can work wonders. And kids with APD can go on to be just as successful as other classmates. Coping strategies and techniques learned in speech therapy can help them go far.

Is There a Relationship between APD and ADHD?

The behaviors of children with APD and attention deficit hyperactivity disorder (ADHD) may be very similar, especially with regard to distractibility. Given what is presently known, APD and ADHD do not appear to be a single developmental disorder. Each can occur independently, or they can coexist. This is a prime example of where the team approach to evaluation is critical, as the team can rule out the presence of ADHD or determine its contribution to the potential educational impact on the child.

Section 34.2

Developmental Apraxia of Speech

This section includes text excerpted from "Apraxia of Speech," National Institute on Deafness and Other Communication Disorders (NIDCD), June 7, 2010. Reviewed October 2016.

What Is Apraxia of Speech?

Apraxia of speech, also known as verbal apraxia or dyspraxia, is a speech disorder in which a person has trouble saying what he or she wants to say correctly and consistently. It is not due to weakness or paralysis of the speech muscles (the muscles of the face, tongue, and lips). The severity of apraxia of speech can range from mild to severe.

What Are the Types and Causes of Apraxia?

There are two main types of speech apraxia: acquired apraxia of speech and developmental apraxia of speech. Acquired apraxia of speech can affect a person at any age, although it most typically occurs in adults. It is caused by damage to the parts of the brain that are involved in speaking, and involves the loss or impairment of existing speech abilities. The disorder may result from a stroke, head injury, tumor, or other illness affecting the brain. Acquired apraxia of speech may occur together with muscle weakness affecting speech production (dysarthria) or language difficulties caused by damage to the nervous system (aphasia).

Developmental apraxia of speech (DAS) occurs in children and is present from birth. It appears to affect more boys than girls. This speech disorder goes by several other names, including developmental verbal apraxia, developmental verbal dyspraxia, articulatory apraxia, and childhood apraxia of speech. DAS is different from what is known as a developmental delay of speech, in which a child follows the "typical" path of speech development but does so more slowly than normal.

The cause or causes of DAS are not yet known. Some scientists believe that DAS is a disorder related to a child's overall language development. Others believe it is a neurological disorder that affects the brain's ability to send the proper signals to move the muscles involved in speech. However, brain imaging and other studies have not found evidence of specific brain lesions or differences in brain structure in children with DAS. Children with DAS often have family members who have a history of communication disorders or learning disabilities. This observation and recent research findings suggest that genetic factors may play a role in the disorder.

What Are the Symptoms of Apraxia?

People with either form of apraxia of speech may have a number of different speech characteristics, or symptoms. One of the most notable symptoms is difficulty putting sounds and syllables together in the correct order to form words. Longer or more complex words are usually harder to say than shorter or simpler words. People with apraxia of speech also tend to make inconsistent mistakes when speaking. For example, they may say a difficult word correctly but then have trouble repeating it, or they may be able to say a particular sound one day and have trouble with the same sound the next day. People with apraxia of speech often appear to be groping for the right sound or word, and may try saying a word several times before they say it correctly. Another common characteristic of apraxia of speech is the incorrect use of "prosody"—that is, the varying rhythms, stresses, and inflections of speech that are used to help express meaning.

Children with developmental apraxia of speech generally can understand language much better than they are able to use language to express themselves. Some children with the disorder may also have other problems. These can include other speech problems, such as dysarthria; language problems such as poor vocabulary, incorrect grammar, and difficulty in clearly organizing spoken information; problems with reading, writing, spelling, or math; coordination or "motor-skill" problems; and chewing and swallowing difficulties.

The severity of both acquired and developmental apraxia of speech varies from person to person. Apraxia can be so mild that a person has trouble with very few speech sounds or only has occasional problems pronouncing words with many syllables. In the most severe cases, a person may not be able to communicate effectively with speech, and may need the help of alternative or additional communication methods.

How Is Apraxia Diagnosed?

Professionals known as speech-language pathologists play a key role in diagnosing and treating apraxia of speech. There is no single factor or test that can be used to diagnose apraxia. In addition, speech-language experts do not agree about which specific symptoms are part of developmental apraxia. The person making the diagnosis generally looks for the presence of some, or many, of a group of symptoms, including those described above. Ruling out other contributing factors, such as muscle weakness or language-comprehension problems, can also help with the diagnosis.

To diagnose developmental apraxia of speech, parents and professionals may need to observe a child's speech over a period of time. In formal testing for both acquired and developmental apraxia, the speech-language pathologist may ask the person to perform speech tasks such as repeating a particular word several times or repeating a list of words of increasing length (for example, love, loving, lovingly). For acquired apraxia of speech, a speech-language pathologist may also examine a person's ability to converse, read, write, and perform non-speech movements. Brain-imaging tests such as magnetic resonance imaging (MRI) may also be used to help distinguish acquired apraxia of speech from other communication disorders in people who have experienced brain damage.

How Is Apraxia Treated?

In some cases, people with acquired apraxia of speech recover some or all of their speech abilities on their own. This is called spontaneous recovery. Children with developmental apraxia of speech will not outgrow the problem on their own. Speech-language therapy is often helpful for these children and for people with acquired apraxia who do not spontaneously recover all of their speech abilities.

Speech-language pathologists use different approaches to treat apraxia of speech, and no single approach has been proven to be the most effective. Therapy is tailored to the individual and is designed to treat other speech or language problems that may occur together with apraxia. Each person responds differently to therapy, and some people will make more progress than others. People with apraxia of speech usually need frequent and intensive one-on-one therapy. Support and encouragement from family members and friends are also important.

In severe cases, people with acquired or developmental apraxia of speech may need to use other ways to express themselves. These might include formal or informal sign language, a language notebook with pictures or written words that the person can show to other people, or an electronic communication device such as a portable computer that writes and produces speech.

Section 34.3

Developmental Disabilities

This section includes text excerpted from "Facts about Developmental Disabilities," Centers for Disease Control and Prevention (CDC), August 31, 2016.

Developmental disabilities are a group of conditions due to an impairment in physical, learning, language, or behavior areas. These conditions begin during the developmental period, may impact day-to-day functioning, and usually last throughout a person's lifetime.

Developmental Milestones

Skills such as taking a first step, smiling for the first time, and waving "bye-bye" are called developmental milestones. Children reach milestones in how they play, learn, speak, behave, and move (for example, crawling and walking).

Children develop at their own pace, so it's impossible to tell exactly when a child will learn a given skill. However, the developmental milestones give a general idea of the changes to expect as a child gets older.

As a parent, you know your child best. If your child is not meeting the milestones for his or her age, or if you think there could be a problem with your child's development, talk with your child's doctor or healthcare provider and share your concerns. Don't wait.

Developmental Monitoring

Your child's growth and development are kept track of through a partnership between you and your healthcare professional. At each well-child visit the doctor looks for developmental delays or problems and talks with you about any concerns you might have. This is called developmental monitoring. Any problems noticed during developmental monitoring should be followed-up with developmental screening.

Children with special healthcare needs should have developmental monitoring and screening just like those without special needs. Monitoring healthy development means paying attention not only to symptoms related to the child's condition, but also to the child's physical, mental, social, and emotional well-being.

Developmental Screening

Well-child visits allow doctors and nurses to have regular contact with children to keep track of—or monitor—your child's health and development through periodic developmental screening. Developmental screening is a short test to tell if a child is learning basic skills when he or she should, or if there are delays. Developmental screening can also be done by other professionals in healthcare, community, or school settings.

The doctor might ask you some questions or talk and play with the child during an examination to see how he or she plays, learns, speaks, behaves, and moves. A delay in any of these areas could be a sign of a problem.

The American Academy of Pediatrics (AAP) recommends that all children be screened for developmental delays and disabilities during regular well-child doctor visits at:

- 9 months
- 18 months
- 24 or 30 months

Additional screening might be needed if a child is at high risk for developmental problems due to preterm birth, low birthweight, or other reasons.

If your child's doctor does not routinely check your child with this type of developmental screening test, you can ask that it be done.

Causes and Risk Factors

Developmental disabilities begin anytime during the developmental period and usually last throughout a person's lifetime. Most developmental disabilities begin before a baby is born, but some can happen after birth because of injury, infection, or other factors.

Most developmental disabilities are thought to be caused by a complex mix of factors. These factors include genetics; parental health and behaviors (such as smoking and drinking) during pregnancy; complications during birth; infections the mother might have during pregnancy or the baby might have very early in life; and exposure of the mother or child to high levels of environmental toxins, such as lead. For some developmental disabilities, such as fetal alcohol syndrome, which is caused by drinking alcohol during pregnancy, we know the cause. But for most, we don't.

Following are some examples of what we know about specific developmental disabilities:

- At least 25% of hearing loss among babies is due to maternal infections during pregnancy, such as cytomegalovirus (CMV) infection; complications after birth; and head trauma.
- Some of the most common known causes of intellectual disability include fetal alcohol syndrome; genetic and chromosomal conditions, such as Down syndrome and fragile X syndrome; and certain infections during pregnancy, such as toxoplasmosis.
- Children who have a sibling are at a higher risk of also having an autism spectrum disorder.
- Low birthweight, premature birth, multiple birth, and infections during pregnancy are associated with an increased risk for many developmental disabilities.
- Untreated newborn jaundice (high levels of bilirubin in the blood during the first few days after birth) can cause a type of brain damage known as kernicterus. Children with kernicterus are more likely to have cerebral palsy, hearing and vision problems, and problems with their teeth. Early detection and treatment of newborn jaundice can prevent kernicterus.

Who Is Affected?

Developmental disabilities occur among all racial, ethnic, and socioeconomic groups. Recent estimates in the United States show that about one in six, or about 15%, of children aged 3 through 17 years have a one or more developmental disabilities, such as:

- ADHD
- autism spectrum disorder
- cerebral palsy
- hearing loss
- intellectual disability
- learning disability

- vision impairment
- and other developmental delays

Living with a Developmental Disability

Children and adults with disabilities need healthcare and health programs for the same reasons anyone else does—to stay well, active, and a part of the community.

Having a disability does not mean a person is not healthy or that he or she cannot be healthy. Being healthy means the same thing for all of us—getting and staying well so we can lead full, active lives. That includes having the tools and information to make healthy choices and knowing how to prevent illness. Some health conditions, such as asthma, gastrointestinal symptoms, eczema and skin allergies, and migraine headaches, have been found to be more common among children with developmental disabilities. Thus, it is especially important for children with developmental disabilities to see a healthcare provider regularly.

Section 34.4

Dyslexia

This section includes text excerpted from "Dyslexia," National Institute of Neurological Disorders and Stroke (NINDS), September 11, 2015.

What Is Dyslexia?

Dyslexia is a brain-based type of learning disability that specifically impairs a person's ability to read. These individuals typically read at levels significantly lower than expected despite having normal intelligence. Although the disorder varies from person to person, common characteristics among people with dyslexia are difficulty with phonological processing (the manipulation of sounds), spelling, and/or rapid visual-verbal responding. In individuals with adult onset of dyslexia, it usually occurs as a result of brain injury or in the context of dementia; this contrasts with individuals with dyslexia who simply were never identified as children or adolescents. Dyslexia can be inherited in some families, and recent studies have identified a number of genes that may predispose an individual to developing dyslexia.

Is There Any Treatment for Dyslexia?

The main focus of treatment should be on the specific learning problems of affected individuals. The usual course is to modify teaching methods and the educational environment to meet the specific needs of the individual with dyslexia.

What Is the Prognosis?

For those with dyslexia, the prognosis is mixed. The disability affects such a wide range of people and produces such different symptoms and varying degrees of severity that predictions are hard to make. The prognosis is generally good, however, for individuals whose dyslexia is identified early, who have supportive family and friends and a strong self-image, and who are involved in a proper remediation program.

What Research Is Being Done?

The National Institute of Neurological Disorders and Stroke (NINDS) and other institutes of the National Institutes of Health (NIH) support dyslexia research through grants to major research institutions across the country. Current research avenues focus on developing techniques to diagnose and treat dyslexia and other learning disabilities, increasing the understanding of the biological and possible genetic bases of learning disabilities, and exploring the relationship between neurophysiological processes and cognitive functions with regard to reading ability.

Section 34.5

Learning Disabilities

This section includes text excerpted from "Learning Disabilities: Condition Information," *Eunice Kennedy Shriver* National Institute of Child Health and Human Development (NICHD), February 28, 2014.

What Are Learning Disabilities?

Learning disabilities are conditions that affect how a person learns to read, write, speak, and calculate numbers. They are caused by differences in brain structure and affect the way a person's brain processes information.

Learning disabilities are usually discovered after a child begins attending school and has difficulties in one or more subjects that do not improve over time. A person can have more than one learning disability.Learning disabilities can last a person's entire life, but they may be alleviated with the right educational supports.

A learning disability is not an indication of a person's intelligence. Also, learning disabilities are not the same as learning problems due to intellectual and developmental disabilities, or emotional, vision, hearing, or motor skills problems.

Common Learning Disabilities

Some of the most common learning disabilities include the following:

- **Dyslexia.** This condition causes problems with language skills, particularly reading. People with dyslexia may have difficulty spelling, understanding sentences, and recognizing words they already know.
- **Dysgraphia.** People with dysgraphia have problems with their handwriting. They may have problems forming letters, writing within a defined space, and writing down their thoughts.

- **Dyscalculia.** People with this math learning disability may have difficulty understanding arithmetic concepts and doing such tasks as addition, multiplication, and measuring.
- **Dyspraxia.** This condition, also termed sensory integration disorder, involves problems with motor coordination that lead to poor balance and clumsiness. Poor hand-eye coordination also causes difficulty with fine motor tasks such as putting puzzles together and coloring within the lines.
- **Apraxia of speech.** Sometimes called verbal apraxia, this disorder involves problems with speaking. People with this disorder have trouble saying what they want to say correctly and consistently.
- **Central auditory processing disorder.** People with this condition have trouble understanding and remembering language-related tasks. They have difficulty explaining things, understanding jokes, and following directions. They confuse words and are easily distracted.
- **Nonverbal learning disorders.** People with these conditions have strong verbal skills but great difficulty understanding facial expression and body language. In addition, they are physically clumsy and have trouble generalizing and following multistep directions.
- **Visual perceptual/visual motor deficit.** People with this condition mix up letters; they might confuse "m" and "w" or "d" and "b," for example. They may also lose their place while reading, copy inaccurately, write messily, and cut paper clumsily.
- **Aphasia.** Aphasia, also called dysphasia, is a language disorder. A person with this disorder has difficulty understanding spoken language, poor reading comprehension, trouble with writing, and great difficulty finding words to express thoughts and feelings. Aphasia occurs when the language areas of the brain are damaged. In adults, it often is caused by stroke, but children may get aphasia from a brain tumor, head injury, or brain infection.

What Are the Indicators of Learning Disabilities?

Many children have difficulty with reading, writing, or other learning-related tasks at some point, but this does not mean they have learning disabilities. A child with a learning disability often has several related signs, and these persist over time. The signs of learning disabilities vary from person to person. Common signs that a person may have learning disabilities include the following:

- Difficulty with reading and/or writing
- Problems with math skills
- Difficulty remembering
- Problems paying attention
- Trouble following directions
- Poor coordination
- Difficulty with concepts related to time
- Problems staying organized

A child with a learning disability also may exhibit one or more of the following:

- Impetuous behavior
- Inappropriate responses in school or social situations
- Difficulty staying on task (easily distracted)
- Difficulty finding the right way to say something
- Inconsistent school performance
- Immature way of speaking
- Difficulty listening well
- Problems dealing with new things in life
- Problems understanding words or concepts

These signs alone are not enough to determine that a person has a learning disability. A professional assessment is necessary to diagnose a learning disability.

Each learning disability has its own signs. Also, not every person with a particular disability will have all of the signs of that disability.

Children being taught in a second language that they are learning sometimes act in ways that are similar to the behaviors of someone with a learning disability. For this reason, learning disability assessment must take into account whether a student is bilingual or a second language learner.

Below are some common learning disabilities and the signs associated with them:

Dyslexia

People with dyslexia usually have trouble making the connections between letters and sounds and with spelling and recognizing words.

People with dyslexia often show other signs of the condition. These may include:

- Failure to fully understand what others are saying
- Difficulty organizing written and spoken language
- Delayed ability to speak
- Poor self-expression (for example, saying "thing" or "stuff" for words not recalled)
- Difficulty learning new vocabulary, either through reading or hearing
- Trouble learning foreign languages
- Slowness in learning songs and rhymes
- Slow reading as well as giving up on longer reading tasks
- Difficulty understanding questions and following directions
- Poor spelling
- Difficulty recalling numbers in sequence (for example, telephone numbers and addresses)
- Trouble distinguishing left from right

Dysgraphia

Dysgraphia is characterized by problems with writing. This disorder may cause a child to be tense and awkward when holding a pen or pencil, even to the extent of contorting his or her body. A child with very poor handwriting that he or she does not outgrow may have dysgraphia.

Other signs of this condition may include:

- A strong dislike of writing and/or drawing
- Problems with grammar
- Trouble writing down ideas

- A quick loss of energy and interest while writing
- Trouble writing down thoughts in a logical sequence
- Saying words out loud while writing
- Leaving words unfinished or omitting them when writing sentences

Dyscalculia

Signs of this disability include problems understanding basic arithmetic concepts, such as fractions, number lines, and positive and negative numbers.

Other symptoms may include:

- Difficulty with math-related word problems
- Trouble making change in cash transactions
- Messiness in putting math problems on paper
- Trouble recognizing logical information sequences (for example, steps in math problems)
- Trouble with understanding the time sequence of events
- Difficulty with verbally describing math processes

Dyspraxia

A person with dyspraxia has problems with motor tasks, such as hand-eye coordination, that can interfere with learning.

Some other symptoms of this condition include:

- Problems organizing oneself and one's things
- Breaking things
- Trouble with tasks that require hand-eye coordination, such as coloring within the lines, assembling puzzles, and cutting precisely
- Poor balance
- Sensitivity to loud and/or repetitive noises, such as the ticking of a clock
- Sensitivity to touch, including irritation over bothersome-feeling clothing

How Many People Are Affected / at Risk for Learning Disabilities?

There is a wide range in estimates of the number of people affected by learning disabilities and disorders. Some of the variation results from differences in requirements for diagnosis in different states.

Some reports estimate that as many as 15% to 20% of Americans are affected by learning disabilities and disorders. In contrast, a major national study found that approximately 5% of children in the United States had learning disabilities. It also found that approximately 4% had both a learning disability and attention deficit hyperactivity disorder (ADHD). Other research, conducted in 2006, estimated that 4.6 million school-age children in the United States have been diagnosed with learning disabilities.

What Causes Learning Disabilities?

Researchers do not know exactly what causes learning disabilities, but they appear to be related to differences in brain structure. These differences are present from birth and often are inherited. To improve understanding of learning disabilities, researchers at the *Eunice Kennedy Shriver* National Institute of Child Health and Human Development (NICHD)

and elsewhere are studying areas of the brain and how they function. Scientists have found that learning disabilities are related to areas of the brain that deal with language and have used imaging studies to show that the brain of a dyslexic person develops and functions differently from a typical brain.

Sometimes, factors that affect a developing fetus, such as alcohol or drug use, can lead to a learning disability. Other factors in an infant's environment may play a role as well. These can include poor nutrition and exposure to toxins such as lead in water or paint. In addition, children who do not receive the support necessary to promote their intellectual development early on may show signs of learning disabilities once they start school.

Sometimes a person may develop a learning disability later in life. Possible causes in such a case include dementia or a traumatic brain injury (TBI).

How Are Learning Disabilities Diagnosed?

Learning disabilities are often identified when a child begins to attend school. Educators may use a process called "response to intervention" (RTI) to help identify children with learning disabilities. Specialized testing is required to make a clear diagnosis, however.

Is There a Cure for Learning Disabilities?

Learning disabilities have no cure, but early intervention can provide tools and strategies to lessen their effects. People with learning disabilities can be successful in school and work and in their personal lives. More information is available about interventions for learning disabilities.

What Are the Treatments for Learning Disabilities?

People with learning disabilities and disorders can learn strategies for coping with their disabilities. Getting help earlier increases the likelihood for success in school and later in life. If learning disabilities remain untreated, a child may begin to feel frustrated with schoolwork, which can lead to low self-esteem, depression, and other problems.

Usually, experts work to help a child learn skills by building on the child's strengths and developing ways to compensate for the child's weaknesses. Interventions vary depending on the nature and extent of the disability.

A child with a learning disability may struggle with low self-esteem, frustration, and other problems. Mental health professionals can help the youngster understand these feelings, develop coping tools, and build healthy relationships.

Children with learning disabilities sometimes have other conditions such as ADHD. These conditions require their own treatments, which may include therapy and medications.

Are There Disorders or Conditions Associated with Learning Disabilities?

Children with learning disabilities may be at greater risk for certain conditions than other youngsters.

One condition found more frequently among children with learning disabilities is attention deficit and hyperactivity disorder (ADHD). A child with ADHD may be very active and impulsive and get distracted easily. ADHD affects about 1 out of 3 children with learning disorders.

Children with disabilities also may develop depression, anxiety, and behavior problems.

Treating conditions associated with a learning disability can help a child feel better overall and become more focused on schoolwork. Treatments may include psychotherapy and medications.

Where Can I Get Help for My Child's Learning Disability?

- **Learning disability evaluation.** If you believe your child may have a reading, writing, or related disability/disorder, you can have him or her professionally evaluated. The National Center for Learning Disabilities provides information about getting your child evaluated at school and questions to ask an evaluator.
- **Parenting.** The National Center for Learning Disabilities provides information on dealing with daily living and parenting a child with a learning disability.
- **Special education services.** The Learning Disabilities Association of America offers extensive information on special education.

Section 34.6

Stuttering

This section includes text excerpted from "Stuttering," National Institute on Deafness and Other Communication Disorders (NIDCD), June 6, 2016.

What Is Stuttering?

Stuttering is a speech disorder characterized by repetition of sounds, syllables, or words; prolongation of sounds; and interruptions in speech known as blocks. An individual who stutters exactly knows what he or she would like to say but has trouble producing a normal flow of speech. These speech disruptions may be accompanied by struggle behaviors, such as rapid eye blinks or tremors of the lips. Stuttering can make it difficult to communicate with other people, which often affects a person's quality of life and interpersonal relationships. Stuttering can also negatively influence job performance and opportunities, and treatment can come at a high financial cost.

Symptoms of stuttering can vary significantly throughout a person's day. In general, speaking before a group or talking on the telephone may make a person's stuttering more severe, while singing, reading, or speaking in unison may temporarily reduce stuttering.

Stuttering is sometimes referred to as stammering and by a broader term, disfluent speech.

Who Stutters?

Roughly 3 million Americans stutter. Stuttering affects people of all ages. It occurs most often in children between the ages of 2 and 6 as they are developing their language skills. Approximately 5 to 10 percent of all children will stutter for some period in their life, lasting from a few weeks to several years. Boys are 2 to 3 times as likely to stutter as girls and as they get older this gender difference increases; the number of boys who continue to stutter is three to four times larger than the number of girls. Most children outgrow stuttering. Approximately 75 percent of children recover from stuttering. For the remaining 25 percent who continue to stutter, stuttering can persist as a lifelong communication disorder.

How Is Speech Normally Produced?

We make speech sounds through a series of precisely coordinated muscle movements involving breathing, phonation (voice production), and articulation (movement of the throat, palate, tongue, and lips). Muscle movements are controlled by the brain and monitored through our senses of hearing and touch.

What Are the Causes and Types of Stuttering?

The precise mechanisms that cause stuttering are not understood. Stuttering is commonly grouped into two types termed developmental and neurogenic.

Developmental Stuttering

Developmental stuttering occurs in young children while they are still learning speech and language skills. It is the most common form of stuttering. Some scientists and clinicians believe that developmental stuttering occurs when children's speech and language abilities are unable to meet the child's verbal demands. Most scientists and clinicians believe that developmental stuttering stems from complex interactions of multiple factors. Recent brain imaging studies have shown consistent differences in those who stutter compared to non stuttering peers. Developmental stuttering may also run in families and research has shown that genetic factors contribute to this type of stuttering. Starting in 2010, researchers at the National Institute on Deafness and Other Communication Disorders (NIDCD) have identified four different genes in which mutations are associated with stuttering.

Neurogenic Stuttering

Neurogenic stuttering may occur after a stroke, head trauma, or other type of brain injury. With neurogenic stuttering, the brain has difficulty coordinating the different brain regions involved in speaking, resulting in problems in production of clear, fluent speech.

At one time, all stuttering was believed to be psychogenic, caused by emotional trauma, but today we know that psychogenic stuttering is rare.

How Is Stuttering Diagnosed?

Stuttering is usually diagnosed by a speech-language pathologist, a health professional who is trained to test and treat individuals with voice, speech, and language disorders. The speech-language pathologist will consider a variety of factors, including the child's case history (such as when the stuttering was first noticed and under what circumstances), an analysis of the child's stuttering behaviors, and an evaluation of the child's speech and language abilities and the impact of stuttering on his or her life.

When evaluating a young child for stuttering, a speech-language pathologist will try to determine if the child is likely to continue his or her stuttering behavior or outgrow it. To determine this difference, the speech-language pathologist will consider such factors as the family's history of stuttering, whether the child's stuttering has lasted 6 months or longer, and whether the child exhibits other speech or language problems.

How Is Stuttering Treated?

Although there is currently no cure for stuttering, there are a variety of treatments available. The nature of the treatment will differ, based upon a person's age, communication goals, and other factors. If you or your child stutters, it is important to work with a speech-language pathologist to determine the best treatment options.

Therapy for Children

For very young children, early treatment may prevent developmental stuttering from becoming a lifelong problem. Certain strategies can help children learn to improve their speech fluency while developing positive attitudes toward communication. Health professionals generally recommend that a child be evaluated if he or she has stuttered for 3 to 6 months, exhibits struggle behaviors associated with stuttering, or has a family history of stuttering or related communication disorders. Some researchers recommend that a child be evaluated every 3 months to determine if the stuttering is increasing or decreasing. Treatment often involves teaching parents about ways to support their child's production of fluent speech. Parents may be encouraged to:

- Provide a relaxed home environment that allows many opportunities for the child to speak. This includes setting aside time to talk to one another, especially when the child is excited and has a lot to say.
- Listen attentively when the child speaks and focus on the content of the message, rather than responding to how it is said or interrupting the child.
- Speak in a slightly slowed and relaxed manner. This can help reduce time pressures the child may be experiencing.
- Listen attentively when the child speaks and wait for him or her to say the intended word. Don't try to complete the child's sentences. Also, help the child learn that a person can communicate successfully even when stuttering occurs.
- Talk openly and honestly to the child about stuttering if he or she brings up the subject. Let the child know that it is okay for some disruptions to occur.

Stuttering Therapy

Many of the current therapies for teens and adults who stutter focus on helping them learn ways to minimize stuttering when they speak, such as by speaking more slowly, regulating their breathing, or gradually progressing from single-syllable responses to longer words and more complex sentences. Most of these therapies also help address the anxiety a person who stutters may feel in certain speaking situations.

Drug Therapy

The U.S. Food and Drug Administration (FDA) has not approved any drug for the treatment of stuttering. However, some drugs that are approved to treat other health problems—such as epilepsy, anxiety, or depression—have been used to treat stuttering. These drugs often have side effects that make them difficult to use over a long period of time.

Electronic Devices

Some people who stutter use electronic devices to help control fluency. For example, one type of device fits into the ear canal, much like a hearing aid, and digitally replays a slightly altered version of the wearer's voice into the ear so that it sounds as if he or she is speaking in unison with another person. In some people, electronic devices may help improve fluency in a relatively short period of time. Additional research is needed to determine how long such effects may last and whether people are able to easily use and benefit from these devices in real-world situations. For these reasons, researchers are continuing to study the long-term effectiveness of these devices.

Self-Help Groups

Many people find that they achieve their greatest success through a combination of self-study and therapy. Self-help groups provide a way for people who stutter to find resources and support as they face the challenges of stuttering.

Chapter 35

Fragile X Syndrome

What Is Fragile X Syndrome?

Fragile X syndrome (FXS) is a genetic disorder. A genetic disorder means that there are changes to the person's genes. FXS is caused by changes in the *fragile X mental retardation 1* (*FMR1*) gene. The *FMR1* gene usually makes a protein called fragile X mental retardation protein (FMRP). FMRP is needed for normal brain development. People who have FXS do not make this protein. People who have other fragile X-associated disorders have changes in their *FMR1* gene but usually make some of the protein.

FXS affects both males and females. However, females often have milder symptoms than males. The exact number of people who have FXS is unknown, but it has been estimated that about 1 in 5,000 males are born with the disorder.

Signs and Symptoms

Signs that a child might have FXS include:

- Developmental delays (not sitting, walking, or talking at the same time as other children the same age);
- Learning disabilities (trouble learning new skills); and

This chapter includes text excerpted from "Facts about Fragile X Syndrome," Centers for Disease Control and Prevention (CDC), June 21, 2016.

- Social and behavior problems (such as not making eye contact, anxiety, trouble paying attention, hand flapping, acting and speaking without thinking, and being very active).

Males who have FXS usually have some degree of intellectual disability that can range from mild to severe. Females with FXS can have normal intelligence or some degree of intellectual disability. Autism spectrum disorders (ASDs) also occur more frequently in people with FXS.

Testing/Diagnosis

FXS can be diagnosed by testing a person's Deoxyribonucleic acid (DNA) from a blood test. A doctor or genetic counselor can order the test. Testing also can be done to find changes in the *FMR1* gene that can lead to fragile X-associated disorders.

A diagnosis of FXS can be helpful to the family because it can provide a reason for a child's intellectual disabilities and behavior problems. This allows the family and other caregivers to learn more about the disorder and manage care so that the child can reach his or her full potential. However, the results of DNA tests can affect other family members and raise many issues. So, anyone who is thinking about FXS testing should consider having genetic counseling prior to getting tested.

Treatments

There is no cure for FXS. However, treatment services can help people learn important skills. Services can include therapy to learn to talk, walk, and interact with others. In addition, medicine can be used to help control some issues, such as behavior problems. To develop the best treatment plan, people with FXS, parents, and healthcare providers should work closely with one another, and with everyone involved in treatment and support—which may include teachers, childcare providers, coaches, therapists, and other family members. Taking advantage of all the resources available will help guide success.

Early Intervention Services

Early intervention services help children from birth to 3 years old (36 months) learn important skills. These services may improve a child's development. Even if the child has not been diagnosed with FXS, he or she may be eligible for services. These services are provided through an early intervention system in each state. Through this system, you can ask for an evaluation. In addition, treatment for particular symptoms, such as speech therapy for language delays, often does not need to wait for a formal diagnosis. While early intervention is extremely important, treatment services at any age can be helpful.

Finding Support

Having support and community resources can help increase confidence in managing FXS, enhance quality of life, and assist in meeting the needs of all family members. It might be helpful for parents of children with FXS to talk with one another. One parent might have learned how to address some of the same concerns another parent has. Often, parents of children with special needs can give advice about good resources for these children.

Remember that the choices of one family might not be best for another family, so it's important that parents understand all options and discuss them with their child's healthcare providers.

- Contact the National Fragile X Foundation at 1-800-688-8765 or ntlfx@fragilex.org to get information about treatments, educational strategies, therapies and intervention.
- Connect with a Community Support Network (CSN) at the National Fragile X Foundation. CSNs are organized and run by parent volunteers and provide support to families.

Chapter 36

Mental Health Disorders in Children

Chapter Contents

Section 36.1

Children's Mental Health: An Overview

This section includes text excerpted from "Children's Mental Health Report," Centers for Disease Control and Prevention (CDC), August 10, 2016.

What Is Childhood Mental Disorder?

The term childhood mental disorder means all mental disorders that can be diagnosed and begin in childhood (for example, attention deficit hyperactivity disorder (ADHD), Tourette syndrome, behavior disorders, mood and anxiety disorders, autism spectrum disorders, substance use disorders, etc.). Mental disorders among children are described as serious changes in the ways children typically learn, behave, or handle their emotions. Symptoms usually start in early childhood, although some of the disorders may develop throughout the teenage years. The diagnosis is often made in the school years and sometimes earlier. However, some children with a mental disorder may not be recognized or diagnosed as having one.

Childhood mental disorders can be treated and managed. There are many evidence-based treatment options, so parents and doctors should work closely with everyone involved in the child's treatment—teachers, coaches, therapists, and other family members. Taking advantage of all the resources available will help parents, health professionals and educators guide the child towards success. Early diagnosis and appropriate services for children and their families can make a difference in the lives of children with mental disorders.

An Important Public Health Issue

Mental health is important to overall health. Mental disorders are chronic health conditions that can continue through the lifespan. Without early diagnosis and treatment, children with mental disorders can have problems at home, in school, and in forming friendships. This can also interfere with their healthy development, and these problems can continue into adulthood.

Children's mental disorders affect many children and families. Boys and girls of all ages, ethnic/racial backgrounds, and regions of the United States experience mental disorders. Based on the National Research Council and Institute of Medicine report (Preventing mental, emotional, and behavioral disorders among young people: progress and possibilities, 2009) that gathered findings from previous studies, it is estimated that 13–20 percent of children living in the United States (up to 1 out of 5 children) experience a mental disorder in a given year and an estimated $247 billion is spent each year on childhood mental disorders. Because of the impact on children, families, and communities, children's mental disorders are an important public health issue in the United States.

Monitoring Children's Mental Health

Public health surveillance—which is the collection and monitoring of information about health among the public over time—is a first step to better understand childhood mental disorders and promote children's mental health. Ongoing and systematic monitoring of mental health and mental disorders will help:

- increase understanding of the mental health needs of children;
- inform research on factors that increase risk and promote prevention;
- find out which programs are effective at preventing mental disorders and promoting children's mental health; and
- monitor if treatment and prevention efforts are effective.

Who Is Affected?

The following are key findings from a Centers for Disease Control and Prevention (CDC) report about mental disorders among children aged 3–17 years:

- Millions of American children live with depression, anxiety, ADHD, autism spectrum disorders, Tourette syndrome or a host of other mental health issues.
- ADHD was the most prevalent current diagnosis among children aged 3–17 years.
- The number of children with a mental disorder increased with age, with the exception of autism spectrum disorders, which was highest among 6 to 11 year old children.

- Boys were more likely than girls to have ADHD, behavioral or conduct problems, autism spectrum disorders, anxiety, Tourette syndrome, and cigarette dependence.
- Adolescent boys aged 12–17 years were more likely than girls to die by suicide.
- Adolescent girls were more likely than boys to have depression or an alcohol use disorder.

Data collected from a variety of data sources between the years 2005–2011 show:

Children aged 3–17 years currently had:

- ADHD (6.8%)
- Behavioral or conduct problems (3.5%)
- Anxiety (3.0%)
- Depression (2.1%)
- Autism spectrum disorders (1.1%)
- Tourette syndrome (0.2%) (among children aged 6–17 years)

Adolescents aged 12–17 years had:

- Illicit drug use disorder in the past year (4.7%)
- Alcohol use disorder in the past year (4.2%)
- Cigarette dependence in the past month (2.8%)

The estimates for current diagnosis were lower than estimates for "ever" diagnosis, meaning whether a child had ever received a diagnosis in his or her lifetime. Suicide, which can result from the interaction of mental disorders and other factors, was the second leading cause of death among adolescents aged 12–17 years in 2010.

Looking to the Future

Public health includes mental health. CDC worked with several agencies to summarize and report this information. The goal is now to build on the strengths of these partnering agencies to develop better ways to document how many children have mental disorders, better understand the impacts of mental disorders, inform needs for treatment and intervention strategies, and promote the mental health of children. This report is an important step on the road to recognizing the impact of childhood mental disorders and developing a public health approach to address children's mental health.

What You Can Do

Parents: You know your child best. Talk to your child's healthcare professional if you have concerns about the way your child behaves at home, in school, or with friends.

Youth: It is just as important to take care of your mental health as it is your physical health. If you are angry, worried or sad, don't be afraid to talk about your feelings and reach out to a trusted friend or adult.

Healthcare professionals: Early diagnosis and appropriate treatment based on updated guidelines is very important. There are resources available to help diagnose and treat children's mental disorders.

Teachers/School Administrators: Early identification is important, so that children can get the help they need. Work with families and healthcare professionals if you have concerns about the mental health of a child in your school.

Section 36.2

Anxiety and Panic Disorders

This section contains text excerpted from the following sources: Text beginning with the heading "What Is Anxiety Disorders?" is excerpted from "Anxiety Disorders," National Institute of Mental Health (NIMH), March 11, 2016; Text beginning with the heading "What Is Panic Disorder?" is excerpted from "Panic Disorder: When Fear Overwhelms," National Institute of Mental Health (NIMH), October 1, 2016.

What Is Anxiety Disorders?

Occasional anxiety is a normal part of life. You might feel anxious when faced with a problem at work, before taking a test, or making an important decision. But anxiety disorders involve more than temporary worry or fear. For a person with an anxiety disorder, the anxiety does not go away and can get worse over time. The feelings can interfere with daily activities such as job performance, school work, and relationships. There are several different types of anxiety disorders. Examples include generalized anxiety disorder, panic disorder, and social anxiety disorder.

Signs and Symptoms

Generalized Anxiety Disorder

People with generalized anxiety disorder display excessive anxiety or worry for months and face several anxiety-related symptoms.

Generalized anxiety disorder symptoms include:

- Restlessness or feeling wound-up or on edge
- Being easily fatigued
- Difficulty concentrating or having their minds go blank
- Irritability
- Muscle tension
- Difficulty controlling the worry
- Sleep problems (difficulty falling or staying asleep or restless, unsatisfying sleep)

Social Anxiety Disorder

People with social anxiety disorder (sometimes called "social phobia") have a marked fear of social or performance situations in which they expect to feel embarrassed, judged, rejected, or fearful of offending others.

Social anxiety disorder symptoms include:

- Feeling highly anxious about being with other people and having a hard time talking to them
- Feeling very self-conscious in front of other people and worried about feeling humiliated, embarrassed, or rejected, or fearful of offending others
- Being very afraid that other people will judge them
- Worrying for days or weeks before an event where other people will be

- Staying away from places where there are other people
- Having a hard time making friends and keeping friends
- Blushing, sweating, or trembling around other people
- Feeling nauseous or sick to your stomach when other people are around

Evaluation for an anxiety disorder often begins with a visit to a primary care provider. Some physical health conditions, such as an overactive thyroid or low blood sugar, as well as taking certain medications, can imitate or worsen an anxiety disorder. A thorough mental health evaluation is also helpful, because anxiety disorders often co-exist with other related conditions, such as depression or obsessive-compulsive disorder.

Risk Factors

Researchers are finding that genetic and environmental factors, frequently in interaction with one another, are risk factors for anxiety disorders. Specific factors include:

- Shyness, or behavioral inhibition, in childhood
- Being female
- Having few economic resources
- Being divorced or widowed
- Exposure to stressful life events in childhood and adulthood
- Anxiety disorders in close biological relatives
- Parental history of mental disorders
- Elevated afternoon cortisol levels in the saliva (specifically for social anxiety disorder)

Treatment and Therapies

Anxiety disorders are generally treated with psychotherapy, medication, or both.

What Is Panic Disorder?

People with panic disorder have sudden and repeated attacks of fear that last for several minutes or longer. These are called panic attacks. Panic attacks are characterized by a fear of disaster or of losing control even when there is no real danger. A person may also have a strong physical reaction during a panic attack. It may feel like having a heart attack. Panic attacks can occur at any time, and many people with panic disorder worry about and dread the possibility of having another attack.

A person with panic disorder may become discouraged and feel ashamed because he or she cannot carry out normal routines like going to the grocery store or driving. Having panic disorder can also interfere with school or work.

Panic disorder often begins in the late teens or early adulthood. More women than men have panic disorder. But not everyone who experiences panic attacks will develop panic disorder.

What Causes Panic Disorder?

Panic disorder sometimes runs in families, but no one knows for sure why some people have it, while others don't. Researchers have found that several parts of the brain are involved in fear and anxiety. Some researchers think that people with panic disorder misinterpret harmless bodily sensations as threats. Researchers are also looking for ways in which stress and environmental factors may play a role.

What Are the Signs and Symptoms of Panic Disorder?

People with panic disorder may have:

- Sudden and repeated attacks of fear
- A feeling of being out of control during a panic attack
- An intense worry about when the next attack will happen
- A fear or avoidance of places where panic attacks have occurred in the past
- Physical symptoms during an attack, such as a pounding or racing heart, sweating, breathing problems, weakness or dizziness, feeling hot or a cold chill, tingly or numb hands, chest pain, or stomach pain.

How Is Panic Disorder Treated?

First, talk to your doctor about your symptoms. Your doctor should do an exam to make sure that another physical problem isn't causing the symptoms. The doctor may refer you to a mental health specialist.

Panic disorder is generally treated with psychotherapy, medication, or both.

Section 36.3

Bipolar Disorder

This section includes text excerpted from "Bipolar Disorder in Children and Teens," National Institute of Mental Health (NIMH), 2015.

What Is Bipolar Disorder?

Bipolar disorder is a serious brain illness. It is also called manic-depressive illness or manic depression. Children with bipolar disorder go through unusual mood changes. Sometimes they feel very happy or "up," and are much more energetic and active than usual, or than other kids their age. This is called a manic episode. Sometimes children with bipolar disorder feel very sad and "down," and are much less active than usual. This is called depression or a depressive episode.

Bipolar disorder is not the same as the normal ups and downs every kid goes through. Bipolar symptoms are more powerful than that. The mood swings are more extreme and are accompanied by changes in sleep, energy level, and the ability to think clearly. Bipolar symptoms are so strong, they can make it hard for a child to do well in school or get along with friends and family members. The illness can also be dangerous. Some young people with bipolar disorder try to hurt themselves or attempt suicide.

Children and teens with bipolar disorder should get treatment. With help, they can manage their symptoms and lead successful lives.

Who Develops Bipolar Disorder?

Anyone can develop bipolar disorder, including children and teens. However, most people with bipolar disorder develop it in their late teen or early adult years. The illness usually lasts a lifetime.

Why Does Someone Develop Bipolar Disorder?

Doctors do not know what causes bipolar disorder, but several things may contribute to the illness. Family genes may be one factor because bipolar disorder sometimes runs in families. However, it is important to know that just because someone in your family has bipolar disorder, it does not mean other members of the family will have it as well.

Another factor that may lead to bipolar disorder is the brain structure or the brain function of the person with the disorder. Scientists are finding out more about the disorder by studying it. This research may help doctors do a better job of treating people. Also, this research may help doctors to predict whether a person will get bipolar disorder. One day, doctors may be able to prevent the illness in some people.

What Are the Symptoms of Bipolar Disorder?

Bipolar "mood episodes" include unusual mood changes along with unusual sleep habits, activity levels, thoughts, or behavior. In a child, these mood and activity changes must be very different from their usual behavior and from the behavior of other children. A person with bipolar disorder may have manic episodes, depressive episodes, or "mixed" episodes. A mixed episode has both manic and depressive symptoms. These mood episodes cause symptoms that last a week or two or sometimes longer. During an episode, the symptoms last every day for most of the day.

Children and teens having a manic episode may:

- Feel very happy or act silly in a way that's unusual for them and for other people their age
- Have a very short temper
- Talk really fast about a lot of different things
- Have trouble sleeping but not feel tired
- Have trouble staying focused
- Do risky things
- Children and teens having a depressive episode may:
- Feel very sad
- Complain about pain a lot, such as stomachaches and headaches

- Sleep too little or too much
- Feel guilty and worthless
- Eat too little or too much
- Have little energy and no interest in fun activities
- Think about death or suicide

Can Children and Teens with Bipolar Disorder Have Other Problems?

Young people with bipolar disorder can have several problems at the same time. These include:

- Substance abuse. Both adults and kids with bipolar disorder are at risk of drinking or taking drugs.
- Attention deficit hyperactivity disorder (ADHD). Children who have both bipolar disorder and ADHD may have trouble staying focused.
- Anxiety disorders, like separation anxiety.

Sometimes behavior problems go along with mood episodes. Young people may take a lot of risks, such as driving too fast or spending too much money. Some young people with bipolar disorder think about suicide. Watch for any signs of suicidal thinking. Take these signs seriously and call your child's doctor.

How Is Bipolar Disorder Diagnosed?

An experienced doctor will carefully examine your child. There are no blood tests or brain scans that can diagnose bipolar disorder. Instead, the doctor will ask questions about your child's mood and sleeping patterns. The doctor will also ask about your child's energy and behavior. Sometimes doctors need to know about medical problems in your family, such as depression or alcoholism. The doctor may use tests to see if something other than bipolar disorder is causing your child's symptoms.

How Is Bipolar Disorder Treated?

Right now, there is no cure for bipolar disorder. Doctors often treat children who have the illness in much the same way they treat adults.

Treatment can help control symptoms. Steady, dependable treatment works better than treatment that starts and stops.

What Can Children and Teens Expect from Treatment?

With treatment, children and teens with bipolar disorder can get better over time. It helps when doctors, parents, and young people work together.

Sometimes a child's bipolar disorder changes. When this happens, treatment needs to change too. For example, your child may need to try a different medication. The doctor may also recommend other treatment changes. Symptoms may come back after a while, and more adjustments may be needed. Treatment can take time, but sticking with it helps many children and teens have fewer bipolar symptoms.

You can help treatment be more effective. Try keeping a chart of your child's moods, behaviors, and sleep patterns. This is called a "daily life chart" or "mood chart." It can help you and your child understand and track the illness. A chart can also help the doctor see whether treatment is working.

How Can I Help My Child or Teen?

Help begins with the right diagnosis and treatment. If you think your child may have bipolar disorder, make an appointment with your family doctor to talk about the symptoms you notice.

If your child has bipolar disorder, here are some basic things you can do:

- Be patient.
- Encourage your child to talk, and listen to your child carefully.
- Be understanding about mood episodes.
- Help your child have fun.
- Help your child understand that treatment can make life better.

How Does Bipolar Disorder Affect Parents and Family?

Taking care of a child or teenager with bipolar disorder can be stressful for you, too. You have to cope with the mood swings and other problems, such as short tempers and risky activities. This can challenge any parent. Sometimes the stress can strain your relationships with other people, and you may miss work or lose free time.

If you are taking care of a child with bipolar disorder, take care of yourself too. Find someone you can talk to about your feelings. Talk with the doctor about support groups for caregivers. If you keep your stress level down, you will do a better job. It might help your child get better too.

Where Do I Go for Help?

If you're not sure where to get help, call your family doctor. You can also check the phone book for mental health professionals. Hospital doctors can help in an emergency. Finally, the Substance Abuse and Mental Health Services Administration (SAMHSA) has an online tool to help you find mental health services in your area.

I Know Someone Who Is in Crisis. What Do I Do?

If you know someone who might be thinking about hurting himself or herself or someone else, get help quickly.

- Do not leave the person alone.
- Call your doctor.
- Call 911 or go to the emergency room.
- Call National Suicide Prevention Lifeline, toll-free: 1-800-273-TALK (8255). The TTY number is 1-800-799-4TTY (4889).

Section 36.4

Depression

This section includes text excerpted from "Depression: What You Need to Know," National Institute of Mental Health (NIMH), December 13, 2015.

Depression Is a Real Illness

Sadness is something we all experience. It is a normal reaction to difficult times in life and usually passes with a little time.

When a person has depression, it interferes with daily life and normal functioning. It can cause pain for both the person with depression and those who care about him or her. Doctors call this condition "depressive disorder," or "clinical depression." It is a real illness. It is not a sign of a person's weakness or a character flaw. You can't "snap out of" clinical depression. Most people who experience depression need treatment to get better.

Signs and Symptoms of Depression

Sadness is only a small part of depression. Some people with depression may not feel sadness at all. Depression has many other symptoms, including physical ones. If you have been experiencing any of the following signs and symptoms for at least 2 weeks, you may be suffering from depression:

- Persistent sad, anxious, or "empty" mood
- Feelings of hopelessness, pessimism
- Feelings of guilt, worthlessness, helplessness
- Loss of interest or pleasure in hobbies and activities
- Decreased energy, fatigue, being "slowed down"
- Difficulty concentrating, remembering, making decisions
- Difficulty sleeping, early-morning awakening, or oversleeping
- Appetite and/or weight changes
- Thoughts of death or suicide, suicide attempts
- Restlessness, irritability
- Persistent physical symptoms

Factors That Play a Role in Depression

Many factors may play a role in depression, including genetics, brain biology and chemistry, and life events such as trauma, loss of a loved one, a difficult relationship, an early childhood experience, or any stressful situation.

Depression can happen at any age, but often begins in the teens or early 20s or 30s. Most chronic mood and anxiety disorders in adults begin as high levels of anxiety in children. In fact, high levels of anxiety as a child could mean a higher risk of depression as an adult.

Depression can co-occur with other serious medical illnesses such as diabetes, cancer, heart disease, and Parkinson disease. Depression can make these conditions worse and vice versa. Sometimes medications taken for these illnesses may cause side effects that contribute to depression. A doctor experienced in treating these complicated illnesses can help work out the best treatment strategy.

Research on depression is ongoing, and one day these discoveries may lead to better diagnosis and treatment.

Types of Depression

There are several types of depressive disorders.

Major depression: Severe symptoms that interfere with the ability to work, sleep, study, eat, and enjoy life. An episode can occur only once in a person's lifetime, but more often, a person has several episodes.

Persistent depressive disorder: A depressed mood that lasts for at least 2 years. A person diagnosed with persistent depressive disorder may have episodes of major depression along with periods of less severe symptoms, but symptoms must last for 2 years.

Some forms of depression are slightly different, or they may develop under unique circumstances. They include:

Psychotic depression, which occurs when a person has severe depression plus some form of psychosis, such as having disturbing false beliefs or a break with reality (delusions), or hearing or seeing upsetting things that others cannot hear or see (hallucinations).

Postpartum depression, which is much more serious than the "baby blues" that many women experience after giving birth, when hormonal and physical changes and the new responsibility of caring for a newborn can be overwhelming. It is estimated that 10 to 15 percent of women experience postpartum depression after giving birth.

Seasonal affective disorder (SAD), which is characterized by the onset of depression during the winter months, when there is less natural sunlight. The depression generally lifts during spring and summer. SAD may be effectively treated with light therapy, but nearly half of those with SAD do not get better with light therapy alone. Antidepressant medication and psychotherapy can reduce SAD symptoms, either alone or in combination with light therapy.

Bipolar disorder is different from depression. The reason it is included in this list is because someone with bipolar disorder experiences episodes of extreme low moods (depression). But a person with bipolar disorder also experiences extreme high moods (called "mania").

Depression Affects People in Different Ways

Not everyone who is depressed experiences every symptom. Some people experience only a few symptoms. Some people have many. The severity and frequency of symptoms, and how long they last, will vary depending on the individual and his or her particular illness. Symptoms may also vary depending on the stage of the illness.

Women

Women with depression do not all experience the same symptoms. However, women with depression typically have symptoms of sadness, worthlessness, and guilt.

Depression is more common among women than among men. Biological, life cycle, hormonal, and psychosocial factors that are unique to women may be linked to their higher depression rate. For example, women are especially vulnerable to developing postpartum depression after giving birth, when hormonal and physical changes and the new responsibility of caring for a newborn can be overwhelming.

Men

Men often experience depression differently than women. While women with depression are more likely to have feelings of sadness, worthlessness, and excessive guilt, men are more likely to be very tired, irritable, lose interest in once-pleasurable activities, and have difficulty sleeping.

Men may turn to alcohol or drugs when they are depressed. They also may become frustrated, discouraged, irritable, angry, and sometimes abusive. Some men may throw themselves into their work to avoid talking about their depression with family or friends, or behave recklessly. And although more women attempt suicide, many more men die by suicide in the United States.

Children

Before puberty, girls and boys are equally likely to develop depression. A child with depression may pretend to be sick, refuse to go to school, cling to a parent, or worry that a parent may die. Because normal behaviors vary from one childhood stage to another, it can be difficult to tell whether a child is just going through a temporary "phase" or is suffering from depression. Sometimes the parents become worried about how the child's behavior has changed, or a teacher mentions that "your child doesn't seem to be himself." In such a case, if a visit to the child's pediatrician rules out physical symptoms, the doctor will probably suggest that the child be evaluated, preferably by a mental health professional who specializes in the treatment of children. Most chronic mood disorders, such as depression, begin as high levels of anxiety in children.

Teens

The teen years can be tough. Teens are forming an identity apart from their parents, grappling with gender issues and emerging sexuality, and making independent decisions for the first time in their lives. Occasional bad moods are to be expected, but depression is different.

Older children and teens with depression may sulk, get into trouble at school, be negative and irritable, and feel misunderstood. If you're unsure if an adolescent in your life is depressed or just "being a teenager," consider how long the symptoms have been present, how severe they are, and how different the teen is acting from his or her usual self. Teens with depression may also have other disorders such as anxiety, eating disorders, or substance abuse. They may also be at higher risk for suicide.

Children and teenagers usually rely on parents, teachers, or other caregivers to recognize their suffering and get them the treatment they need. Many teens don't know where to go for mental health treatment or believe that treatment won't help. Others don't get help because they think depression symptoms may be just part of the typical stress of school or being a teen. Some teens worry what other people will think if they seek mental healthcare.

Depression often persists, recurs, and continues into adulthood, especially if left untreated. If you suspect a child or teenager in your life is suffering from depression, speak up right away.

Depression Is Treatable

Depression, even the most severe cases, can be treated. The earlier treatment begins, the more effective it is. Most adults see an improvement in their symptoms when treated with antidepressant drugs, talk therapy (psychotherapy), or a combination of both.

If you think you may have depression, start by making an appointment to see your doctor or healthcare provider. This could be your primary doctor or a health provider who specializes in diagnosing and treating mental health conditions (psychologist or psychiatrist). Certain medications, and some medical conditions, such as viruses or a thyroid disorder, can cause the same symptoms as depression. A doctor can rule out these possibilities by doing a physical exam, interview, and lab tests. If the doctor can find no medical condition that may be causing the depression, the next step is a psychological evaluation.

Quick Tip: Making an Appointment

If you still need to make an appointment, here are some things you could say during the first call: "I haven't been myself lately, and I'd like to talk to the provider about it," or "I think I might have depression, and I'd like some help."

Talking to Your Doctor

How well you and your doctor talk to each other is one of the most important parts of getting good healthcare. But talking to your doctor isn't always easy. It takes time and effort on your part as well as your doctor's.

To prepare for your appointment, make a list of:

- Any symptoms you've had, including any that may seem unrelated to the reason for your appointment
- When did your symptoms start?
- How severe are your symptoms?
- Have the symptoms occurred before?
- If the symptoms have occurred before, how were they treated?
- Key personal information, including any major stresses or recent life changes
- All medications, vitamins, or other supplements that you're taking, including how much and how often
- Questions to ask your health provider

If you don't have a primary doctor or are not at ease with the one you currently see, now may be the time to find a new doctor. Whether you just moved to a new city, changed insurance providers, or had a bad experience with your doctor or medical staff, it is worthwhile to spend time finding a doctor you can trust.

Tests and Diagnosis

Your doctor or healthcare provider will examine you and talk to you at the appointment. Your doctor may do a physical exam and ask questions about your health and symptoms. There are no lab tests that can specifically diagnose depression, but your doctor may also order some lab tests to rule out other conditions.

Ask questions if the doctor's explanations or instructions are unclear, bring up problems even if the doctor doesn't ask, and let the doctor know if you have concerns about a particular treatment or change in your daily life.

Your doctor may refer you to a mental health professional, such as a psychiatrist, psychologist, social worker, or mental health counselor, who should discuss with you any family history of depression or other mental disorder, and get a complete history of your symptoms. The mental health professional may also ask if you are using alcohol or drugs, and if you are thinking about death or suicide.

You Are Not Alone

Major depressive disorder is one of the most common mental disorders in the United States. You are not alone.

Sometimes living with depression can seem overwhelming, so build a support system for yourself. Your family and friends are a great place to start. Talk to trusted family members or friends to help them understand how you are feeling and that you are following your doctor's recommendations to treat your depression.

In addition to your treatment, you could also join a support group. These are not psychotherapy groups, but some may find the added support helpful. At the meetings, people share experiences, feelings, information, and coping strategies for living with depression.

Remember: Always check with your doctor before taking any medical advice that you hear in your group.

You can find a support group through many professional, consumer, advocacy, and service-related organizations.

Some of these partners sponsor support groups for different mental disorders including depression. You can also find online support groups, but you need to be careful about which groups you join. Check and make sure the group is affiliated with a reputable health organization, moderated professionally, and maintains your anonymity.

If unsure where to start, talk to someone you trust who has experience in mental health—for example, a doctor, nurse, social worker, or religious counselor. Some health insurance providers may also have listings of hospitals offering support groups for depression.

If You Think a Loved One May Have Depression

If you know someone who is depressed, it affects you too. The most important thing you can do is to help your friend or relative get a diagnosis and treatment. You may need to make an appointment and go with him or her to see the doctor. Encourage your loved one to stay in treatment or to seek different treatment options if no improvement occurs after 6 to 8 weeks.

To help your friend or relative:

- Offer emotional support, understanding, patience, and encouragement.
- Talk to him or her, and listen carefully.
- Never dismiss feelings, but point out realities and offer hope.
- Never ignore comments about suicide and report them to your loved one's therapist or doctor.
- Invite your loved one out for walks, outings, and other activities. Keep trying if he or she declines, but don't push him or her to take on too much too soon.
- Provide assistance in getting to doctors' appointments.
- Remind your loved one that with time and treatment, the depression will lift.

Caring for someone with depression is not easy. Someone with depression may need constant support for a long period of time. Make sure you leave time for yourself and your own needs. If you feel you need additional support, there are support groups for caregivers too.

Section 36.5

Obsessive-Compulsive Disorder

This section includes text excerpted from "Obsessive-Compulsive Disorder," National Institute of Mental Health (NIMH), January 2016.

What Is Obsessive-Compulsive Disorder (OCD)?

Obsessive-Compulsive Disorder (OCD) is a common, chronic and long-lasting disorder in which a person has uncontrollable, recurring thoughts (obsessions) and behaviors (compulsions) that he or she feels the urge to repeat over and over.

Signs and Symptoms of OCD

People with OCD may have symptoms of obsessions, compulsions, or both. These symptoms can interfere with all aspects of life, such as work, school, and personal relationships.

Obsessions are repeated thoughts, urges, or mental images that cause anxiety. Common symptoms include:

- Fear of germs or contamination
- Unwanted forbidden or taboo thoughts involving sex, religion, and harm
- Aggressive thoughts towards others or self
- Having things symmetrical or in a perfect order

Compulsions are repetitive behaviors that a person with OCD feels the urge to do in response to an obsessive thought. Common compulsions include:

- Excessive cleaning and/or handwashing
- Ordering and arranging things in a particular, precise way
- Repeatedly checking on things, such as repeatedly checking to see if the door is locked or that the oven is off
- Compulsive counting

Not all rituals or habits are compulsions. Everyone double checks things sometimes. But a person with OCD generally:

- Can't control his or her thoughts or behaviors, even when those thoughts or behaviors are recognized as excessive
- Spends at least 1 hour a day on these thoughts or behaviors
- Doesn't get pleasure when performing the behaviors or rituals, but may feel brief relief from the anxiety the thoughts cause
- Experiences significant problems in their daily life due to these thoughts or behaviors

Some individuals with OCD also have a tic disorder. Motor tics are sudden, brief, repetitive movements, such as eye blinking and other eye movements, facial grimacing, shoulder shrugging, and head or shoulder jerking. Common vocal tics include repetitive throat-clearing, sniffing, or grunting sounds.

Symptoms may come and go, ease over time, or worsen. People with OCD may try to help themselves by avoiding situations that trigger their obsessions, or they may use alcohol or drugs to calm themselves. Although most adults with OCD recognize that what they are doing doesn't make sense, some adults and most children may not realize that their behavior is out of the ordinary. Parents or teachers typically recognize OCD symptoms in children.

If you think you have OCD, talk to your doctor about your symptoms. If left untreated, OCD can interfere in all aspects of life.

Risk Factors of OCD

OCD is a common disorder that affects adults, adolescents, and children all over the world. Most people are diagnosed by about age 19, typically with an earlier age of onset in boys than in girls, but onset after age 35 does happen.

The causes of OCD are unknown, but risk factors include:

Genetics

Twin and family studies have shown that people with first-degree relatives (such as a parent, sibling, or child) who have OCD are at a higher risk for developing OCD themselves. The risk is higher if the first-degree relative developed OCD as a child or teen. Ongoing research continues to explore the connection between genetics and OCD and may help improve OCD diagnosis and treatment.

Brain Structure and Functioning

Imaging studies have shown differences in the frontal cortex and subcortical structures of the brain in patients with OCD. There appears to be a connection between the OCD symptoms and abnormalities in certain areas of the brain, but that connection is not clear. Research is still underway. Understanding the causes will help determine specific, personalized treatments to treat OCD.

Environment

People who have experienced abuse (physical or sexual) in childhood or other trauma are at an increased risk for developing OCD.

In some cases, children may develop OCD or OCD symptoms following a streptococcal infection—this is called Pediatric Autoimmune Neuropsychiatric Disorders Associated with Streptococcal Infections (PANDAS).

Treatments and Therapies

OCD is typically treated with medication, psychotherapy or a combination of the two. Although most patients with OCD respond to treatment, some patients continue to experience symptoms.

Sometimes people with OCD also have other mental disorders, such as anxiety, depression, and body dysmorphic disorder, a disorder in which someone mistakenly believes that a part of their body is abnormal. It is important to consider these other disorders when making decisions about treatment.

Part Five

Additional Help and Information

Chapter 37

Glossary of Terms Related to Childhood Diseases and Disorders

acute otitis media: Ear infection, usually caused by bacteria; when the middle ear becomes infected and swollen, trapping fluid and mucus behind the eardrum.

adenoid: Small pad of infection-fighting tissue located near the eustachian tube.

adenovirus: A member of a family of viruses that can cause infections in the respiratory tract, eye, and gastrointestinal tract. Forms of adenoviruses that do not cause disease are used in gene therapy.

adrenal gland: A small gland that makes steroid hormones, adrenaline, and noradrenaline. These hormones help control heart rate, blood pressure, and other important body functions. There are two adrenal glands, one on top of each kidney. Also called suprarenal gland.

allergy: A condition in which the body has an exaggerated response to a substance (e.g., food or drug). Also known as hypersensitivity.

antibody: A protein found in the blood that is produced in response to foreign substances (e.g., bacteria or viruses) invading the body.

This glossary contains terms excerpted from documents produced by several sources deemed reliable.

Antibodies protect the body from disease by binding to these organisms and destroying them.

arthritis: A disease that causes inflammation and pain in the joints.

asthma: A chronic medical condition where the bronchial tubes (in the lungs) become easily irritated. This leads to constriction of the airways resulting in wheezing, coughing, difficulty breathing, and production of thick mucus.

autism: A chronic developmental disorder usually diagnosed between 18 and 30 months of age.

autosomal: Describes genetic material (chromosomes or genes) that are not gender-related.

bacteria: Tiny one-celled organisms present throughout the environment that require a microscope to be seen. While not all bacteria are harmful, some cause disease.

biopsy: The removal of cells or tissues for examination by a pathologist. The pathologist may study the tissue under a microscope or perform other tests on the cells or tissue. There are many different types of biopsy procedures. The most common types include: (1) incisional biopsy, in which only a sample of tissue is removed; (2) excisional biopsy, in which an entire lump or suspicious area is removed; and (3) needle biopsy, in which a sample of tissue or fluid is removed with a needle.

carrier: A person who has a mutated (changed) copy of a gene. This change may cause a disease in that person or in his or her children.

cholesteatoma: Accumulation of dead cells in the middle ear, caused by repeated middle ear infections.

chromosome: Part of a cell that contains genetic information. Except for sperm and eggs, all human cells contain 46 chromosomes.

chronic otitis media with effusion: Repeated occurrences of otitis media with effusion (ear infection), in which fluid remains in the middle ear after the infection is gone.

cognition: Thinking skills that include perception, memory, awareness, reasoning, judgment, intellect, and imagination.

computerized tomography (CT) scan: A series of detailed pictures of areas inside the body taken from different angles. The pictures are created by a computer linked to an X-ray machine.

Crohn's disease: A chronic medical condition characterized by inflammation of the bowel.

cystic fibrosis: A common hereditary disease in which exocrine (secretory) glands produce abnormally thick mucus. This mucus can cause problems in digestion, breathing, and body cooling.

diabetes: A chronic health condition where the body is unable to produce insulin and properly break down sugar (glucose) in the blood.

dysarthria: Group of speech disorders caused by disturbances in the strength or coordination of the muscles of the speech mechanism as a result of damage to the brain or nerves.

dysphagia: Any impairment of the voice or speaking ability.

encephalopathy: A general term describing brain dysfunction.

endocrine system: A system of glands and cells that make hormones that are released directly into the blood and travel to tissues and organs all over the body. The endocrine system controls growth, sexual development, sleep, hunger, and the way the body uses food.

epilepsy: A group of disorders marked by problems in the normal functioning of the brain. These problems can produce seizures, unusual body movements, a loss of consciousness or changes in consciousness, as well as mental problems or problems with the senses.

exposure: Contact with infectious agents (bacteria or viruses) in a manner that promotes transmission and increases the likelihood of disease.

fever: An increase in body temperature above normal (98.6° F), usually caused by disease.

gastric reflux: The backward flow of stomach acid contents into the esophagus (the tube that connects the mouth to the stomach). Also called esophageal reflux and gastroesophageal reflux.

genetic counseling: A communication process between a specially trained health professional and a person concerned about the genetic risk of disease. The person's family and personal medical history may be discussed, and counseling may lead to genetic testing.

haemophilus influenzae type b (hib): A bacterial infection that may result in severe respiratory infections, including pneumonia, and other diseases such as meningitis.

hepatitis: Disease of the liver causing inflammation. Symptoms include an enlarged liver, fever, nausea, vomiting, abdominal pain, and dark urine.

hereditary: Transmitted from parent to child by information contained in the genes.

immune system: The complex system in the body responsible for fighting disease. Its primary function is to identify foreign substances in the body (bacteria, viruses, fungi, or parasites) and develop a defense against them.

incubation period: The time from contact with infectious agents (bacteria or viruses) to onset of disease.

infection: Invasion and multiplication of germs in the body. Infections can occur in any part of the body and can spread throughout the body. The germs may be bacteria, viruses, yeast, or fungi.

inflammatory bowel disease (ibd): A general term for any disease characterized by inflammation of the bowel. Examples include colitis and Crohn's disease.

influenza: A highly contagious viral infection characterized by sudden onset of fever, severe aches and pains, and inflammation of the mucous membrane.

Kallmann syndrome: Disorder that can include several characteristics such as absence of the sense of smell and decreased functional activity of the gonads (organs that produce sex cells), affecting growth and sexual development.

magnetic resonance imaging (MRI): A procedure in which radio waves and a powerful magnet linked to a computer are used to create detailed pictures of areas inside the body. These pictures can show the difference between normal and diseased tissue.

otitis media: A viral or bacterial infection that leads to inflammation of the middle ear. This condition usually occurs along with an upper respiratory infection.

otoscope: Ear infection in which fluid remains trapped behind the eardrum inside the middle ear after the infection is over.

parasitic: Having to do with or being a parasite (an animal or plant that gets nutrients by living on or in an organism of another species).

pathogens: Organisms (e.g., bacteria, viruses, parasites, and fungi) that cause disease in human beings.

pertussis (whooping cough): Bacterial infectious disease marked by a convulsive spasmodic cough, sometimes followed by a crowing intake of breath.

pinkeye: A condition in which the conjunctiva (membranes lining the eyelids and covering the white part of the eye) become inflamed or infected. Also called conjunctivitis.

pneumonia: Inflammation of the lungs characterized by fever, chills, muscle stiffness, chest pain, cough, shortness of breath, rapid heart rate, and difficulty breathing.

prosody: The rhythm, speed, pitch, and tone of spoken language.

Reye syndrome: Encephalopathy (general brain disorder) in children following an acute illness such as influenza or chickenpox. This condition may result in coma or death.

sarcoma: A cancer of the bone, cartilage, fat, muscle, blood vessels, or other connective or supportive tissue.

seizure: Sudden, uncontrolled body movements and changes in behavior that occur because of abnormal electrical activity in the brain.

spasmodic dysphonia: Momentary disruption of voice caused by involuntary movements of one or more muscles of the larynx or voice box.

stuttering: Frequent repetition of words or parts of words that disrupts the smooth flow of speech.

tinnitus: Sensation of a ringing, roaring, or buzzing sound in the ears or head. It is often associated with many forms of hearing impairment and noise exposure.

tumor: An abnormal mass of tissue that results when cells divide more than they should or do not die when they should. Tumors may be benign (not cancer) or malignant (cancer). Also called neoplasm.

ultrasound: A procedure in which high-energy sound waves are bounced off internal tissues or organs and make echoes. The echo patterns are shown on the screen of an ultrasound machine, forming a picture of body tissues called a sonogram. Also called ultrasonography.

Usher syndrome: Hereditary disease that affects hearing and vision and sometimes balance.

vaccine: A product that produces immunity therefore protecting the body from the disease. Vaccines are administered through needle injections, by mouth, and by aerosol.

vertigo: Illusion of movement; a sensation as if the external world were revolving around an individual (objective vertigo) or as if the individual were revolving in space (subjective vertigo).

virus: A tiny organism that multiplies within cells and causes disease such as chickenpox, measles, mumps, rubella, pertussis, and hepatitis. Viruses are not affected by antibiotics, the drugs used to kill bacteria.

Chapter 38

Resource List for Parents and Caregivers

General Health Organizations

American Academy of Pediatrics (AAP)
National Headquarters
141 N.W. Pt. Blvd.
Elk Grove Village, IL 60007-1098
Phone: 847-434-4000
Fax: 847-434-8000
Toll-Free: 800-433-9016
Website: www.aap.org
E-mail: csc@aap.org

Centers for Disease Control and Prevention (CDC)
1600 Clifton Rd.
Atlanta, GA 30329-4027
Toll-Free: 800-CDC-INFO (800-232-4636)
TTY: 888-232-6348
Website: www.cdc.gov
E-mail: cdcinfo@cdc.gov

Cleveland Clinic
9500 Euclid Ave.
Cleveland, OH 44195-0001
Phone: 216-444-2200
Fax: 216-445-8160
Toll-Free: 800-223-2273
Website: www.clevelandclinicmeded.com

Resources in this chapter were compiled from several sources deemed reliable; all contact information was verified and updated in October 2016.

Eunice Kennedy Shriver *National Institute of Child Health and Development (NICHD) Information Resource Center*
P.O. Box 3006
Rockville, MD 20847
Toll-Free Fax: 866-760-5947
Toll-Free: 800-370-2943
Toll-Free TTY: 888-320-6942
Website: www.nichd.nih.gov
E-mail: NICHDInformationResourceCenter@ mail.nih.gov

National Heart, Lung, and Blood Institute (NHLBI)
NHLBI Health Information Center
P.O. Box 30105
Bethesda, MD 20824-0105
Phone: 301-592-8573
Fax: 301-592-8563
TTY: 240-629-3255
Website: www.nhlbi.nih.gov
E-mail: nhlbiinfo@nhlbi.nih.gov

National Institute of Allergy and Infectious Diseases (NIAID)
Office of Communications and Government Relations
5601 Fishers Ln. MSC 9806
Bethesda, MD 20892-9806
Phone: 301-402-1663
Fax: 301-402-0120
Toll-Free: 866-284-4107
Toll-Free TDD: 800-877-8339
Website: www.niaid.nih.gov
E-mail: ocpostoffice@niaid.nih.gov

National Institute of Diabetes and Digestive and Kidney Diseases (NIDDK)
Office of Communications and Public Liaison
31 Center Dr. MSC 2560
Bldg. 31 Rm. 9A06
Bethesda, MD 20892-2560
Phone: 301-496-3583
Website: www.niddk.nih.gov

National Organization for Rare Disorders (NORD)
55 Kenosia Ave.
Danbury, CT 06810
Phone: 203-744-0100
Fax: 203-263-9938
Website: www.rarediseases.org
E-mail: orphan@rarediseases.org / RN@rarediseases.org

The Nemours Foundation / KidsHealth®
1600 Rockland Rd.
Wilmington, DE 19803
Phone: 302-651-4046
Website: www.kidshealth.org
E-mail: info@KidsHealth.org

U.S. Department of Health and Human Services (HHS)
200 Independence Ave. S.W.
Washington, DC 20201
Toll-Free: 877-696-6775
Website: www.hhs.gov

U.S. Environmental Protection Agency (EPA)
Ariel Rios Bldg.
1200 Pennsylvania Ave. N.W.
Washington, DC 20460
Phone: 202-272-0167
TTY: 202-272-0165
Website: www.epa.gov

U.S. Food and Drug Administration (FDA)
10903 New Hampshire Ave.
Silver Spring, MD 20993
Toll-Free: 888-INFO-FDA (888-463-6332)
Website: www.fda.gov

Weight-Control Information Network (WIN)
1 WIN Way
Bethesda, MD 20892-3665
Phone: 202-828-1025
Fax: 202-828-1028
Toll-Free: 877-946-4627
Website: www.win.niddk.nih.gov
E-mail: win@info.niddk.nih.gov

Allergies and Asthma

Asthma and Allergy Foundation of America (AAFA)
8201 Corporate Dr. Ste. 1000
Ste. 1000
Landover, MD 20785
Toll-Free: 800-7-ASTHMA (800-727-8462)
Website: www.aafa.org
E-mail: info@aafa.org

Arthritis and Musculoskeletal Diseases

American College of Rheumatology (ACR)
2200 Lake Blvd. N.E.
Atlanta, GA 30319
Phone: 404-633-3777
Fax: 404-633-1870
Website: www.rheumatology.org
E-mail: acr@rheumatology.org

Arthritis Foundation
1355 Peachtree St. N.E.
Ste. 600
Atlanta,GA 30309
Phone: 404-872-7100
Toll-Free: 844-571-4357
Website: www.arthritis.org

National Institute of Arthritis and Musculoskeletal and Skin Diseases (NIAMS)
1 AMS Cir.
Bethesda, MD 20892-3675
Phone: 301-495-4484
Fax: 312-718-6366
Toll-Free: 877-22-NIAMS (877-226-4267)
TYY: 301-565-2966
Website: www.niams.nih.gov
E-mail: NIAMSinfo@mail.nih.gov

Cancer

American Cancer Society (ACS)
250 Williams St. N.W.
Atlanta, GA 30303
Toll-Free: 800-ACS-2345 (800-227-2345)
Toll-Free TTY: 866-228-4327
Website: www.cancer.org

Leukemia and Lymphoma Society (LLS)
3 International Dr. Ste. 200
Rye Brook, NY 10573
Phone: 914-949-5213
Fax: 914-949-6691
Toll-Free: 800-955-4LSA (800-955-4572)
Website: www.lls.org
E-mail: infocenter@lls.org

National Cancer Institute (NCI)
NCI Public Inquiries Office
9609 Medical Center Dr.
BG 9609 MSC 9760
Bethesda, MD 20892-9760
Toll-Free: 800-422-6237 (800-4-CANCER)
Website: www.cancer.gov

National Children's Cancer Society (NCCS)
5740 Westbourne Ave.
Columbus, OH 43213
Phone: 855-501-7712
Website: www.nccsservices.com
E-mail: info@nccsservices.com

Pediatric Brain Tumor Foundation (PBTF)
302 Ridgefield Ct.
Asheville, NC 28806
Fax: 828-665-6894
Toll-Free: 800-253-6530
Website: www.pbtfus.org
E-mail: info@pbtfus.org

Cardiovascular Disorders

American Heart Association (AHA)
7272 Greenville Ave.
Dallas, TX 75231
Toll-Free: 800-AHA-USA1 (800-242-8721)
Website: www.heart.org

National Hemophilia Foundation (NHF)
7 Penn Plaza
Ste.1204
New York, NY 10001
Phone: 212-328-3700
Fax: 212-328-3777
Toll-Free: 800-42-HANDI (800-424-2634)
Website: www.hemophilia.org
E-mail: handi@hemophilia.org

Developmental Disorders

Attention Deficit Disorder Association (ADDA)
P.O. Box 7557
Wilmington, DE 19803-9997
Fax: 800-939-1019
Website: www.add.org
E-mail: info@add.org

Autism Society of America (ASA)
4340 E.W. Hwy
Ste. 350
Bethesda, MD 20814
Phone: 301-657-0881
Toll-Free: 800-3-AUTISM (800-328-8476)
Website: www.autism-society.org
E-mail: info@autism-society.org

Autism Speaks
1 E. 33rd St. 4th Fl.
New York, NY 10016
Phone: 212-252-8584
Fax: 212-252-8676
Website: www.autismspeaks.org
E-mail: contactus@autismspeaks.org

Learning Disabilities Association of America (LDA)
4156 Library Rd.
Pittsburgh, PA 15234-1349
Phone: 412-341-1515
Fax: 412-344-0224
Website: www.ldaamerica.org
E-mail: info@ldaamerica.org

National Center for Learning Disabilities (NCLD)
32 Laight St.
2nd Fl.
New York, NY 10013
Phone: 212-545-7510
Fax: 212-545-9665
Toll-Free: 888-575-7373
Website: www.ncld.org

Diabetes

American Diabetes Association (ADA)
Attention: Center for Information
1701 N. Beauregard St.
Alexandria, VA 22311
Toll-Free: 800-DIABETES (800-342-2383)
Website: www.diabetes.org
E-mail: AskADA@diabetes.org

Juvenile Diabetes Research Foundation International (JDRF)
26 Broadway
New York, NY 10004
Fax: 212-785-9595
Toll-Free: 800-533-CURE (800-533-2873)
Website: www.jdrf.org
E-mail: info@jdrf.org

National Diabetes Education Program (NDEP)
1 Diabetes Way
Bethesda, MD 20814-9692
Phone: 301-496-3583
Toll-Free: 888-693-NDEP (888-693-6337 to order materials)
Website: www.ndep.nih.gov
E-mail: ndep@mail.nih.gov

National Diabetes Information Clearinghouse (NDIC)
1 Information Way
Bethesda, MD 20892-3560
Fax: 703-738-4929
Toll-Free: 800-860-8747
Toll-Free TTY: 866-569-1162
Website: diabetes.niddk.nih.gov
E-mail: ndic@info.niddk.nih.gov

Foodborne Illnesses

Center for Food Safety and Applied Nutrition (CFSAN)
5001 Campus Dr.
College Park, MD 20740-3835
Toll-Free: 888-SAFEFOOD (888-723-3366)
Website: www.fda.gov
E-mail: consumers@fda.gov

U.S. Department of Agriculture (USDA)
1400 Independence Ave. S.W.
Washington, DC 20250
Phone: 202-720-2791 (Information Hotline)
Toll-Free: 888-674-6854 (Meat and Poultry Hotline)
Website: www.usda.gov

Gastrointestinal and Digestive Disorders

American College of Gastroenterology (ACG)
6400 Goldsboro Rd., Ste. 200
Bethesda, MD 20817
Phone: 301-263-9000
Website: www.acg.gi.org
E-mail: info@acg.gi.org

American Gastroenterological Association (AGA)
4930 Del Ray Ave.
Bethesda, MD 20814
Phone: 301-654-2055
Fax: 301-654-5920
Website: www.gastro.org
E-mail: member@gastro.org

Celiac Disease Foundation (CDF)
20350 Ventura Blvd Ste. 240
Woodland Hills, CA 91364
Phone: 818-716-1513
Fax: 818-267-5577
Website: www.celiac.org
E-mail: cdf@celiac.org

Celiac Support Association (CSA)
P.O. Box 254
Seward, NE 68434
Phone: 402-643-4101
Fax: 402-643-4108
Toll-Free: 877-CSA-4CSA (877-372-4272)
Website: www.csaceliacs.org
E-mail: celiacs@csaceliacs.org

Crohn's and Colitis Foundation of America (CCFA)
733 3rd Ave.
Ste. 510
New York, NY 10017
Phone: 800-932-2423
Fax: 212-779-4098
Website: www.ccfa.org
E-mail: info@ccfa.org

Cyclic Vomiting Syndrome Association (CVSA)
P.O. Box 270341
Milwaukee, WI 53227
Phone: 414-342-7880
Fax: 414-342-8980
Website: www.cvsaonline.org
E-mail: cvsa@cvsaonline.org

Digestive Disease National Coalition (DDNC)
507 Capitol Ct. N.E.
Ste. 200
Washington, DC 20002
Phone: 202-544-7497
Fax: 202-546-7105
Website: www.ddnc.org
E-mail: psurio@hmcw.org

Food Allergy Research and Education (FARE)
7925 Jones Branch Dr.
Ste. 1100
McLean, VA 22102
Phone: 703-691-3179
Fax: 703-691-2713
Toll-Free: 1-800-929-4040
Website: www.foodallergy.org

International Foundation for Functional Gastrointestinal Disorders (IFFGD)
P.O. Box 170864
Milwaukee, WI 53217
Phone: 414-964-1799
Website: www.iffgd.org

National Digestive Diseases Information Clearinghouse (NDDIC)
2 Information Way
Bethesda, MD 20892-3570
Phone: 301-654-3810
Toll-Free: 800-891-5389
Website: www.digestive.niddk.nih.gov
E-mail: nddic@info.niddk.nih.gov

North American Society for Pediatric Gastroenterology, Hepatology, and Nutrition (NASPGHAN)
714 N. Bethlehem Pike, Ste. 300
Ambler, PA 19002
Phone: 215-641-9800
Fax: 215-641-1995
Website: www.naspghan.org
E-mail: naspghan@naspghan.org

Pediatric Adolescent Gastroesophageal Reflux Association (PAGER)
P.O. Box 7728
Silver Spring, MD 20907
Phone: 301-601-9541
Website: www.reflux.org
E-mail: gergroup@aol.com

Growth Disorders

Human Growth Foundation (HGF)
997 Glen Cove Ave., Ste. 5
Glen Head, NY 11545
Phone: 1-800-451-6434
Fax:1-516-671-4055
Toll-Free: 1-800-451-6434
Website: www.hgfound.org
E-mail: hgf1@hgfound.org

MAGIC Foundation
6645 W. N. Ave.
Oak Park, IL 60302
Phone: 708-383-0808
Toll-Free: 800-3-MAGIC-3
(800-362-4423)
Website: www.magicfoundation.org
E-mail: contactus@magicfoundation.org

Hearing Disorders

National Institute on Deafness and Other Communication Disorders (NIDCD)
Information Clearinghouse
31 Center Dr. MSC 2320
Bethesda, MD 20892-2320
Phone: 301-827-8183
Fax: 301-402-0018
Toll-Free: 800-241-1044
Toll-Free TTY: 800-241-1055
Website: www.nidcd.nih.gov
E-mail: nidcdinfo@nidcd.nih.gov

Injury Prevention

Safe Kids Worldwide
1255 23rd St. N.W.
Ste. 400
Washington, DC 20037-1151
Phone: 202-662-0600
Fax: 202-393-2072
Website: www.safekids.org
E-mail: gkarton@safekids.org

Kidney and Urological Disorders

American Society of Pediatric Nephrology (ASPN)
3400 Research Forest Dr.
Ste. B-7
The Woodlands, TX 77381
Phone: 346-980-9752
Fax: 346-980-9752
Website: www.aspneph.com
E-mail: info@aspneph.com

American Urological Association Foundation (AUA)
1000 Corporate Blvd.
Linthicum, MD 21090
Phone: 410-689-3700
Fax: 410-689-3998
Toll-Free: 800-828-7866
Website: www.auanet.org
E-mail: auafoundation@auafoundation.org

National Association for Continence (NAFC)
P.O. Box 1019
Charleston, SC 29402-1019
Phone: 843-377-0900
Fax: 843-377-0905
Toll-Free: 800-BLADDER
(800-252-3337)
Website: www.nafc.org
E-mail: memberservices@nafc.org

The Urology Care Foundation
1000 Corporate Blvd.
Linthicum, MD 21090
Phone: 410-689-3998
Fax: 410-689-3800
Toll-Free: 800-828-7866
Website: www.urologyhealth.org
E-mail: info@UrologyCareFoundation.org

Liver Disorders

Alpha-1 Foundation
2937 SW 27th Ave. Ste. 302
Miami, FL 33133
Phone: 305-567-9888
Fax: 305-567-1317
Toll-Free: 800-785-3177
Website: www.alpha1.org
E-mail: info@alpha-1foundation.org

American Association for the Study of Liver Diseases (AASLD)
1001 N. Fairfax St. Ste. 400
Alexandria, VA 22314
Phone: 703-299-9766
Fax: 703-299-9622
Website: www.aasld.org
E-mail: aasld@aasld.org

American Liver Foundation (ALF)
39 Broadway Ste. 2700
New York, NY 10006
Phone: 212-668-1000
Fax: 212-483-8179
Toll-Free: 800-GO-LIVER (800-465-4837)
Website: www.liverfoundation.org
E-mail: info@liverfoundation.org

Hepatitis Foundation International (HFI)
8121 Georgia Ave.
Ste. 350
Silver Spring, MD 20910
Phone: 301-565-9410
Fax: 301-622-4702
Toll-Free: 800-891-0707
Website: www.hepatitisfoundation.org
E-mail: info@hepatitisfoundation.org

Mental Health

American Academy of Child and Adolescent Psychiatry (AACAP)
3615 Wisconsin Ave. N.W.
Washington, DC 20016-3007
Phone: 202-966-7300
Fax: 202-966-2891
Website: www.aacap.org
E-mail: communications@aacap.org

Mental Health America (MHA)
2000 N. Beauregard St.
6th Fl.
Alexandria, VA 22311
Phone: 703-684-7722
Fax: 703-684-5968
Toll-Free: 800-969-6642
Toll-Free TTY: 800-433-5959
Toll-Free Crisis Line: 800-273-TALK (800-273-8255)
Website: www.mentalhealthamerica.net
E-mail: info@mentalhealthamerica.net

National Association for Children's Behavioral Health (NACBH)
1025 Connecticut Ave. N.W. Ste. 1012
Washington, DC 20036
Phone: 202-857-9735
Fax: 202-362-5145
Website: www.nacbh.org

National Federation of Families for Children's Mental Health (FFCMH)
9605 Medical Center Dr.
Ste. 280
Rockville, MD 20850
Phone: 240-403-1901
Fax: 240-403-1909
Website: www.ffcmh.org
E-mail: ffcmh@ffcmh.org

National Institute of Mental Health (NIMH)
6001 Executive Blvd.
Rm. 8184, MSC 9663
Bethesda, MD 20892-9663
Phone: 301-443-4513
Fax: 301-443-4279
Toll-Free: 866-615-NIMH (866-615-6464)
Toll-Free TTY: 866-415-8051
TTY: 301-443-8431
Website: www.nimh.nih.gov
E-mail: nimhinfo@nih.gov

Muscular Dystrophy

Muscular Dystrophy Association (MDA)
National Headquarters
3300 E. Sunrise Dr.
Tucson, AZ 85718-3208
Phone: 520-529-2000
Fax: 520-529-5300
Toll-Free: 800-572-1717
Website: www.mda.org
E-mail: mda@mdausa.org

Neurological Disorders

Charlie Foundation to Help Cure Pediatric Epilepsy
515 Ocean Ave. Ste. 602 N.
Santa Monica, CA 90402
Phone: 310-393-2347
Website: www.charliefoundation.org

Epilepsy Foundation
8301 Professional Pl.
Landover, MD 20785-7223
Phone: 866-330-2718
Fax: 301-459-1569
Toll-Free: 800-EFA-1000 (800-332-1000)
Website: www.epilepsyfoundation.org
E-mail: ContactUs@efa.org

Pediatric Brain Foundation (PBF)
1726 Franceschi Rd.
Santa Barbara, CA 93103-1870
Phone: 805-898-4442
Fax: 805-898-4448
Toll-Free: 866-CNS-5580 (866-267-5580)
Website: www.cnsfoundation.org
E-mail: info@cnsfoundation.org

Scoliosis

National Scoliosis Foundation (NSF)
5 Cabot Pl.
Stoughton, MA 02072
Phone: 781-341-6333
Fax: 781-341-8333
Toll-Free: 800-NSF-MYBACK (800-673-6922)
Website: www.scoliosis.org
E-mail: nsf@scoliosis.org

Skin Disorders

American Academy of Dermatology (AAD)
930 E. Woodfield Rd.
Schaumburg, IL 60618-4014
Phone: 847-240-1280
Fax: 847-240-1859
Toll-Free: 866-503-SKIN (866-503-7546)
Website: www.aad.org
E-mail: MRC@aad.org

Sleep Disorders

National Sleep Foundation (NSF)
1010 N. Glebe Rd. Ste. 310
Arlington, VA 22201
Phone: 703-243-1697
Website: www.sleepfoundation.org
E-mail: nsf@sleepfoundation.org

Vision Disorders

Lighthouse International
111 E. 59th St.
New York, NY 10022-1202
Phone: 212-821-9200
Fax: 212-821-9707
Toll-Free: 800-829-0500
Website: lighthouse.org
E-mail: info@lighthouse.org

National Eye Institute (NEI)
Information Office
31 Centers Dr. MSC 2510
Bethesda, MD 20892-2510
Phone: 301-496-5248
Website: nei.nih.gov
E-mail: 2020@nei.nih.gov

Index

Index

Page numbers followed by 'n' indicate a footnote. Page numbers in *italics* indicate a table or illustration.

A

B

C

E

G

H

I

N

P

Q

T

U

V

W

X

Y

Z